产科学聚焦

Obstetrics

INfocus

产科学聚焦

Obstetrics

IN*focus*

原　著　David K James
Alec McEwan

主　译　郑建华
黄明莉

译　者　黄可金　黄明莉　刘运铎
彭春杰　贲　崴　曲晓力
郑建华

北京大学医学出版社
Peking University Medical Press

Obstetrics in Focus, 1st edition
David K James , Alec McEwan
ISBN-13: 978-0-443-07435-6
ISBN-10: 0-443-07435-6

Authorized Simplified Chinese translation from English language edition published by the Proprietor.
978-981-259-564-5
981-259-564-3

Elsevier (Singapore) Pte Ltd.
3 Killiney Road, #08-01 Winsland House I, Singapore 239519
Tel: (65) 6349-0200, Fax: (65) 6733-1817
First Published 2007
2007 年初版

北京市版权局著作权合同登记号：图字：01-2006-1816

图书在版编目（CIP）数据

产科学聚焦 /（英）詹姆斯（James, D. K.），（英）麦克尤恩（McEwan, A.）原著；郑建华，黄明莉译.
北京：北京大学医学出版社，2006.12
书名原文：Obstetrics in Focus
ISBN 7-81071-986-6

I.产… II.①詹… ②麦… ③郑… ④黄…
III.产科学—汉、英 IV. R714

中国版本图书馆 CIP 数据核字（2006）第 141309 号

产科学聚焦

主　　译：郑建华　黄明莉
出版发行：北京大学医学出版社 (电话：010-82802230)
地　　址：(100083) 北京市海淀区学院路 38 号　北京大学医学部院内
网　　址：http://www.pumpress.com.cn
E-mail：booksale@bjmu.edu.cn
印　　刷：莱芜市圣龙印务有限责任公司
经　　销：新华书店
责任编辑：刘燕　　**责任校对**：杜悦　　**责任印制**：郭桂兰
开　　本：880mm × 1100mm　1/32　**印张**：9　**字数**：291 千字
版　　次：2007 年 1 月第 1 版　2007 年 1 月第 1 次印刷
书　　号：ISBN 7-81071-986-6
定　　价：69.90 元

序

本产科图书以简明扼要的版式书写，配有提问与回答，我们希望将会引起产科培训中的医学生、护士、助产士的兴趣。照片图示了各种情况下的重要内容，因为学生看到的情况范围非常有限，并与机会有关。因此我们侧重于能够用照片和扫描清楚地展示的情况，我们希望图片同提问与回答一样，能够对学生们有所帮助并且激励学生。

David James

Alec McEwan

致谢

我们非常感谢为这本图书提供一些图示的人员：G.M. Stirrat 教授、B.Spiedal 博士、P.Savage 先生、P.Burton 博士、R.Slade 博士、D. Warnock 博士、A.Jeffcote 博士、N.Hunter 博士、C.Harman 博士、J.Haworth 博士、H. Andrews 博士、D. Freer 小姐、S.Rosevear 博士、C.Kennedy 博士、J.Zuccollo 博士、J.Pardey 博士、W.Irving 教授、T.Jaspan 博士、J. Padfield 博士、E. Bradley 夫人、G. Ender 教授、M.R. Howard博士以及P.J. Hamilton博士。我们尤其感激Bristol Southmead医院医学图片系的N. Bowyer先生和Nottingham女王医学中心的产科N. Bullimore先生给予的建议以及图片准备过程中的实际帮助。

DJ AM

译者前言

《产科学聚焦》一书包含了大量的临床照片，行文简洁流畅，易懂易记，具有很高的实用性。各章节篇幅不长，虽无深奥理论，但重点突出，概念清晰准确，诊疗方法详实，包括了产科领域最新进展，有助于提高产科医师的诊疗水平。

本书是英汉对照版本，在获取医学的同时还可以提高专业英语水平，既可供医学生、研究生、住院医师、全科医师学习和提高，也可作为专科医生参考借鉴之用。

在翻译此书的过程中我们尽量做到词准意达，但是由于水平有限，可能存在不妥之处，请各位同仁赐教指正。

郑建华

2007 年 1 月

于哈尔滨医科大学第一附属医院

目录

Contents

Contents

早期妊娠

受精与植入

卵子与精子受精发生在输卵管的外侧三分之一（壶腹部）。在36～48小时之后受精卵分裂达到了四个细胞的阶段（图1）。胚胎细胞在72～96小时（16个细胞）到达子宫，在宫腔内保持自由的状态大约4～5天。

植入发生在受精后的6～9天。初级绒毛大约在13～15天发育。在末次月经第一天后的4～5周，妊娠囊可以通过阴道超声检查看到（那就是受孕后的2～3周）（图2），在这之后很快又有卵黄囊。

妊娠的早期诊断

人绒毛膜促性腺激素（hCG）是一种糖蛋白激素，由胎盘的滋养层细胞分泌。在孕妇的尿液及血清中出现，是妊娠诊断的确定性检测。

应用单克隆抗体的分析是迅速、简单而敏感的，现在能够达到敏感度为25～50mU/ml的hCG水平，大约为受孕后的10～14天。

预产期（expected date of delivery, EDD）是末次月经（last menstrual period，LMP）头一天之后的280天（Naegele准则）。正常妊娠的时间在不同的种族之间有一定的差异，但是仅仅是若干天的时间。

这种从末次月经计算预产期的方法是假设受孕的时间发生在末次月经后的两周。当月经周期更长（比如35天、42天）或月经周期不规则，受孕可以发生在更晚的时间。并且，有时候患者对末次月经的记忆也不准确。因为在最初的16周的时间里，胎儿的大小变异很小，超声检查通过测量顶臀长（图3）或者双顶径可能有助于确定预产期。

以后，由于遗传以及环境的因素比如母体患有糖尿病、感染、应用药物以及先兆子痫，可以引起胎儿大小的明显差异，这使得通过超声的方法检测晚期妊娠的方法变得不再准确。

1 Early pregnancy

Fertilization and implantation

Fertilization of the ovum by sperm occurs in the outer third of the fallopian tube. The division of the conceptus reaches a four-cell stage after 36-48 h (Fig 1). The blastocyst arrives in the uterus at 72-96 h (16 cells) and remains free in the uterine cavity for 4-5 days.

Implantation occurs 6-9 days after fertilization. Primitive chorionic villi develop at 13-15 days. The gestation sac is visible on vaginal ultrasound 4-5 weeks after the first day of the last menstrual period (i.e. 2-3 weeks postconception) (Fig 2), and a yolk sac soon after this.

Early diagnosis of pregnancy

Human chorionic gonadotrophin (hCG) is a glycoprotein hormone secreted by the trophoblastic cells of the placenta. It is present in the urine and serum of pregnant women and is the definitive test for diagnosing pregnancy.

Assays using monoclonal antibodies are quick, simple and sensitive and can now reliably detect as little as 25-50 mU/mL of hCG-the level found approximately 10-14 days after conception.

The expected date of delivery (EDD) is 280 days after the first day of the last menstrual period (LMP) (Naegele's rule). There is some ethnic variation in the length of normal pregnancy but only by a few days.

This method of calculating the EDD from the LMP assumes conception was 2 weeks after the LMP. Conception is likely to occur later with a long cycle (e.g. 35, 42 days), irregular periods, or recent oral contraceptive use. Also, memory of the date of the LMP is often poor. Because fetal size shows little variability in the first 16 weeks of pregnancy, ultrasound may help clarify the EDD in such cases by measuring either the crown-rump length (Fig 3) or biparietal diameter.

Later, genetic and environmental factors such as maternal diabetes, infections, drug use and pre-eclampsia cause significant variation in fetal size at any particular gestation, making 'late' dating by ultrasound imprecise.

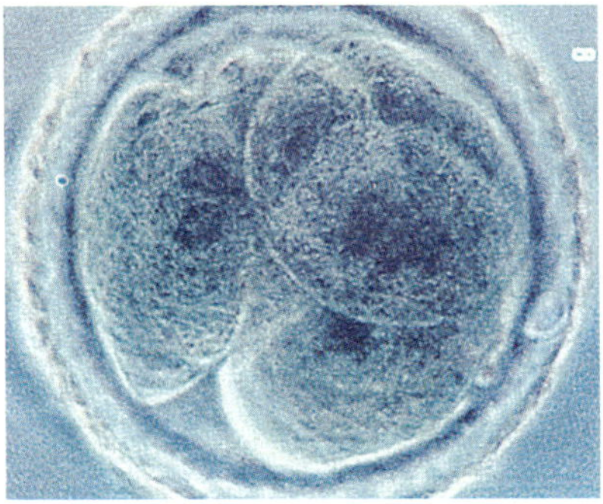

图 1　胚泡：四细胞阶段
Blastocyst: four-cell stage

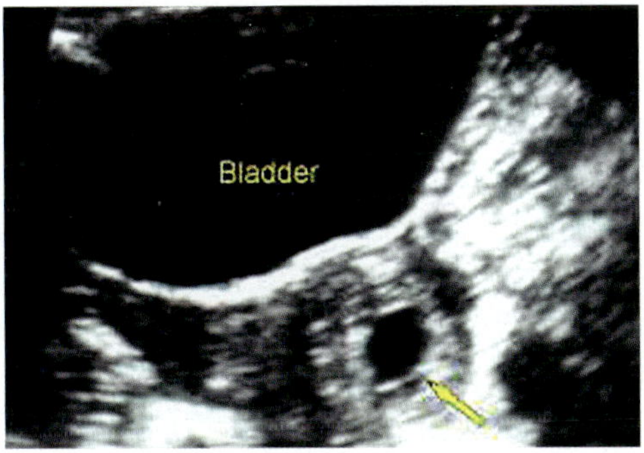

图 2　宫内妊娠囊的超声学检查（5 周）（箭头所指）
Ultrasound of intrauterine gestation sac (5 weeks) (arrowed)

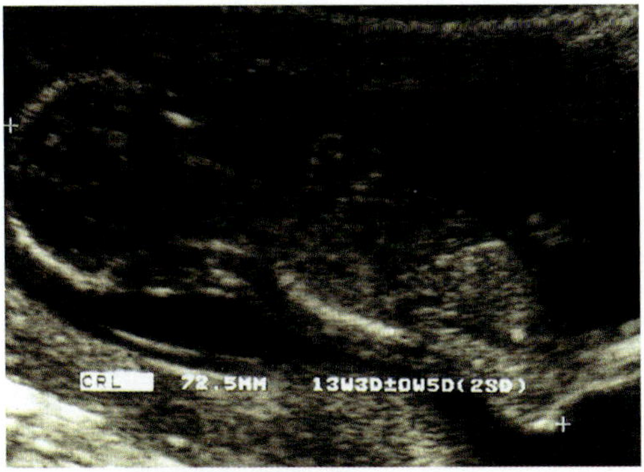

图 3　超声检查顶臀长
Ultrasound of crown-rump length

保健的目的

在绝大多数的情况下，妊娠是一个正常的生理过程，对母亲或孩子都有很小的风险。然而，在一些情况下有不利结局的很大风险。产前保健的目的是：

- 提供建议、放心、教育、对孕妇及其家庭的支持。
- 解决妊娠期间的小疾病。
- 提供全面的健康筛查。
- 预防、发现及处理对孕妇及胎儿产生不利影响的因素。

通过反复的采集病史、产前检查，回顾妊娠期间风险水平，对“常规”的保健进行调整。

就诊

最近由 National Institute of Clinical Excellence（NICE）发布的指南建议低危妊娠的产前检查次数应该减少（初次就诊在 8 ～ 14 周，随后的就诊时间在 20、24、28、30、32、34、36、38、40 和 41 周）。这种保健可单由全科医生和社区的助产士提供或者与产科医生检查相联合（“分担保健”）。

病史

在第一次就诊时记录以下数据：母亲的年龄、婚姻状态、种族背景、月经、医疗、精神病史、手术史、产科史、家族史和社会史，以及其他问题的任何细节。应用毒品、酗酒和吸烟史都应记录在案。使用结构性的母亲情况的记录（通常由孕妇保管），减少了漏掉高危因素的机会。在随后的检查中，任何新出现的问题都记录下来，同时记录下自觉胎动情况。

在妊娠期间的生理改变可以引起多种症状。多数器官或系统可受累：胃肠道（恶心、呕吐、食管炎、便秘、痔疮、牙龈增生）（图 4）；泌尿生殖系（尿频）；乳腺（麻刺感、增大、乳头色素沉着）（图5）；皮肤（色素沉着增加）（图 6）；心脏和呼吸（心悸），

Normal pregnancy and care

Aims of care

Pregnancy in most cases will be a normal event with low risk of harm to mother or baby. For a few, however, there is a greater risk of adverse outcomes. The aims of antenatal care are:

- To provide advice, reassurance, education and support for the woman and her family.
- To deal with minor ailments of pregnancy.
- To provide general health screening.
- To prevent, detect and manage those factors that adversely affect the health of mother and/or baby.

By repeated history-taking, examination and investigations the level of risk in a pregnancy is regularly reviewed and modifications to 'routine' care are made in the light of this.

Visits

Recent evidence-based guidelines from the National Institute of Clinical Excellence (NICE) have recommended a reduction in the number of antenatal appointments in low-risk pregnancies (first visit at 8-14 weeks, followed by visits at 20, 24, 28, 30, 32, 34, 36, 38, 40 and 41 weeks). Care is provided either solely by the general practitioner and community midwife or in combination with a consultant obstetrician ('shared care').

History

At the first ('booking') visit, the following data are recorded: maternal age, marital status, ethnic background, menstrual, medical, psychiatric, surgical, obstetric, family and social histories and details of any other problems. Drug intake, alcohol and smoking habits are also documented. The use of structured maternity records (usually carried by pregnant women) reduces the chances that identifiable risk factors will be missed. At subsequent visits any new problems are noted, together with maternal perception of fetal movements.

Physiological changes occurring in pregnancy may cause a multitude of symptoms. Most organ systems may be involved: gastrointestinal (nausea, vomiting, oesophagitis, constipation, haemorrhoids, gum hypertrophy) (Fig 4); urogenital (urinary frequency); breasts (tingling, enlargement, nipple pigmentation) (Fig 5); skin (increased pigmentation) (Fig 6); cardiorespiratory (palpitations,

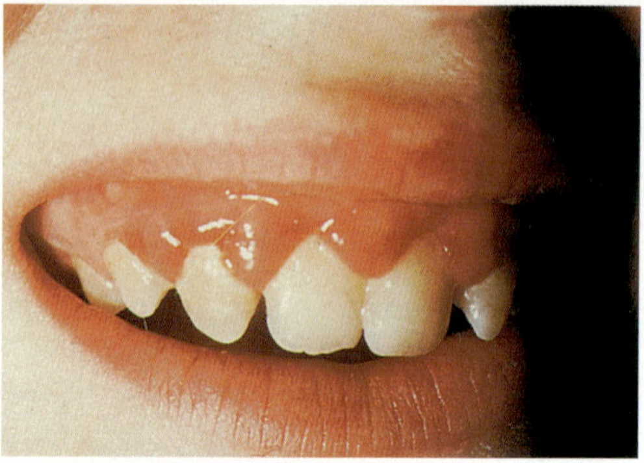

图 4　牙龈增生
Gum hypertrophy

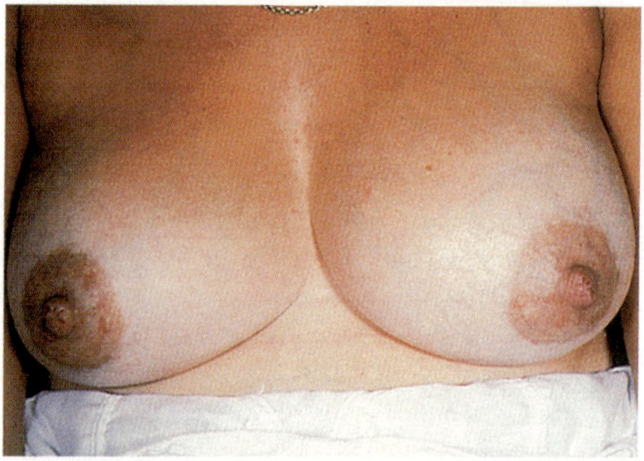

图 5　乳房改变
Breast changes

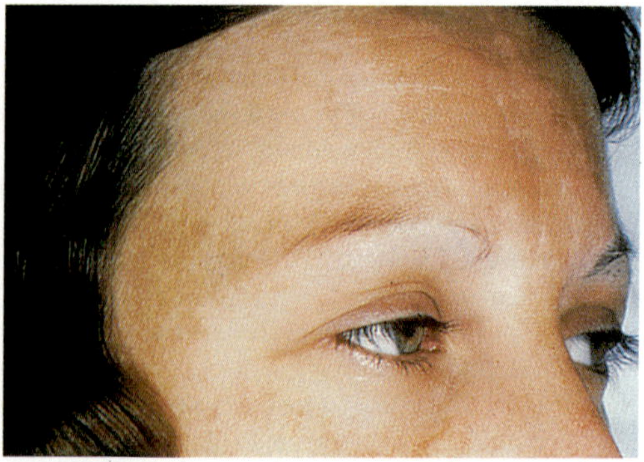

图 6　黄褐斑（面部色素沉着）
Chloasma（facial pigmentation）

呼吸困难；神经系统（腕管综合征）。其他的症状可能代表病理情况（比如头痛和腹痛，分辨这两种情况可能是困难的）。

检查

在预约的就诊中，体重质量指数的计算以及血压（bloocd pressure，BP）的测量都是非常重要的。心脏、呼吸、乳房以及盆腔的检查仅限于那些有高危因素或症状的患者。在所有的就诊中都应该记录血压和子宫的大小。在妊娠晚期应记录胎位、胎先露、胎儿头部入盆的情况，胎心情况应该进行听诊。

体征

妊娠早期的体征包括乳房的改变（增大、色素沉着、静脉充血和蒙氏结节）（图5），和生殖器改变（阴道和宫颈的淡蓝色着色、变软和子宫的增大）。其他的体征还有牙龈增生（图 4）、黄褐斑（图 6）、妊娠纹（图 7）、腹白线色素沉着、脐色素沉着和脐外翻（图 8）、淋巴结病、甲状腺增大和静脉曲张（图 9）。

化验

初次就诊时，进行尿分析（检查糖、蛋白、酮体）和中段尿培养。采血进行全血的计数和检查、ABO和Rh 血型分析、抗体筛查、风疹抗体状态和梅毒的血清血检查、乙型肝炎和HIV的检查。如果妇女是美国黑人/加勒比海人、地中海人或从远东来的，建议进行血红蛋白电泳。在妊娠 16 周时可以进行生化筛查检测，在检查胎儿的神经管缺陷或唐氏综合征。有一些医疗单位通过在 11 ～ 13 周时胎儿颈背半透明测量进行唐氏筛查（图 29）。在随后的每次检查中都进行尿分析检查，在 28 和 34 周时重复进行血红蛋白及红细胞抗体筛查。

breathlessness); and neurological (carpal tunnel syndrome). Other symptoms may indicate pathology (e.g. headaches and abdominal pain; distinguishing the two may be difficult).

Examination

At the booking visit, calculation of the body mass index and measurement of the blood pressure (BP) are important. Cardiorespiratory, breast and pelvic examinations are only necessary in those with risk factors or symptoms. At all visits, BP and uterine size are recorded. In later pregnancy, the fetal lie and presentation and the engagement of the fetal head are noted and the fetal heart is auscultated.

Signs

Early signs of pregnancy include changes in the breasts (enlargement, pigmentation, venous engorgement and Montgomery's tubercles) (Fig 5) and genitalia (bluish coloration of vaginal skin and cervix, softening and enlargement of uterus). Other signs include gum hypertrophy (Fig 4), chloasma (Fig 6), striae gravidarum (Fig 7), linea nigra, umbilical pigmentation and eversion (Fig 8), lymphadenopathy, thyroid enlargement and varicose veins (Fig 9).

Investigations

At the first visit, urinalysis is undertaken (testing for glucose, protein, ketones) and a midstream sample of urine is sent for culture. Blood is taken for complete blood count and film, ABO and rhesus typing, antibody screening, rubella antibody status and serological tests for syphilis, hepatitis B and HIV. Haemoglobin electrophoresis is indicated if the woman is Afro-American/Caribbean, Mediterranean, or from the Far East. At 16 weeks, biochemical screening tests may be performed for fetal neural tube defects and Down syndrome. Some units offer screening for Down syndrome by fetal nuchal translucency measurement at 11-13 weeks (Fig 29). Urinalysis is performed at all subsequent visits, and haemoglobin and red cell antibody screening is repeated at 28 and 34 weeks.

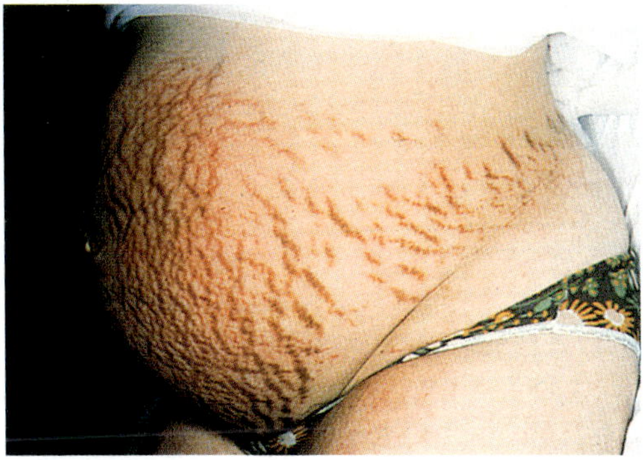

图 7　妊娠纹
Striae gravidarum

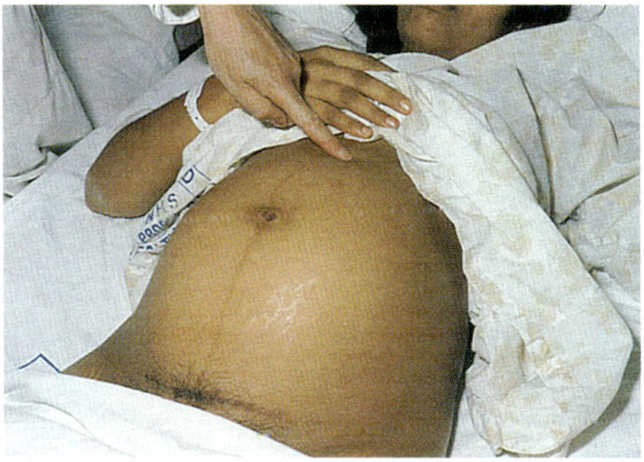

图 8　腹白线色素沉着和脐部色素沉着及脐外翻
Linea nigra and umbilical pigmentation and eversion

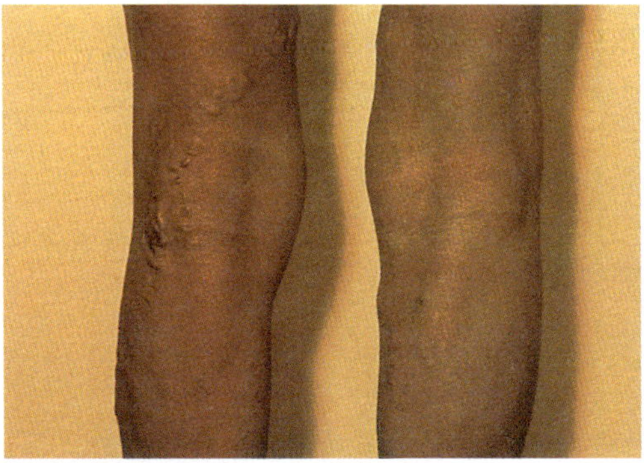

图 9　曲张的静脉
Varicose veins

流产

定义

如果在妊娠24周（美国为20周）之前排出妊娠组织，在这种情况下胎儿在娩出后没有生命迹象。大多数的流产发生在最初的12周。临床检测到的妊娠大约有15% ~ 20% 发生流产。习惯性流产的定义为三次或更多的自发性流产。

分类

- *先兆流产*：阴道流血，但是妊娠继续。
- *难免流产*：阴道流血，子宫收缩（疼痛）以及宫颈口开，但是妊娠组织没有排出。
- *不完全流产*：妊娠组织已经通过阴道排出，但是子宫还没有排空。宫颈口是开的（图10）。
- *完全流产*：所有的妊娠组织都被排出，子宫排空，宫颈口关闭。
- *稽留流产*：通过超声检查诊断。坐高（顶臀径）≥ 6mm 的胎儿没有看见心跳（图11）。
- *Anembryonic 妊娠（枯萎卵）*：在超声上表现为 ≥ 20mm 的空的妊娠囊。

病因

经常没有明显的原因。但是如果调查，胎儿的异常（尤其是染色体的异常）是最通常的原因。其他的原因包括磷脂综合征（比如狼疮）、血栓形成倾向、多囊卵巢综合征、先天性子宫异常、细胞毒性药物、宫颈松弛（妊娠中期妊囊丢失）。

临床特征

停经、腹绞痛（40%）、流血（量有不同)(98%)、休克(5%)、宫颈口扩张以及妊娠组织排出（15%），偶尔通过超声发现。

处理

在妊娠早期诊断可能有困难，反复的检查是必要的。处理方法有保守的方法、药物的方法（应用抗孕激素药物）或手术（图12）。选择何种方法应根据临床特征以及患者的意愿。

Miscarriage

Definition

Expulsion of the products of conception before the 24th week of pregnancy (20th week in USA) in which the fetus shows no signs of life after delivery. Most miscarriages occur in the first 12 weeks. Miscarriage occurs in 15-20% of clinically detected pregnancies. Recurrent miscarriage is defined as three or more consecutive spontaneous miscarriages.

Classification

- *Threatened*: vaginal bleeding but pregnancy continues.
- *Inevitable*: vaginal bleeding, uterine contractions (pain) and an open cervical os, but before the passage of products of conception.
- *Incomplete*: pregnancy tissues have been passed per vaginum, but the uterus is not yet empty. The cervical os is open (Fig 10).
- *Complete*: all the products of conception have been expelled, the uterus is empty and the cervix is closed.
- *Missed*: an ultrasound diagnosis. No heart beat is visible in a fetus with a crown-rump length of ⩾ 6 mm (Fig 11).
- *Anembryonic pregnancy (blighted ovum)*: an empty gestation sac measuring ⩾ 20 mm on ultrasound.

Aetiology

Often no cause is apparent. However, if investigated, fetal abnormalities (especially chromosomal) are the most common cause. Others include phospholipid syndromes (e.g. lupus), thrombophilias, polycystic ovary syndrome, congenital uterine anomalies, cytotoxic drugs, cervical incompetence (second trimester losses).

Clinical features

Amenorrhea, colicky pain (40%), bleeding (variable in amount) (98%), shock (5%), cervical dilation and passage of products (15%), chance ultrasound finding.

Management

Making a diagnosis may be difficult at early gestations and repeated scanning is often necessary. Management can be conservative, medical (using antiprogestogens) or surgical (Fig 12). The choice is determined by the clinical features and patient's wishes.

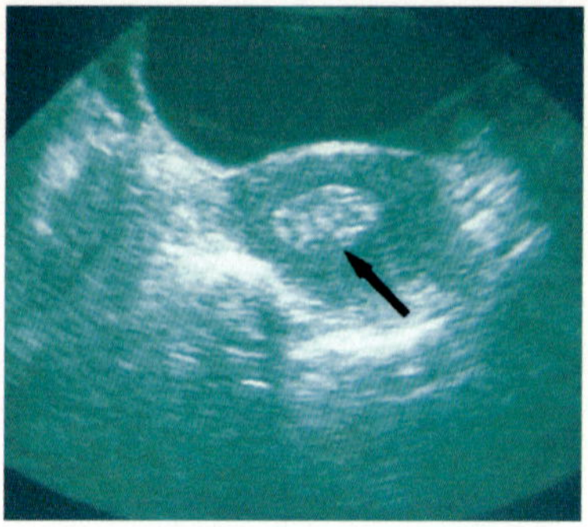

图 10　妊娠组织滞留的不完全流产
Incomplete miscarriage with retained products of conception

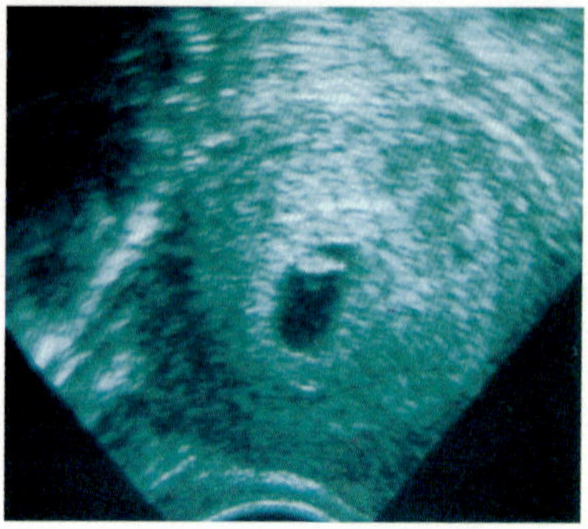

图 11　稽留流产的阴道超声
Vaginal ultrasound of missed miscarriage

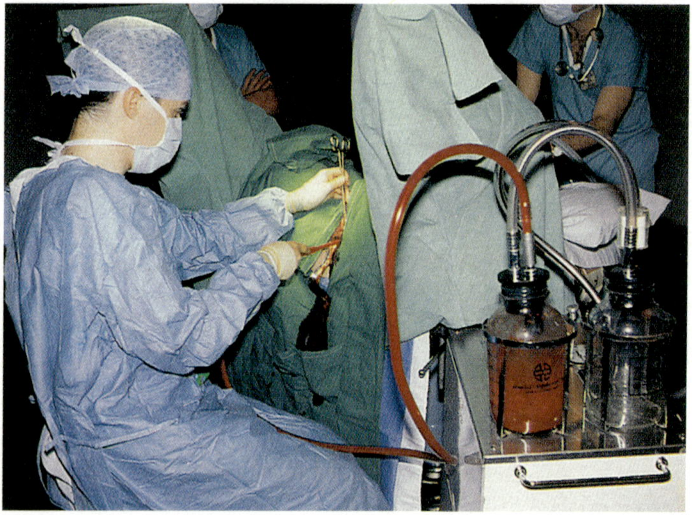

图 12　滞留的妊娠组织通过手术排空
Surgical evacuation of retained products of conception

异位妊娠

定义

妊娠囊的植入没有在正常的宫腔（图13），1%的妊娠可以出现。最常发生的位置是输卵管的壶腹部（图14）。其他的位置包括卵巢和腹部。

病因学

高危因素包括输卵管损坏（继发于盆腔感染、输卵管重建手术以及前次的异位妊娠）、宫腔内避孕措施的应用以及辅助生殖技术。

临床特征

症状　下腹痛（通常是单侧的）、流血（通常是暗红色阴道点滴出血）、头晕和肩顶部疼痛（腹腔内出血引起的膈下刺激征）。

体征　低血压和心跳加快（与可见的出血程度不成比例），宫颈触痛，附件区触痛以及有时有包块。输卵管破裂将会引起突然的疼痛，然后发生休克及虚脱。

检查

联合应用超声检查和血清hCG测定，避免过度应用腹腔镜来诊断。当hCG水平高于1500IU/L时，宫腔内的妊娠囊应该能够看见。绝大多数的宫腔内妊娠hCG的水平在48小时会上升超过66%以上。绝大多数的异位妊娠不会有这种情况。

处理

取决于临床表现、阴道超声的发现和血清hCG的水平。选择包括：

药物：对于症状轻、没有心血管损害、小的异位妊娠，顺应性好的妇女可以应用肌内注射甲氨蝶呤的方法保守治疗。

手术：最常见的处理是应用腹腔镜或开腹输卵管切开（保守性的手术）或输卵管切除（将受到影响的输卵管切除）（图15）。如果另一侧表现正常，目前赞成应用输卵管切除，因为输卵管切开有持续性的滋养细胞存活的风险以及将来再次异位妊娠的发病率高。

Ectopic pregnancy

Definition

Implantation of a pregnancy in a site other than the normal uterine cavity (Fig 13). Occurs in 1% of pregnancies. The most common site is the ampullary portion of the fallopian tube (Fig 14). Other sites include the ovary and abdomen.

Aetiology

Risk factors include tubal damage (secondary to pelvic infection, tubal reconstructive surgery and a previous ectopic pregnancy), use of intrauterine contraceptive devices and assisted reproductive techniques.

Clinical features

Symptoms Lower abdominal pain (usually unilateral), bleeding (often dark red vaginal 'spotting'), dizziness and shoulder tip pain (subdiaphragmatic irritation by intraperitoneal blood).

Signs Hypotension and tachycardia out of proportion to the visible bleeding, cervical excitation, adnexal tenderness and sometimes a mass. Tubal rupture will produce sudden pain followed by shock and collapse.

Investigations

A combination of transvaginal ultrasound scanning and measurement of serum human chorionic gonadotrophin (hCG) levels avoids excessive use of laparoscopy for making the diagnosis. An intrauterine gestation sac should be visible with hCG levels greater than 1500 IU/L. The majority of intrauterine ongoing pregnancies will demonstrate a greater than 66% rise in hCG levels over 48 h. Most ectopic pregnancies do not.

Management

Depends on clinical features, vaginal ultrasound findings and serum hCG levels. Options include:

- *Medical*. Intramuscular methotrexate is reserved for compliant women with minimal symptoms, no cardiovas cular compromise and small ectopics.
- *Surgical*. The most common treatment is laparoscopic or open salpingotomy (conservative surgery) or salpingectorny (removal of the affected tube) (Fig15). Salpingectomy is currently favoured if the other tube appears normal because salpingotomy carries a risk of persistent trophoblast and higher future ectopic rate.

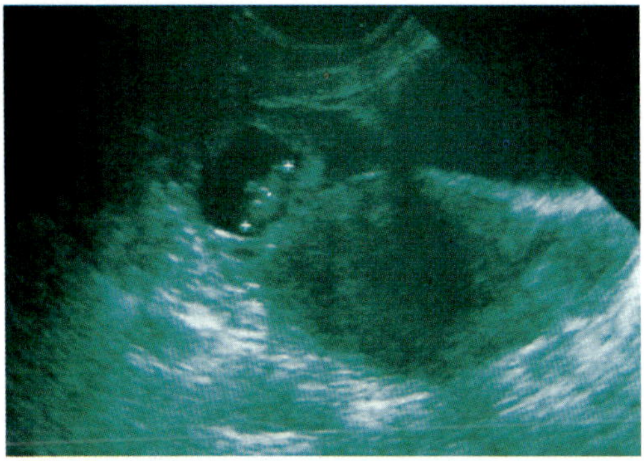

图 13　阴道超声显示异位妊娠（胎儿在上方，在空子宫的左侧）
Vaginal ultrasound showing ectopic pregnancy with the fetus above and to the left of the empty uterus

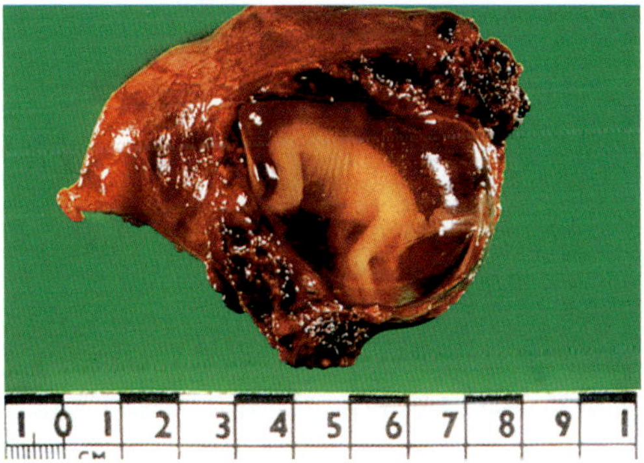

图 14　异位妊娠的病理标本
Pathology specimen of ectopic pregnancy

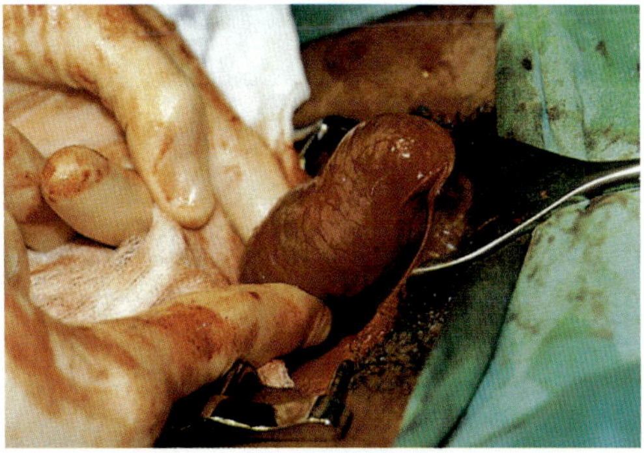

图 15　腹腔镜下输卵管异位妊娠
Tubal ectopic pregnancy at laparotomy

滋养细胞疾病

定义
在胎盘发生的肿瘤。

发生率
在远东的发生率是1/600。但是在西方国家为1/2000。

病理学
绒毛变得非常水肿。大部分是良性的（水泡状胎块），但是有假恶性的特征，能够侵入子宫肌层和造成系统的播散。在“完全性”葡萄胎（图16）不出现胎儿。染色体是双倍体（46条染色体），但是染色体是完全的父系来源。在罕见的情况下，完全性葡萄胎能够变成恶性的（绒癌）。“部分性”葡萄胎（图17）总是发现与三倍体胎儿（69条染色体）有关，额外的染色体来自于父亲。部分性葡萄胎通常不会变成恶性。

临床特征
子宫流血，夸大的妊娠特征，子宫比预计的大许多，通过阴道排出葡萄粒样组织。先兆子痫和甲状腺毒症可以使临床征象更为复杂。

诊断
经常在认为是不完全性流产清宫时发现。超声学表现为特征性的胎盘“落雪”图像，以及较高的hCG水平，事先倾向于此诊断。

检查
组织进行组织学及染色体检查；胸片；血清hCG；甲状腺、肝和肾功能；全血细胞计数；ABO和Rh血型。

处理
通过负压吸引和刮宫清空子宫。然后在三个国家滋养叶细胞疾病中心之一进行尿和/或血液的hCG水平检测。hCG水平不下降或者下降后又再次升高提示清宫不全、侵犯肌层、转移或恶变。经常采用甲氨蝶呤化疗进行治疗，极少采用子宫切除术。强烈建议应该至少一年内避孕。

Trophoblastic disease

Definition

Neoplasia occurring in the placenta.

Incidence

1 in 600 pregnancies in the Far East, but 1 in 2000 in the West.

Pathology

The villi become grossly hydropic. The majority are benign (hydatidiform mole) but have pseudomalignant properties, capable of myometrial invasion and systemic dissemination. In a 'complete' mole (Fig 16) no fetus is present. The karyotype is diploid (46 chromosomes) but the chromosomes are totally paternal in origin. Rarely, a complete mole can become malignant (choriocarcinoma). A 'partial' mole (Fig 17) is always found in association with a triploid fetus (69 chromosomes) with the extra set of chromosomes being of paternal origin. Partial moles do not normally become malignant.

Clinical features

Uterine bleeding, exaggerated features of pregnancy, a larger than expected uterus and the passage of grape-like tissue per vaginum. Pre-eclampsia and thyrotoxicosis may complicate the clinical picture.

Diagnosis

Often made at curettage for presumed incomplete miscarriage. A characteristic placental 'snowstorm' appearance on ultrasound (Fig 18) and very high hCG levels often point to the diagnosis beforehand.

Investigations

Tissue for histology and karyotype; chest radiograph; serum hCG; thyroid, liver and renal function; complete blood count; ABO and rhesus group.

Management

The uterus is emptied by suction and curettage. Subsequent monitoring of urinary and/or serum hCG levels is supervised by one of the three national trophoblast centres. Levels that fail to fall or subsequently rise again suggest incomplete evacuation, invasion, metastasis or malignant change. Chemotherapy with methotrexate is usually curative and hysterectomy is rarely indicated. Avoidance of pregnancy for at least a year is strongly advised.

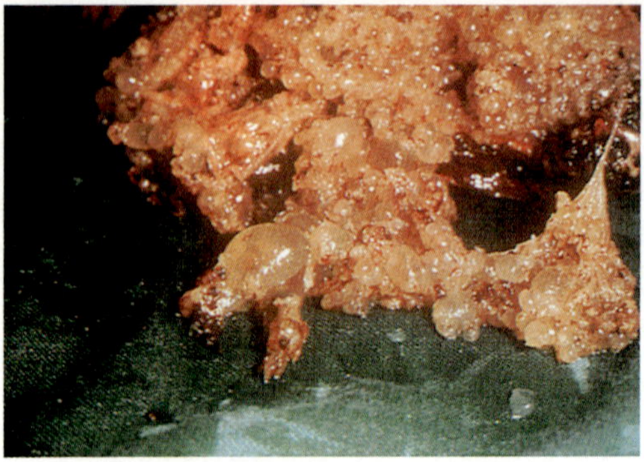

图 16　完全性葡萄胎
Complete mole

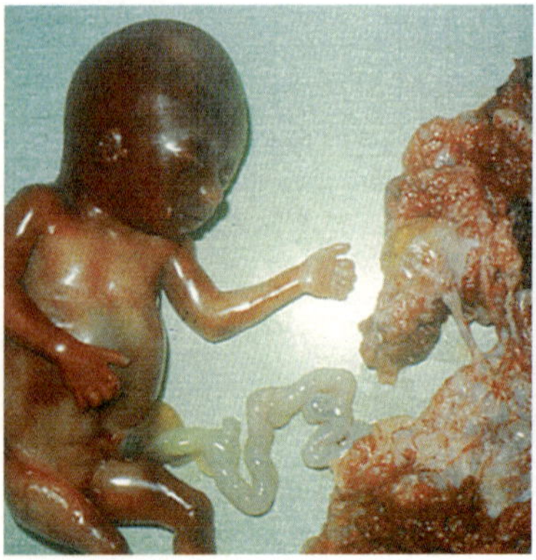

图 17　部分性葡萄胎伴有三倍体的胎儿
Partial mole with triploid fetus

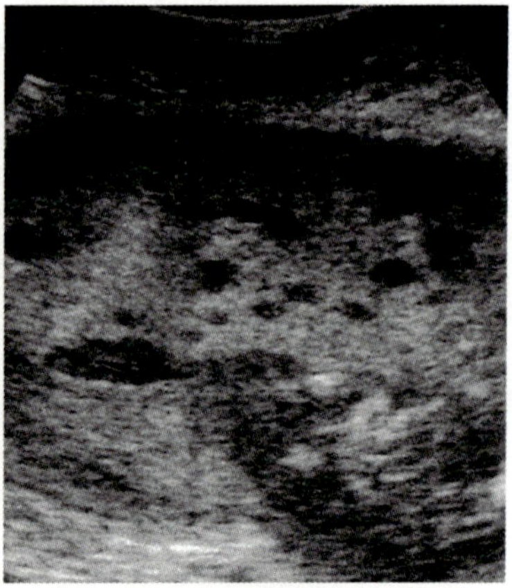

图 18　部分性葡萄胎的超声图像（胎盘的多处无回声区，但胎儿也存在）。
Ultrasound picture of a partial mole (multiple echolucent areas in the placenta but with fetal Parts also)

风疹

母亲

潜伏期2～3周。表现为皮疹（图19）、淋巴结炎、发热、不适、结膜炎以及咳嗽。依靠发现风疹特异性IgM抗体（在3个月后下降）或IgG滴度的升高进行诊断。从咽部涂片可以培养出病毒。

没有免疫的妇女应该进行分娩后疫苗。在妊娠早期无意的疫苗注射与先天性的疾病没有关系。

婴孩

如果妊娠最初三个月发生感染，大约有80%～90%会发生幸存者的损害，包括眼睛（图20）和心脏损害、头小畸形、智力发育迟缓、血小板减少性紫癜、肝脾大以及发育受限。妊娠4～6个月的感染会引起10%～15%发生感觉神经性耳聋。

弓形体病

母亲

经常是没有症状的。高危因素包括与猫接触、食用欠熟的肉。通过血清学检查发现弓形虫特异的IgM抗体进行诊断。

婴孩

少数的胎儿（20%）会发生感染，其中大约有15%发生先天性的异常。包括生长受限、脉络视网膜炎、脑积水和颅内钙化。血小板减少性紫癜、肝脾大、黄疸、发热、肺炎抽搐在出生时可能明显。

肉芽肿性疾病（图21）、拟孢囊和钙化发生在中枢神经系统、眼睛、肺、心脏、肝、脾和肾。

梅毒

母亲

在母体发生疾病的阶段不同，胎儿感染的风险也不同：一期（下疳）和二期（散布的淋巴结炎和皮疹）感染90%，潜伏感染40%；三期感染（梅毒性树胶肿、

Rubella

Mother

Incubation period of 2-3 weeks. Maculopapular rash (Fig 19), lymphadenopathy, fever, malaise, conjunctivitis and cough. Diagnosed by finding rubella-specific IgM antibody (falls after 3 months) or rising titres of IgG. Virus can be cultured from a throat swab.

Non-immune women should be offered postnatal vaccination. Inadvertent vaccination in early pregnancy has not been associated with congenital disease.

Baby

First trimester fetal infection carries an 80-90% risk of damage in survivors, including eye (Fig 20) and cardiac defects, microcephaly, mental retardation, thrombocytopenic purpura, hepatosplenomegaly and growth restriction. Second trimester infection causes sensorineural deafness in 10-15%.

Toxoplasmosis

Mother

Often asymptomatic. Risk factors include contact with cats and ingestion of undercooked meat. Diagnosed by finding toxoplasma-specific IgM on serological testing.

Baby

Fetal infection occurs in a minority of cases (20%) with 15% developing congenital abnormalities, including growth restriction, chorioretinitis, hydrocephalus and intracranial calcification. Thrombocytopenic purpura, hepatosplenomegaly, jaundice, fever, pneumonitis and convulsions may be apparent at birth.

Granulomatous lesions (Fig 21), pseudocysts and calcification occur in the central nervous system, eyes, lungs, heart, liver, spleen and kidneys.

Syphilis

Mother

The risk of fetal infection varies with stage of maternal disease: 90% with primary (chancre) and secondary (disseminated lymphadenopathy and rash) infection; 40% with latent infection; and 10% with late (gummas,

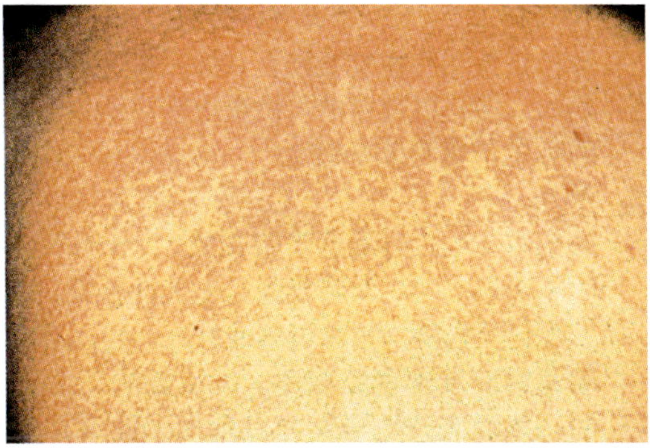

图 19　母亲的风疹皮疹（德国风疹）
Maternal rubella rash (German measles)

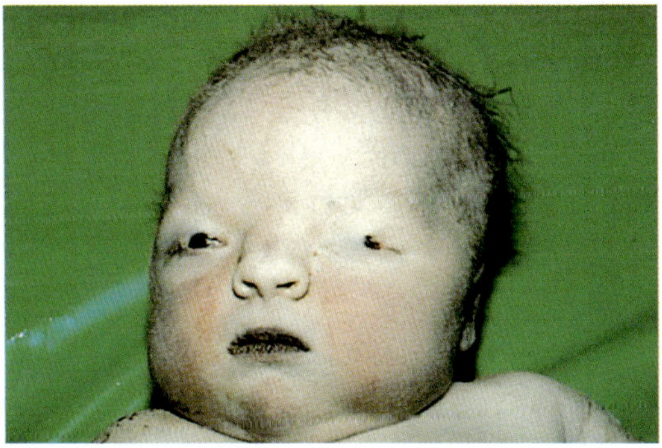

图 20　风疹导致的微小眼炎
Rubella-induced microphthalmia

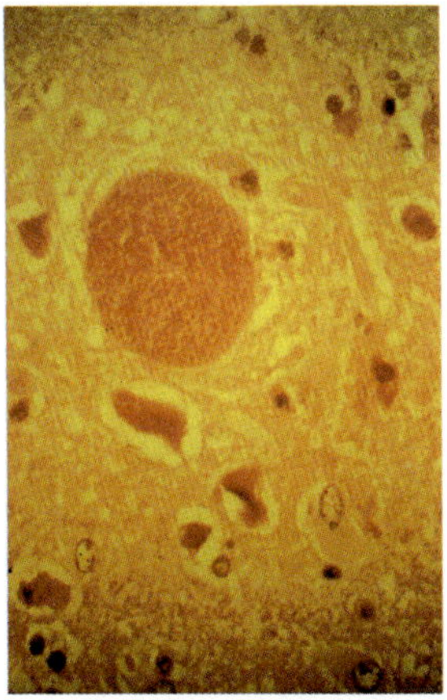

图 21　胎儿大脑内的弓形体
Toxoplasma body within the fetal brain

神经系统和心血管系统）10%。通过分离出病原体（一期和二期）以及血清学检查进行诊断。血清学检查阳性的母亲用青霉素治疗。

婴儿

大约有1/4的梅毒感染胎儿死亡，1/4发生早产或胎儿生长受限，一半发生新生儿先天性感染。相关的超声学发现包括水肿、羊水过多或肝大。可以直接检测羊水或胎儿血液发现密螺旋体。大多数的新生儿是没有症状的，然而有一些早期会出现先天性梅毒（皮疹、肝脾大、淋巴结炎、水肿）。用青霉素治疗。

巨细胞病毒

母亲

大多数的患者没有症状。如果可疑巨细胞病毒(cytomegalovirus, CMV)，从宫颈或尿有可能分离出巨细胞病毒。CMV能够再活动，引起对胎儿的较小程度的危害。

婴孩

30% ~ 40% 的原发母体感染能够感染胎儿。在这些被感染的胎儿中，5% ~ 7% 在出生时有症状，伴有血小板减少性紫癜（图22）、肝脾大、脉络膜视网膜炎、微小眼炎、肾炎、小头畸形、耳聋、智力迟缓、大脑钙化和生长受限。分离出病毒可以做出诊断。

组织学上，CMV感染的细胞经常会有胞质内包涵体（被溶酶体包围的病毒颗粒）（图23）。

细小病毒

母亲

发热、不适，感染后关节痛罕见。20%的成年人感染后没有症状。

婴孩

胎儿感染能够引起生长不全危象，伴有贫血、心肌炎以及胎儿水肿（图24）。如在妊娠4 ~ 6个月时感染，胎儿死亡率可以达到1/10，发生在暴露于病毒4 ~ 6周后。20周后的危险就明显降低。胎儿贫血可以通过宫腔内输血治疗。

neurological and cardiovascular) infection. Diagnosis is by isolation of the organism (primary and secondary) and serological tests. Seropositive mothers are usually treated with penicillin.

Baby

A quarter of fetal syphilis infections end in fetal loss, a quarter in preterm labour or fetal growth restriction and half in a congenitally infected neonate. Associated ultrasound findings may include hydrops, polyhydramnios or hepatomegaly. Amniotic fluid or fetal blood can be tested directly for *Treponema pallidum.* Most newborns are asymptomatic; however a few will manifest early congenital syphilis (rash, hepatosplenomegaly, lymphadenopathy, oedema). Treatment is with penicillin.

Cytomegalovirus

Mother

Almost always asymptomatic. If cytomegalovirus (CMV) is suspected, then isolation of the virus from cervix or urine is possible. CMV can reactivate, posing minimal risk to the fetus.

Baby

The fetus becomes infected in 30-40% of primary maternal infections. Of those infected, 5-7% will be symptomatic at birth, with thrombocytopenic purpura (Fig 22), hepatosplenomegaly, chorioretinitis, microphthalmia, nephritis, microcephaly, deafness, mental retardation, cerebral calcifications and growth restriction. Diagnosis is by isolation of the virus.

Histologically, CMV-infected cells frequently have cytoplasmic inclusions (virus particles surrounded by lysosomes) (Fig 23).

Parvovirus

Mother

Fever, malaise and rarely postinfectious arthralgia. 20% of adult infections are asymptomatic.

Baby

Fetal infection can cause an aplastic crisis, with anaemia, myocarditis and hydrops fetalis (Fig 24). In the second trimester, fetal loss rates may reach 1 in 10, occurring 4-6 weeks after exposure. The risk after 20 weeks is significantly less. Fetal anaemia can be treated with intrauterine transfusions.

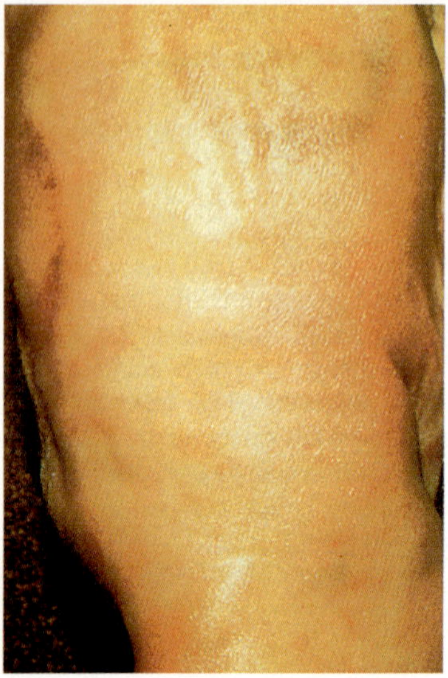

图 22 巨细胞病毒（CMV）：躯干的皮肤表现
Cytomegalovirus (CMV)：cutaneous manifestations in the trunk

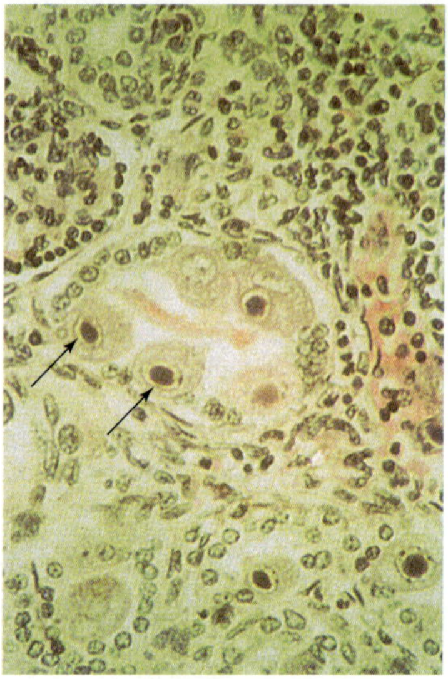

图 23 巨细胞病毒（CMV）：在胎儿肾内的包涵体
Cytomegalovirus (CMV)：inclusion bodies found within the fetal kidney

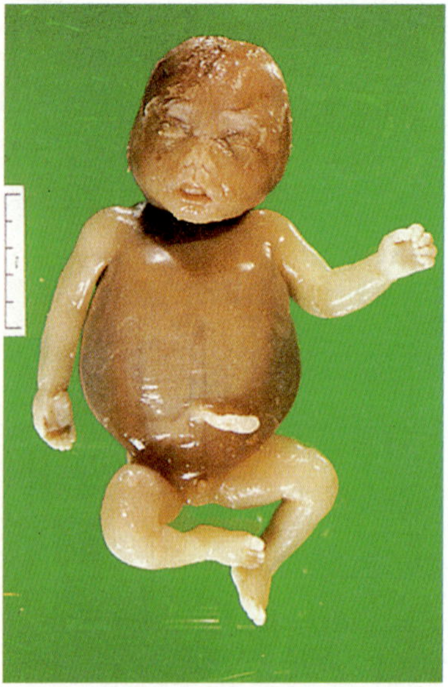

图 24 胎儿细小病毒感染引起水肿
Fetal parvovirus infection causing hydrops

水痘

母亲

症状包括发热、不适和斑丘疹，会变得播散及有小泡。潜伏期大约是10～20天，是通过呼吸道飞沫传播。个体是在皮疹出现前的48小时发生感染。大约有10%的成人出现肺炎，大约有6%是致命性的。母亲的感染可以通过水痘免疫球蛋白预防，疾病本身可以通过应用阿昔洛韦改善。

婴孩

当母体的感染发生早于孕20周，先天性水痘症状在1%～2%的妊娠发生。包括小头畸形、脑皮层萎缩、肢体发育不全（图25）以及严重的皮肤瘢痕。水痘免疫球蛋白有可能减低其风险性。围产期的感染可以引起一系列的新生儿水痘感染症状[播散的皮疹（图26）、血小板减少、肝脾大、黄疸、脑膜脑炎]。无症状的新生儿以后可能表现出“卵石症”，代表宫腔内获得的感染再次活动（图27）。

利斯特杆菌病

母亲

感染利斯特杆菌经常是没有症状的，偶尔会产生伴有腹痛和腹泻的流感样表现。应该避免食用未经过高热杀菌的食物和生的蔬菜。治疗是应用氨苄青霉素。

婴孩

先天性的感染仅发生在有大量的病原微生物的情况。在早期妊娠时可能发生流产，以后可以发生死产。存活者可能发生早期的或晚期的疾病表现。在前者播散性败血症引起皮肤（图28）、肺、肝和神经系统疾病（死亡率90%）。晚期的感染表现可能在出生后获得，表现脑膜炎，伴有智力发育迟缓和/或脑水肿（死亡率40%）。

Varicella zoster (chickenpox)

Mother

Symptoms include fever, malaise and a pruritic maculopapular rash which becomes widespread and vesicular. Incubation period is 10-20 days and transmission is through respiratory droplets. Individuals are infectious 48 h before the rash appears. A pneumonitis occurs in 10% of adults and is said to be fatal in as many as 6%. Maternal infection may be prevented by administration of varicella immunoglobulin (VZIG) and the disease itself ameliorated by the use of aciclovir.

Baby

The congenital varicella syndrome occurs in 1-2% of pregnancies when maternal infection occurs at less than 20 weeks' gestation. It comprises microcephaly, cortical atrophy, limb hypoplasia (Fig 25) and severe skin scarring; VZIG probably reduces this risk. Peripartum infection may result in a serious neonatal varicella infection (widespread skin rash (Fig 26), thrombocytopenia, hepatosplenomegaly, jaundice, meningoencephalitis). Asymptomatic newborns may later present with 'shingles', representing a reactivation of their in utero infection (Fig 27).

Listeriosis

Mother

Infection with *Listeria monocytogenes* is usually asymptomatic, occasionally producing a flu-like illness with abdominal pain and diarrhoea. Eating unpasteurized dairy products and raw vegetables should be avoided. Treatment is with ampicillin.

Baby

Congenital infection only occurs with very heavy colonization. Miscarriage may occur in early pregnancy, stillbirth later on. Survivors develop either an early- or late-onset disease pattern. In the former, diffuse septicaemia causes cutaneous (Fig 28), pulmonary, hepatic and neurological lesions (mortality 90%). Late-onset infection, possibly acquired after birth, is characterized by meningitis, with mental retardation and/or hydrocephalus (mortality 40%).

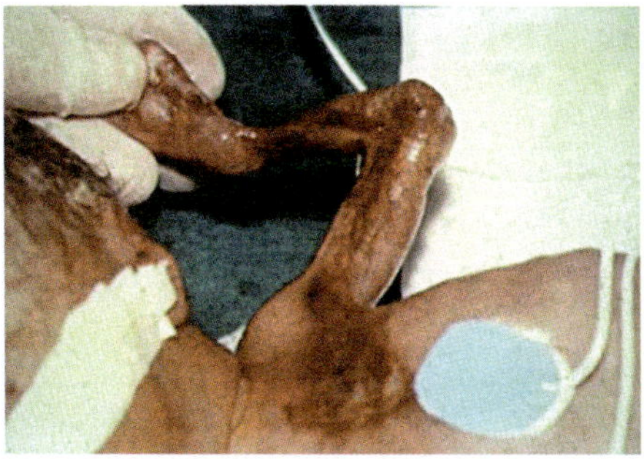

图 25 继发于胎儿水痘感染的肢体发育不全
（Gisela Enders，institute for Virology，Infectiology and Epidemiology，Stuttgart 同意出版）。
Limb hypoplasia secondary to fetal varicella infection. Reproduced with permission from Gisela Enders, Institute for Virology, Infectiology and Epidemiology, Stuttgart

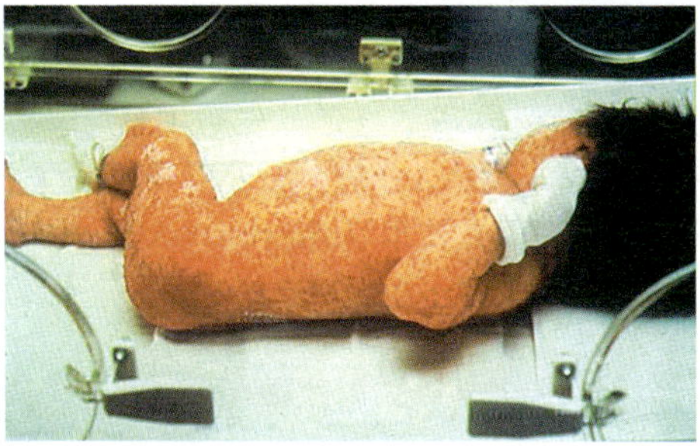

图 26 播散的新生儿水痘
Disseminated neonatal varicella

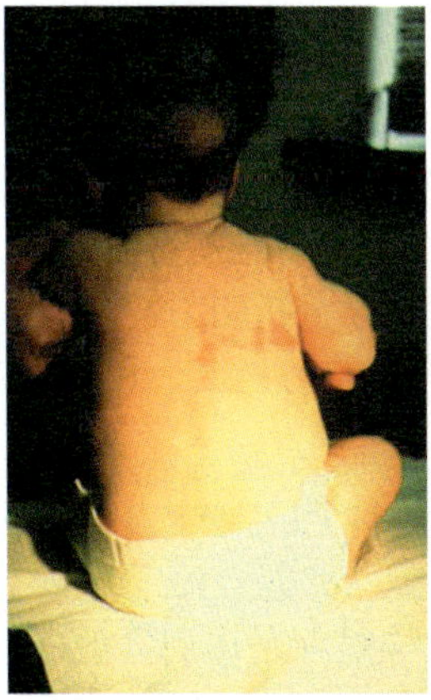

图 27 疱疹（卵石征）
Herpes zoster
（'shingles'）

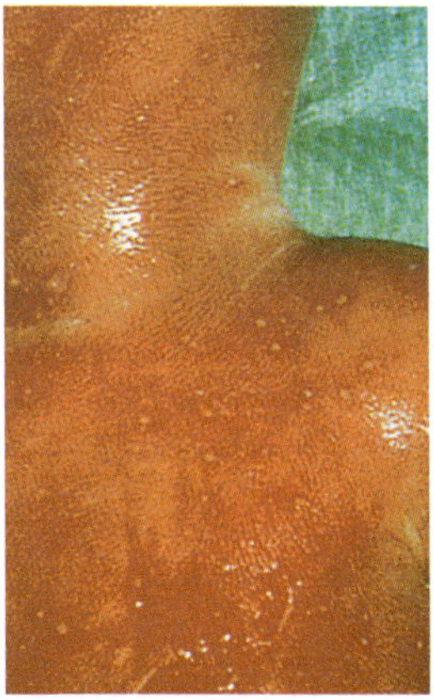

图 28 利斯特杆菌病：皮肤表现
Listeriosis: cutaneous mamifestations

产前诊断

概要

在过去的 20 年里，产前诊断有了巨大的进步。

胎儿图像

超声分辨率明显的提高（图29），对疑难病例可以应用 MRI（第 7 章）。

产科操作

这些操作在超声的监控下进行，包括绒毛膜绒毛取样（胎盘活检）、羊膜腔穿刺术、胎儿血样化验以及胎儿组织活检。

实验室技术

包括对中期细胞直接的或在胎儿细胞培养后进行的染色体检查、DNA分析、酶分析及血液学指标的测量。原位杂交荧光技术（fluorescence in situ hybridization, FISH）（图30）是一种相对较新的分子技术，用来计算分裂间期的细胞的染色体；24～48小时之内可以排除或确认重要的非整倍体状态。

绒毛膜绒毛检查

步骤

通过经腹或经宫颈能够进行细胞的活检或吸取（图31）。前者更加经常被应用。

绒毛膜绒毛（图 32）可以用来进行染色体分析、DNA分析（比如囊纤维化、血红蛋白变异、Duchenne 肌肉营养不良）和酶学分析(出生时代谢异常)。

风险

风险取决于妊娠的时间。妊娠越早，流产的风险越高（比如妊娠 11 周大约是 2%，妊娠 16 周大约是 1%）。另外的风险包括破膜、感染、Rh 致敏作用和子宫损伤。绒毛膜绒毛取样很少在10周之前进行，因为存在着肢体缺损的风险。

Prenatal diagnosis

General

Over the past 20 years, dramatic advances have been made in prenatal diagnosis.

Fetal imaging

The resolution of ultrasound (Fig 29) has improved significantly and MRI can be used for difficult cases (see Ch 7).

Obstetric procedures

These are performed under ultrasound control and include chorionic villus sampling (placental biopsy), amniocentesis, fetal blood sampling and fetal tissue biopsy.

Laboratory methods

These include chromosome analysis (karyotyping) of metaphase cells either directly or after fetal cell culture, DNA analysis, enzyme assay and measurement of haematological values. Fluorescence in situ hybridization (FISH) (Fig 30) is a relatively new molecular technique used for counting chromosomes in interphase cells; major aneuploidies can be excluded or confirmed within 24-48 h.

Chorionic villus sampling

Procedures

Biopsy or aspiration of cells can be achieved using transabdominal (Fig 31) or transcervical routes, the former being more commonly practised.

Chorionic villi (Fig 32) may be used for chromosome analysis, DNA analysis (e.g. cystic fibrosis, haemoglobinopathies, Duchenne muscular dystrophy) and enzymology (inborn errors of metabolism).

Risks

The risk is dependent on gestational age. The earlier in pregnancy, the higher the risk of miscarriage (e.g. about 2% at 11 weeks and about 1% at 16 weeks). Additional risks include membrane rupture, infection, rhesus sensitization and uterine trauma. Chorionic villus sampling is rarely performed before 10 weeks because of the risk of limb defects.

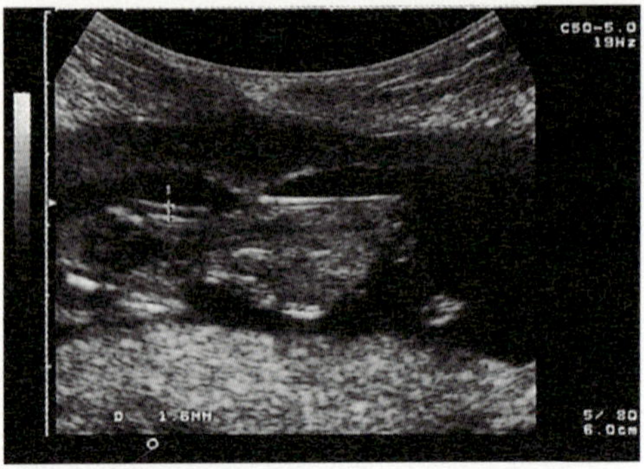

图 29　颈背半透明

Nuchal translucency

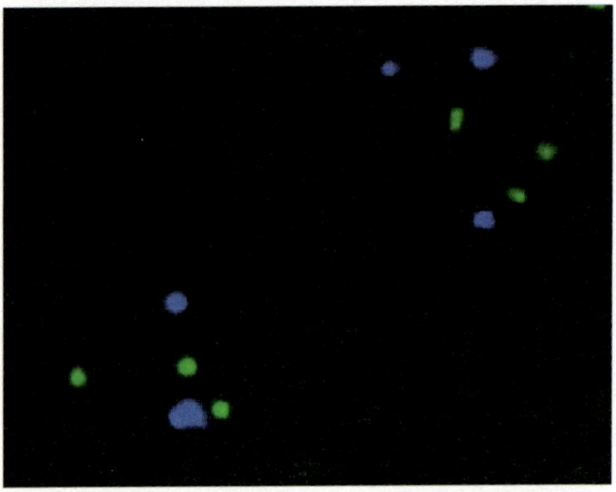

图 30　FISH 检查显示两个三倍体细胞（每个染色体复制 3 倍）

FISH study showing two triploid cells (three copies of each chromosome)

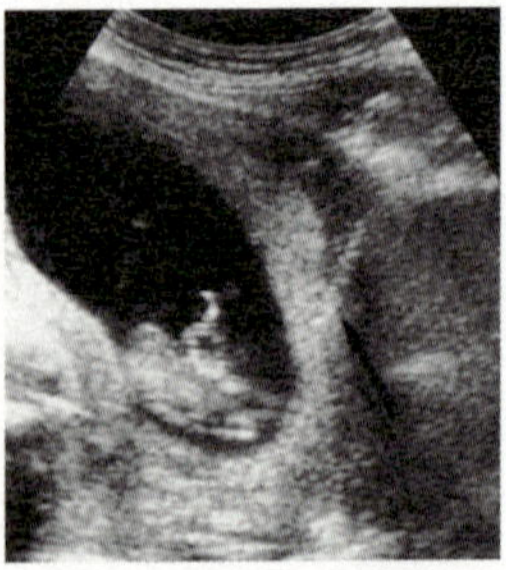

图 31　经腹绒毛膜绒毛取样(箭头)

Transabdominal chorionic villus sampling (needle arrowed)

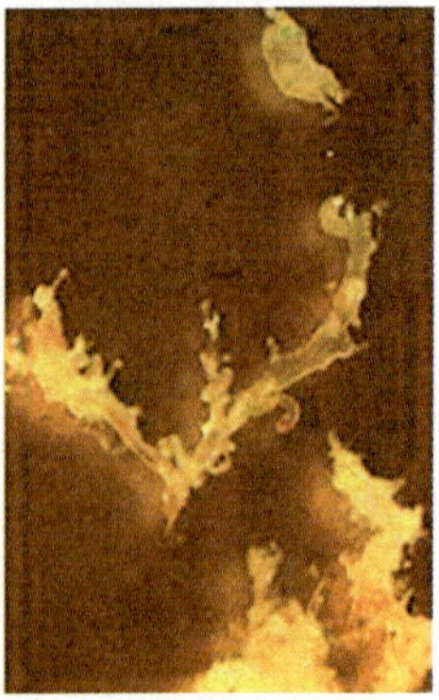

图 32　绒毛膜绒毛低倍镜视野

Low-power view of chorionic villi

羊膜腔穿刺术

步骤

在超声的引导下用 18-20- 脊髓针经腹穿刺入羊膜腔获取羊水（图 33 ~ 35）。在妊娠的头三个月之后进行操作，通常在 16 周。

适应证

染色体分析（用于染色体异常、X 连锁疾病的检查）、出生时代谢异常（酶、细胞或上清液的代谢物）、DNA 分析（如果有特殊情况下用的基因探针）以及以后在妊娠期进行 Rh 溶血疾病的评价（见第 9 章）。

风险

15 周之后的羊膜腔穿刺术大约有 1.0% 的风险会发生流产。如果在妊娠的更早期进行，则有更大的风险发生呼吸窘迫及姿态畸形（postural deformility）。在妊娠更晚期进行羊膜腔穿刺术有可能引起胎膜早破、绒毛膜羊膜炎和早产。Rh致敏作用可以发生在任何的时间（在上述的任何侵入性技术应用的同时），并且Rh阴性的妇女必须接受Kleihauer检测，以及接受抗D免疫球蛋白。

胎儿血标本和其他的技术

在妊娠18周之后可以通过脐带抽取胎儿血液，虽然有时也采取其他的部位（比如脐静脉的肝内部分）（图 36）。采用胎儿血液可以用来诊断/检测遗传性血红蛋白异常、胎儿病毒感染、Rh疾病、难以解释的水肿以及胎儿贫血。风险包括流产、损伤、失血、胎儿死亡、胎膜早破、早产以及Rh致敏。由于分子遗传学技术的进步，胎儿皮肤和肝的活检已经很少进行，这种技术的进步能够从胎盘获取的组织得到诊断，而无需对受影响器官进行组织学检查。

Amniocentesis

Procedure

Amniotic fluid is obtained by inserting an 18-20-gauge spinal needle into the amniotic cavity transabdominally under ultrasound guidance (Figs 33-35). It is performed after the first trimester, usually at 16 weeks.

Indications

Chromosome analysis (for chromosomal abnormalities, fetal sexing in X-linked conditions), inborn errors of metabolism (enzymes, metabolites using cells or supernatant), DNA analysis (if there is a gene probe for a specific condition) and later in pregnancy for assessment of rhesus disease (see Ch 9).

Risks

Amniocentesis after 15 weeks carries a miscarriage risk of 1.0%. If performed at earlier gestations there is a greater risk of respiratory distress and postural deformities. Amniocentesis at later gestations may cause preterm rupture of membranes, chorioamnionitis and preterm labour. Rhesus sensitization can occur at any time (as with any of these invasive techniques) and rhesus-negative women must have a Kleihauer test performed and anti-D immunoglobulin given.

Fetal blood sampling and other techniques

Fetal blood can be aspirated from the umbilical cord after 18 weeks' gestation, although alternative sites are sometimes chosen (e.g. intrahepatic part of the umbilical vein) (Fig 36). Fetal blood may be required to diagnose/ investigate inherited haemoglobin disorders, inborn errors of metabolism, chromosomal anomalies, fetal viral infections, rhesus disease, unexplained hydrops and fetal anaemia. Risks include miscarriage, trauma, blood loss, fetal death, preterm rupture of membranes and labour, and rhesus sensitization. Fetal skin and liver biopsy are now rarely required due to advances in molecular genetics, which allow diagnosis of many conditions from placental tissue without the need for histological examination of the affected organs.

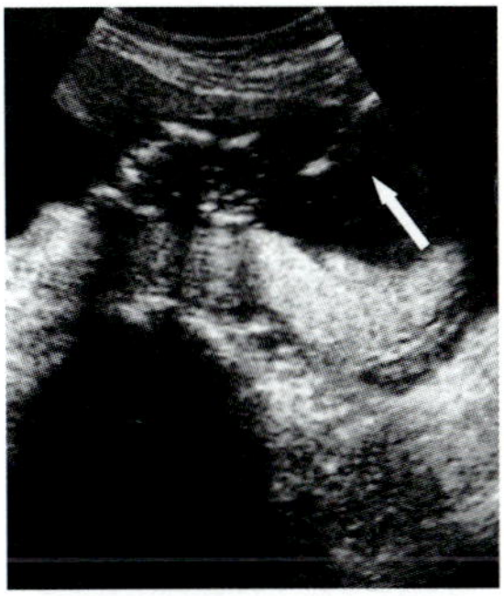

图 33 羊膜腔穿刺术超声学图像（箭头指示）

Ultrasound picture of amniocentesis (needle arrowed)

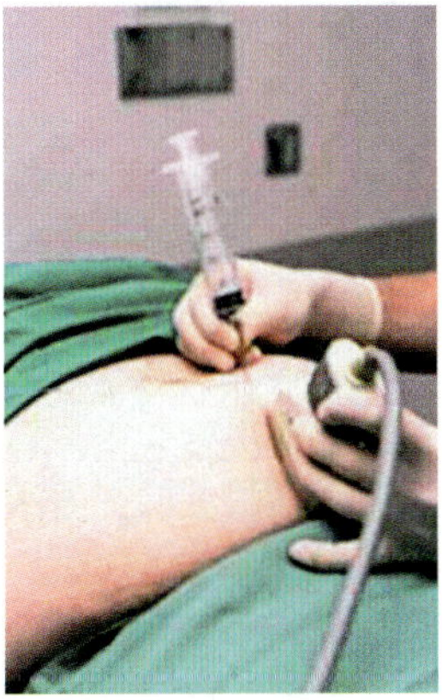

图 34 羊膜腔穿刺术：在超声引导下进行羊膜腔穿刺术

Amniocentesis: insertion of the needle under ultrasound guidance

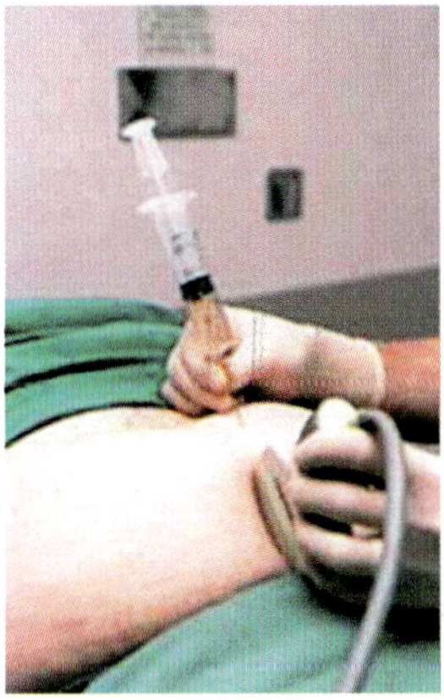

图 35 羊膜腔穿刺术：吸取羊水

Amniocentesis: aspiration of liquor

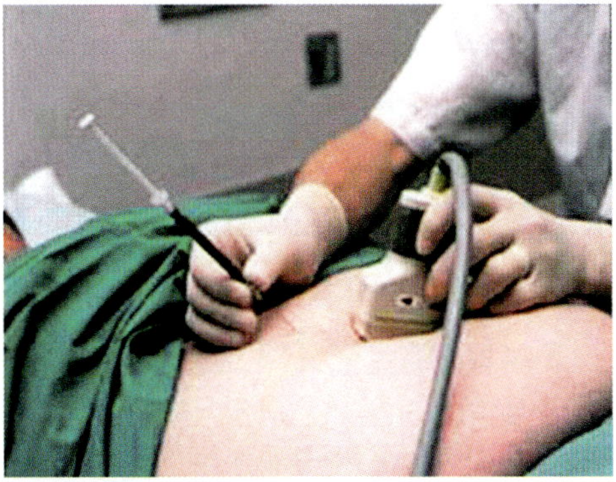

图 36 胎儿血液取样

Fetal blood sampling

Down 综合征（21 三倍体）

发生率

700例活胎分娩大约有1例发生，随着母亲年龄的增加发生率也随之增加（在25岁时为1/2000，在35岁时为1/365，在40岁时为1/100）。发生的风险决定于母亲的年龄，除非存在着罕见的父母平衡性易位。

病因

94%的病例是21三体（图37）。非平衡性易位占3%（其中有一半发生了“重排”），剩余的3%发生了镶嵌现象。

临床特征

下述情况风险增高：胎儿死亡、发育受限、特征性的张力减退的脸部（图38）、短头畸形、单掌皱褶、心脏缺陷（40%）、十二指肠闭锁、不同程度的智力水平，通常是中等程度的学习困难。

出生前的筛查

不同的方法具有不同的敏感性和阳性的预测价值。通用的是“二次检验”，在妊娠15～19周用母亲的血液进行。低于平均水平的甲胎蛋白以及更高水平的hCG预示着较高的风险。基于年龄和标志物，对高于1/250风险的妇女可提供一种诊断性的检测（见下）。加入了用于分析的非结合雌激素和抑制素的三倍体和四倍体检测提高了检查的敏感性。最近，在妊娠11～13周进行的颈背半透明度扫描结合头三个月的生物化学标志物检查为Down综合征提供了一种更为敏感的检测工具（见图29）。超过37岁的妇女，或者既往有过异常妊娠的妇女，经常会被直接提供诊断性检测（羊膜腔穿刺或绒毛膜绒毛取样）。

Edward 综合征（18 三倍体）

发生率

3000活胎分娩中发生1例，随着母亲年龄增加发生率增高。

病因

18三倍体（图39）。

Down syndrome (trisomy 21)

Incidence

Occurs in 1 in 700 live births and shows increasing incidence with older mothers (1 in 2000 at age 25, 1 in 365 at age 35 and 1 in 100 at age 40). Recurrence risk is usually determined by maternal age unless a rare parental balanced translocation exists.

Aetiology

Trisomy 21 in 94% of cases (Fig 37). Unbalanced translocation in 3% (half of which arise 'de novo') and mosaics in the remaining 3%.

Clinical features

Elevated risk of fetal loss, growth restriction, characteristic hypotonic facies (Fig 38), brachycephaly, single palmar creases, cardiac defects (40%), duodenal atresia, variable intellect, usually moderate learning difficulties.

Antenatal screening

Various methods exist, with differing sensitivities and positive predictive values. Universally available is the 'double test', performed at 15-19 weeks on maternal blood. Lower than average levels of α -fetoprotein and higher levels of hCG confer a higher risk. Women with a risk greater than 1 in 250 calculated on the basis of their age and these markers are offered a diagnostic test (see below). The 'triple' and 'quadruple' tests add in unconjugated estriol and inhibin to the assay, improving sensitivity of detection. More recently, nuchal translucency scanning at 11-13 weeks combined with first trimester biochemical markers has proved to be a more-sensitive screening tool for Down syndrome (see Fig 29). Women over the age of 37, or those with previously abnormal pregnancies, are often offered direct access to diagnostic tests (amniocentesis or chorionic villus sampling).

Edward syndrome (trisomy 18)

Incidence

1 in 3000 live births; risk increases with maternal age.

Aetiology

Trisomy 18 (Fig 39).

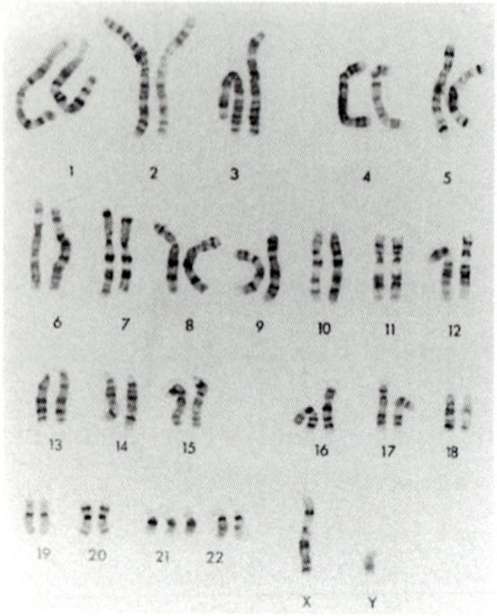

图 37　21 三倍体染色体核型
Trisomy 21 karyotype

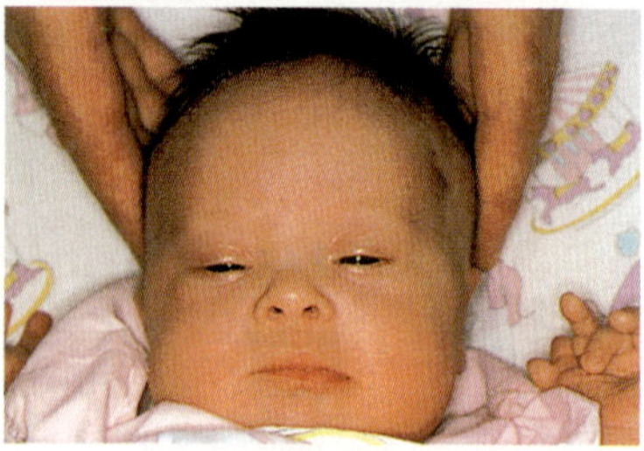

图 38　有 Down 综合征的婴儿（21 三倍体）
Baby with Down syndrome (trisomy 21)

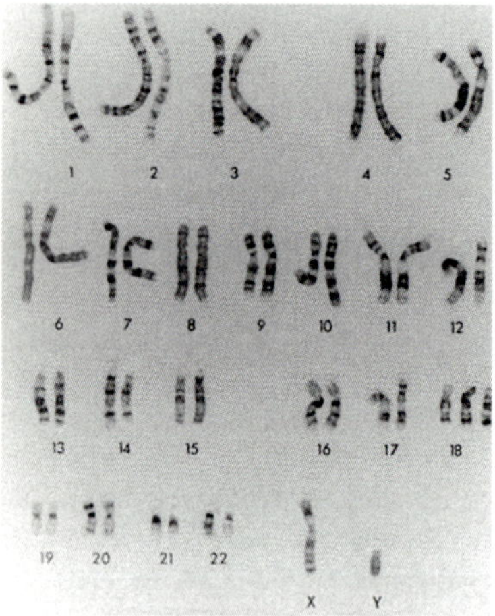

图 39　18 三倍体染色体核型
Trisomy 18 karyotype

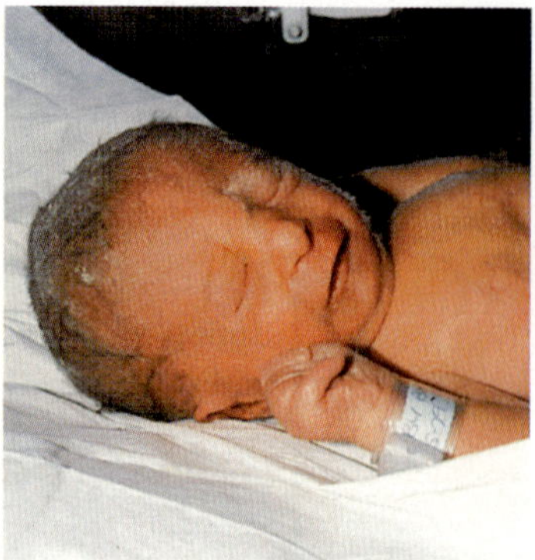

图 40　有 Edward 综合征的婴儿
Baby with Edward syndrome

临床特征

流产/胎儿死亡、生长受限、严重的学习障碍、心脏缺陷、肺发育不全、屈曲畸形、伴手指重叠的紧握的拳（图40）、摇椅脚、脐疝、脉络膜丛囊泡、泌尿生殖器异常。大多数在数月内死亡，存活1年的不超过10%。

Patau 综合征（13 三倍体）

发病率

不常见。发生率很低。母亲年龄增加则发生率增加。

病因

13 染色体三倍体（图 41）。

临床特征

流产/胎儿死亡、生长受限、脸部眼和前脑中线缺陷、前脑无裂畸形、唇腭裂（图 42）。严重的学习困难、耳聋、摇椅脚、多指 / 趾畸形、先天性心脏缺陷、隐睾。存活 1 年的不超过 20%。

Turner 综合征 （45，XO）

发病率

5000例活产中有1例。经常是散发的（比如与年龄和家族史无关）。

病因学

单 X 染色体。

临床特征

Turner综合征可以表现为流产或胎儿死亡，经常伴有囊性水囊瘤（图43）或者水肿（图44）。一般的特征包括发育受限、蹼颈、具有宽大乳头的宽阔的胸部、低发际线、短颈、肘外翻。10%的患者有主动脉缩窄，智力上的轻微损害也是特征性的。

Turner 综合征的妇女身高矮，第二性征发育缺陷。她们有条索状卵巢，并且是不育。需要雌激素替代治疗。

Clinical features

Miscarriage/fetal death, growth restriction, severe learning defects, cardiac defects, hypoplastic lungs, flexion deformities, clenched fists with overlapping fingers (Fig 40), rocker-bottom feet, exomphalos, choroid plexus cysts, urogenital abnormalities. The majority die within a few months; less than 10% survive a year.

Patau syndrome (trisomy 13)

Incidence

Uncommon. Low recurrence risk. Risk increases with maternal age.

Aetiology

Trisomy 13 (Fig 41).

Clinical features

Miscarriage/fetal death, growth restriction, midline defects of the face, eyes and forebrain, holoprosencephaly, cleft lip and palate (Fig 42). Severe learning difficulties, deafness, rocker-bottom feet, polydactyly, congenital heart defects and cryptorchidism. Less than 20% survive the first year of life.

Turner syndrome (45,XO)

Incidence

Occurs in 1 in 5000 live births. Incidence is usually sporadic (i.e. not related to age or family history).

Aetiology

Single X chromosome.

Clinical features

Turner syndrome can present as miscarriage or fetal death, often with a cystic hygroma (Fig 43) or hydrops (Fig 44). Common features include growth restriction, neck webbing, broad chest with widely spaced nipples, low hairline and short neck and cubitus valgus. Coarctation of the aorta is found in 10% and a mild impairment of intellect is said to be characteristic.

Women with Turner syndrome are of short stature and experience failure of secondary sexual development. They have streak ovaries and are infertile. Oestrogen replacement is required.

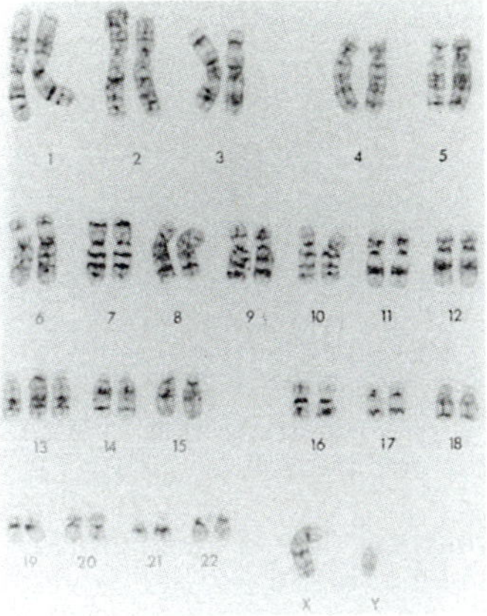

图 41　13 三倍体染色体核型
Trisomy 13 karyotype

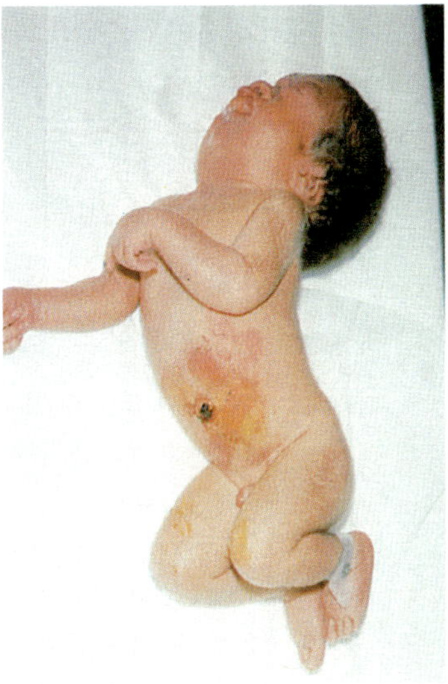

图 42　Patau 综合征的新生儿（13 三倍体）
Newborn with Patau syndrome (trisomy 13)

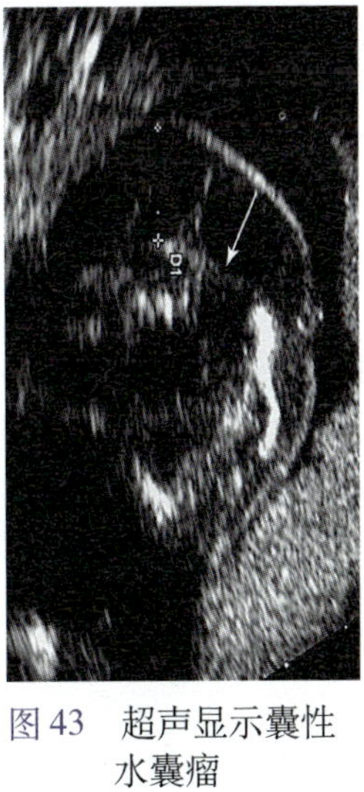

图 43　超声显示囊性水囊瘤
Ultrasound showing a cystic hygroma

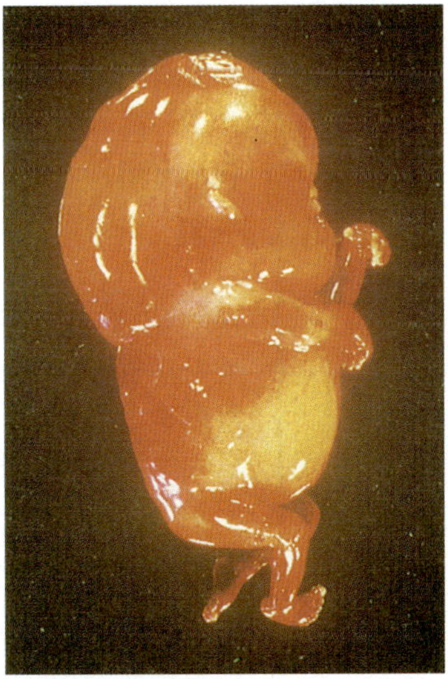

图 44　Turner 综合征的胎儿（45，XO）
Fetus with Turner syndrome (45,XO)

胎儿图像

超声

概要

大多数的英国妊娠妇女在妊娠的前半期都有常规的扫描。

原则

所有的超声检查工作都遵循相同的基础原则。将探头放在母亲的腹部，或者放在阴道，应用一层胶以确保良好的接触。

在对结构的分辨上超声同声纳或雷达的原理相同。诊断性图像应用 1ms 脉冲的超声（通常为 3.5mHz)，接着以1ms的间断探测返回的声波。通过快速连续的序列发放发射器，获得了实时的图像（图45)。

通过对多普勒超声增加探测血流的机制，使得获得实时彩色血流图像成为可能（图 46)。

更加近期的技术上的进步导致了三维超声图像的产生。这些对于确定精细的表面的异常（比如面部的裂）有用处。

应用

决定胎儿的生存能力及判断胎儿的异常、异位妊娠、多胎妊娠及滋养层疾病。在妊娠的前半期，超声被用来判断妊娠的时间长短，在妊娠的后半期被用来判断胎盘的位置以及胎先露部，记录胎儿的生长、行为以及测量羊水的体积。对于侵入性的措施比如羊水穿刺，超声是必须的辅助手段。

胎儿影像的其他方法

胎儿镜（直接的内镜检查）具有侵入性、风险性，使用于特殊的指征（如对于双胎输血综合征胎盘血管的激光消融）。在对胎儿中枢神经系统异常提供更加详细的评估中，胎儿的MRI检查越来越流行（图47)。

Ultrasound

General

The majority of pregnant women in the UK have a routine scan in the first half of pregnancy.

Principles

All ultrasound machines work on the same basic principle. A probe is applied to the maternal abdomen or into the vagina, using a film of gel to ensure good contact.

The identification of structures in the ultrasound beam occurs by the same principle as sonar or radar. Diagnostic imaging uses a 1 ms pulse of ultrasound (usually 3.5 mHz) followed by a 1 ms gap for detection of the returning sound wave. By sequencing the firing of the transmitters in rapid succession, a real-time image is obtained (Fig 45).

By incorporating a mechanism for detecting blood flow by Doppler ultrasound it is possible to obtain a real-time image with a colour picture of blood flow (Fig 46).

More recent advances in technology have resulted in three-dimensional ultrasound images. These are useful in clarifying the detail of subtle surface abnormalities (e.g. facial clefts).

Applications

Determination of fetal viability and diagnosis of fetal abnormality, ectopic pregnancy, multiple pregnancy and trophoblastic disease. In the first half of pregnancy, it is used to assess gestational age; in the latter half of pregnancy for determining placental site and fetal presentation, documenting fetal growth and behaviour and measuring liquor volume. It is a mandatory adjunct for invasive procedures such as amniocentesis.

Other methods of fetal imaging

Fetoscopy (direct endoscopy) is invasive, risky and reserved for specific indications (e.g. laser ablation of placental vessels in the twin-twin transfusion syndrome). Fetal MRI is becoming increasingly popular in providing a more detailed assessment of central nervous system abnormalities (Fig 47).

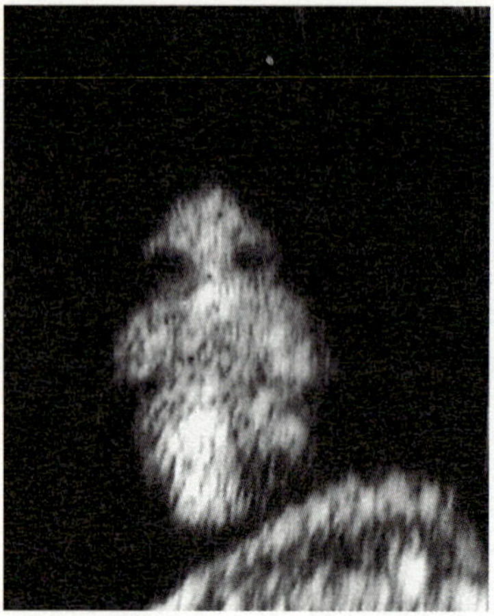

图 45　超声图像显示胎儿面部（鼻孔、唇和下巴）
Ultrasound image showing fetal face (nostrils, lips and chin)

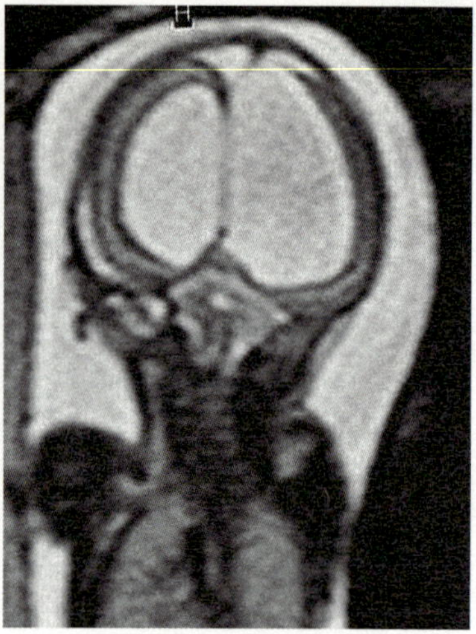

图 47　胎儿 MRI 显示脑室扩大
Fetal MRI showing ventriculomegaly

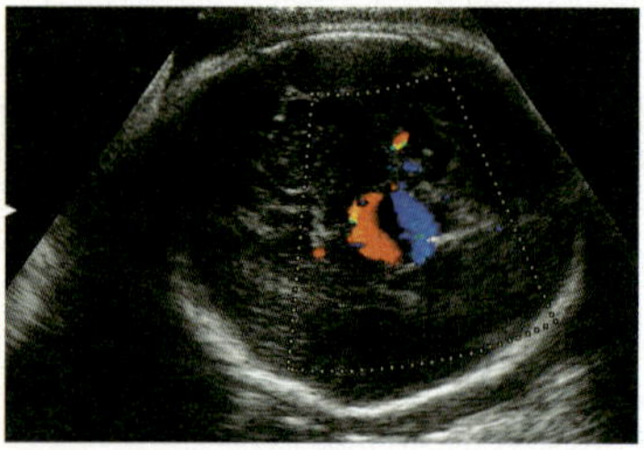

a

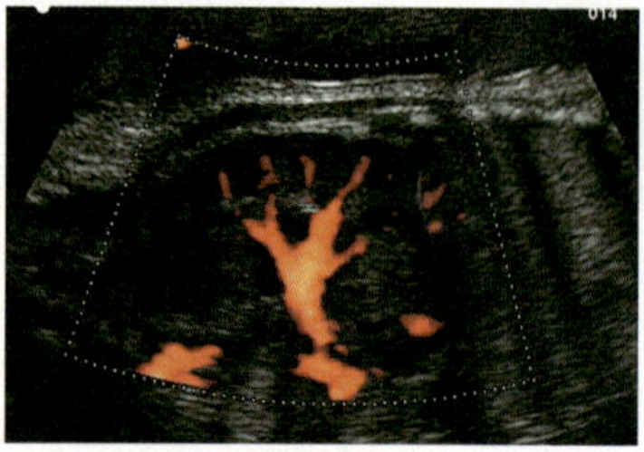

b

图 46（a）应用彩色多普勒超声证实通过心脏的血流；(b) Power 多普勒显示肾血管解剖
(a) Ultrasound using colour Doppler to demonstrate blood flow through the heart；(b) Power Doppler showing renal vascular anatomy

神经管缺陷（neural tube defects, NTD）

类型

脊柱裂（脊髓脊膜膨出、脑脊膜膨出）、无脑畸形、脑膨出。

发病率

英国总发病率大约是1/1000，但是有地域上的差异。在英国由于出生前筛查项目的推行（见下）以及对受影响妊娠的终止，在过去的20年里登记的先天性异常出生率下降了90%。

病因学

遗传因素以及叶酸缺乏联合造成。

预防

没有个人或者家族性NTD病史的妇女应该在妊娠前至少服用400 μg的叶酸达2个月，一直持续到妊娠最初三个月结束。有明显病史、家族史的妇女或者应用叶酸拮抗剂（如抗惊厥药）的妇女，在围妊娠期应该用5mg的叶酸。

产前筛查

在妊娠16～18周时对妇女提供血清甲胎蛋白(AFP)筛查。低于人群平均值的2.3～2.5倍提示发生NTD的风险较低。增高的数值使得NTD更容易发生，但是其他的原因也可以引起AFP的数值升高，包括胎儿腹壁缺损、多胎妊娠、不正确妊娠周数估计以及在妊娠时流血。当甲胎蛋白值升高时，需要进行更加详细的检查（图48）。可以应用MRI对疑难的病例进行更进一步的评估（图49）。

临床特征

- *脊柱裂*：充满液体的囊内经常包含神经组织和有潜在缺损的脊柱弓，94%的病例位于腰骶部（图50）。残疾的程度可以有所不同，包括引起下肢的瘫痪、尿便失禁、肢体畸形、臀部错位、泌尿系感染和脑积水（70%）。
- *无脑畸形*：前脑和颅窝缺失，面部变形（图51）。不能成活。
- *脑膨出*：脑膜及大脑通过颅骨（通常是枕骨）疝出（图52）。

Neural tube defects (NTD)

Types

Spina bifida (meningomyelocele, meningocele), anencephaly, encephalocele.

Incidence

Overall UK occurrence is about 1 in 1000, but there is geographical variation. In the UK, the incidence in registered births has fallen by 90% over the past two decades due to antenatal screening programmes (see below) and termination of affected pregnancies.

Aetiology

Combination of genetic factors and folic acid deficiency.

Prevention

Women with no personal or family history of NTD should take 400 μg of folic acid for at least 2 months preconceptually and to the end of the first trimester. Women with a previous or family history, or taking folate antagonists (e.g. anticonvulsants), should take 5 mg of folic acid in the periconceptual period.

Antenatal screening

Women are offered serum α -fetoprotein (AFP) screening at 16-18 weeks. A value of less than 2.3-2.5 times the population median indicates a low risk of NTD. A raised value makes NTD more likely, but other causes include fetal abdominal wall defects, multiple pregnancy, incorrect gestational age and bleeding in pregnancy. When the AFP value is raised, a detailed scan is undertaken (Fig 48). MRI can be used to further evaluate difficult cases (Fig 49).

Clinical features

- *Spina bifida*: a fluid-filled sac often containing neural tissue and an underlying defect of the spinal arch; 94% of cases are lumbosacral (Fig 50). The degree of handicap varies and can include paralysis of the lower limb, urinary and fecal incontinence, limb deformities, hip dislocations, urinary infections and hydrocephalus (70%).
- *Anencephaly*: absence of the forebrain and skull vault, facial distortion (Fig 51). It is incompatible with life.
- *Encephalocele*: herniation of the meninges and brain through the skull (usually occipital) (Fig 52).

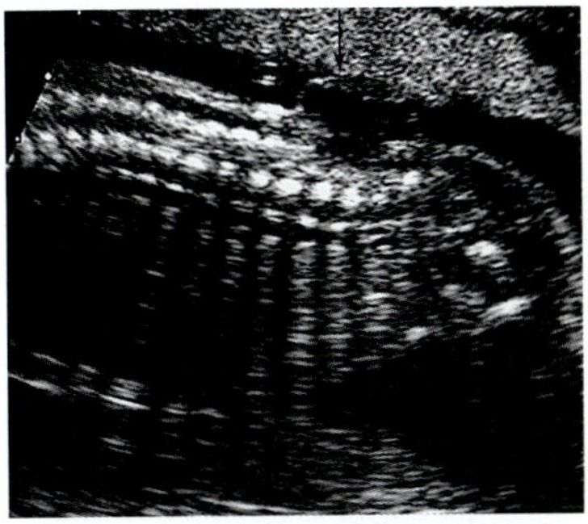

图 48　超声影像显示腰骶部脑脊膜膨出（脊柱裂）
Ultrasound image showing lumbosacral meningocele (spina bifida)

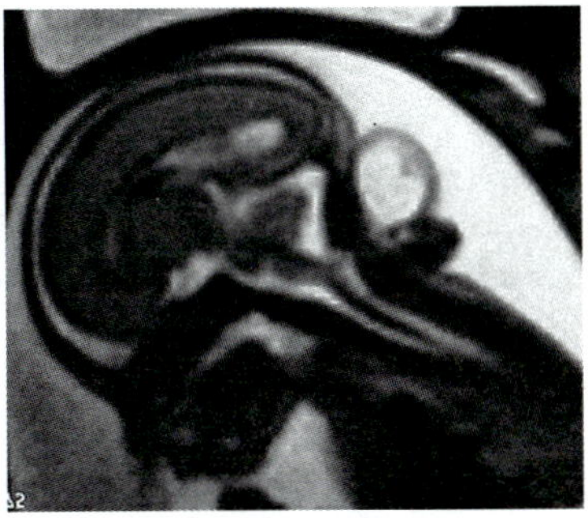

图 49　宫颈部脑脊膜 MRI 图像
MRI of cervical meningocele

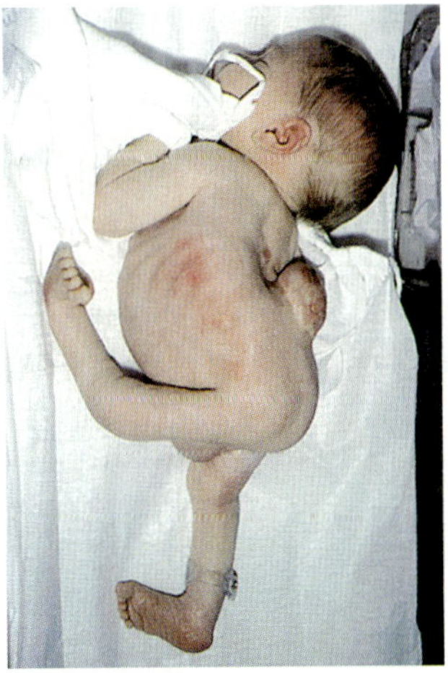

图 50　脊柱裂的新生儿
Newborn with spina bifida

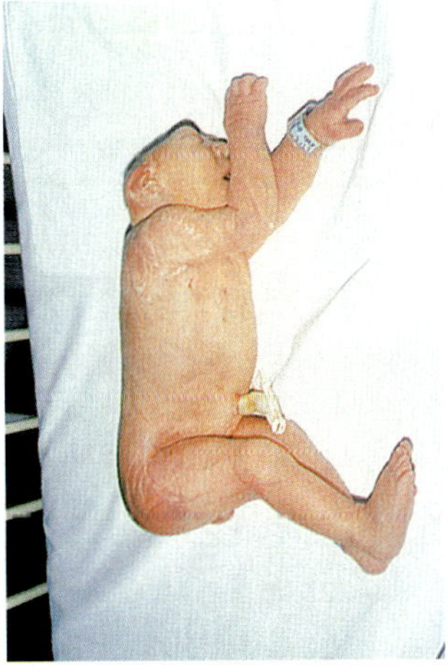

图 51　无脑儿
Anencephalic baby

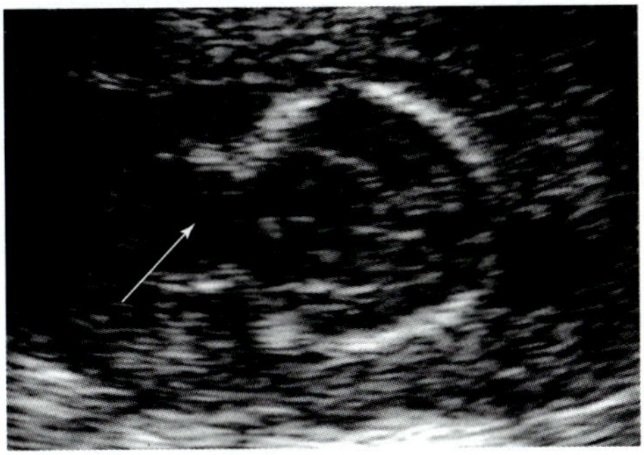

图 52　枕骨脑膨出的超声图像
Ultrasound image of occipita encephalocele

颅骨 / 脑缺陷

脑室扩大 / 脑积水

定义

脑室扩大是脑室腔扩大伴有过多的脑室内脑脊液（图 53）。如果引起了颅骨的增大则称为脑积水（图 54）。

病因学

可以单独发生或者继发于管腔狭窄、脑室内出血、胎儿病毒感染（如巨细胞病毒）或神经管缺陷。也同样与非整倍体有关。通过超声联合其他的检查方法（如病毒检查、染色体核型分析）可以做出诊断。不应该与前脑无裂畸形或脑穿通畸形相混淆（图 55）。

MRI 有助于确认异常。

预后

情况存在差异，在产前预测比较困难。较差的预后与其他异常的存在、伴有皮质变薄的严重的脑室增大、颅骨的加速增长有关。

在出生后可能需要脑室分流，即便如此孩子也可能会有不可逆的残疾。在产前发现的脑室轻微增大可能会有正常的后果。然而脑室增大的程度与预后并不一定密切相符。如果有潜在的所谓重要异常（比如神经管缺陷或非整倍体），给出预后就相对容易多了。

小头畸形

定义

头围低于平均值的 3 个标准差或更低。

病因

常不明，但是有可能为家族性的。病理性原因包括先天的病毒感染（比如风疹病毒）、出生时的代谢异常、母亲的苯丙酮尿症和很多遗传异常综合征。预后与发病原因有关。

Skull/brain defects

Ventriculomegaly/hydrocephalus

Definition

Ventriculomegaly is enlargement of the cerebral ventricles with excessive intraventricular cerebrospinal fluid (Fig 53). If this causes enlargement of the skull it is known as hydrocephalus (Fig 54).

Aetiology

May occur in isolation or be secondary to aqueduct stenosis, intraventricular haemorrhage, fetal viral infection (e.g. cytomegalovirus) or neural tube defects. It is also associated with aneuploidy. Diagnosis is made by a combination of ultrasound with other investigations (e.g. viral studies, karyotyping). It should not be confused with conditions such as holoprosencephaly or porencephaly (Fig 55).

MRI may be helpful in clarifying the abnormality.

Prognosis

This varies and can be difficult to predict antenatally. Poor prognostic factors include the presence of other anomalies, severe ventriculomegaly with cortical thinning, and an accelerating rate of growth of the skull.

Ventricular shunts may be required after birth and even then the child may be irreversibly handicapped. Mild cases of ventriculomegaly detected antenatally may have a normal outcome. The degree of ventriculomegaly does not closely match outcome, however. If there is an underlying named major abnormality (such as NTD or aneuploidy), giving a prognosis is somewhat easier.

Microcephaly

Definition

A head circumference 3 standard deviations or more below the mean.

Aetiology

Often unknown, but may be familial. Pathological causes include congenital viral infections (e.g. rubella), inborn errors of metabolism, maternal phenylketonuria and many genetic malformation syndromes. Prognosis depends on the cause.

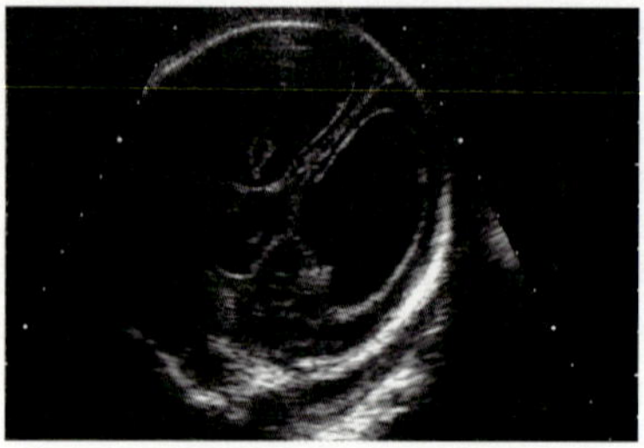

图 53　头部超声检查显示脑室增大
Coronal ultrasound scan
showing ventriculomegaly

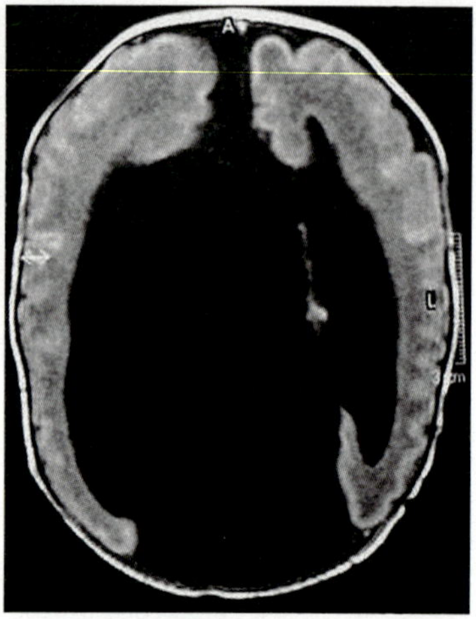

图 55　胎儿 MRI 显示脑穿通畸形
Fetal MRI showing
porencephaly

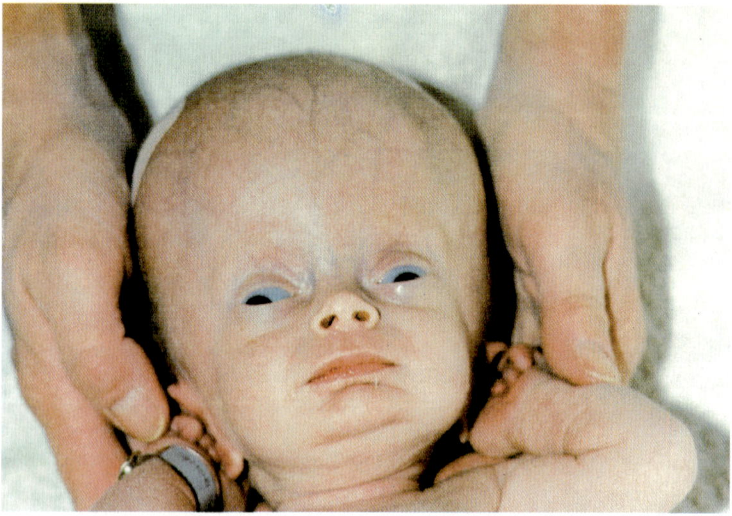

图 54　脑积水的婴儿
Baby with hydrocephalus

腹壁缺损

腹裂和脐疝

病理学

不常见。在胎儿发育过程中旋转失败或者消化道折返入腹腔。腹裂有可能与环境毒素相关，脐疝有可能与非整倍体相关。

特征

腹裂和脐疝都与母亲增高的血清 AFP 水平相关，依靠超声诊断。

- *腹裂*：缺损的腹壁与脐带插入的位置分离（图56、57）。腹腔内脏疝出，腹膜覆盖物缺失。它通常是一种独立的缺陷。
- *脐疝*：腹腔内脏通过脐的缺陷疝出（图 58，59）。通常腹膜的覆盖物仍旧保留，脐带直接插入到囊内。其他的先天异常是常见的（心脏、肠管和染色体）。可以通过胎盘活检或血液采样进行染色体组型分析。

处理

如果有其他的异常或者异常的染色体核型，可以选择终止妊娠。否则在出生后尽可能早地进行手术闭合。新生儿有可能发生低体温和/或者脱水。手术有可能需要两步，先将腹腔内容物暂时闭合于一个人工囊内。分娩的方式并不能影响到预后。

梨状腹综合征

病因学

不常见，仅有散发。有可能是由于子宫内继发于尿道梗阻的极度增大膀胱的减压。

特征

腹壁肌肉组织表现为梨状腹。通常可见睾丸未降和肾异常，后者决定了结果。如果是非致命性的，腹壁在婴儿期进行重建。

Abdominal wall defects

Gastroschisis and exomphalos

Pathology

Uncommon. Failure of rotation and re-entry of gut into abdominal cavity during fetal development. Gastroschisis is possibly linked to environmental toxins; exomphalos is associated with aneuploidy.

Features

Both gastroschisis and exomphalos are associated with elevated maternal serum AFP and are diagnosed by ultrasound.

- *Gastroschisis*: defect of the abdominal wall separate from the insertion of the umbilical cord (Figs 56, 57). The abdominal viscera herniate and the peritoneal covering is lost. Usually an isolated defect.
- *Exomphalos*: herniation of the abdominal viscera through a defect at the umbilicus (Figs 58, 59). Usually the peritoneal covering is preserved and the umbilical cord is inserted on to the sac. Other congenital abnormalities are common (cardiac, bowel and chromosomal). Karyotyping by placental biopsy or blood sampling is advisable.

Management

Termination may be chosen if there are other anomalies or an abnormal karyotype. Otherwise, surgical closure is undertaken as soon as possible after birth. The neonate is at risk of hypothermia and/or dehydration. The operation may have to be a two-stage procedure, with the abdominal contents initially being enclosed in a temporary artificial sac. Mode of delivery does not influence the prognosis.

Prune belly syndrome

Aetiology

Uncommon, with only sporadic occurrence. Probably results from the in utero decompression of a massively enlarged bladder secondary to urethral obstruction.

Features

Deficient abdominal wall musculature, giving a rugose prune belly appearance. Undescended testes and renal anomalies are usually found and the latter determine outcome. If non-lethal, the abdominal wall is reconstructed in infancy.

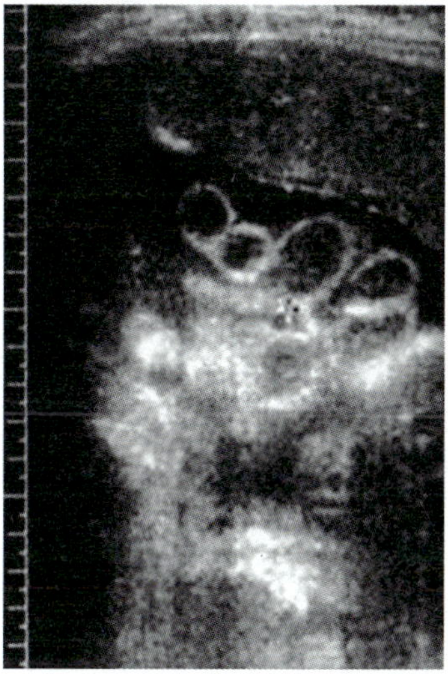

图 56 超声图像显示腹裂（在羊膜腔内肠管自由漂浮的光环）
Ultrasound picture showing gastroschisis (loops of bowel floating free in amniotic cavity)

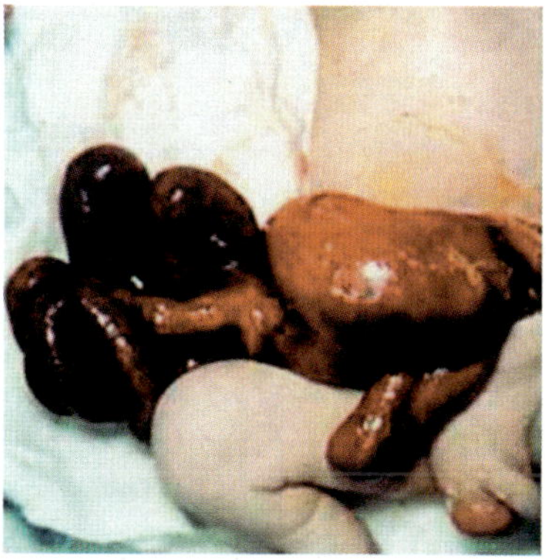

图 57 腹裂在出生后
Gastroschisis after birth

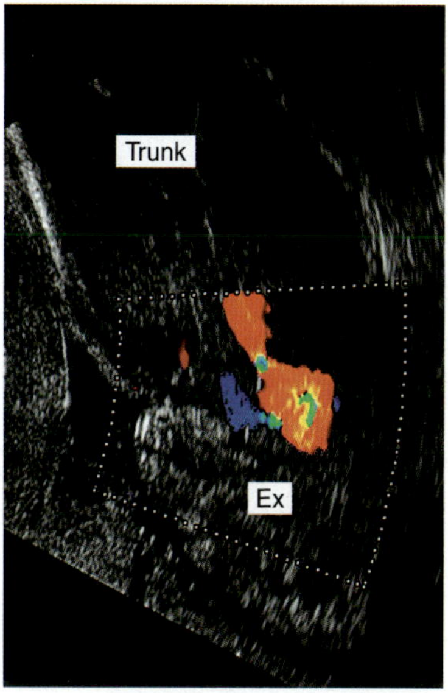

图 58 超声图像显示脐疝
Ultrasound image showing exomphalos (Ex)

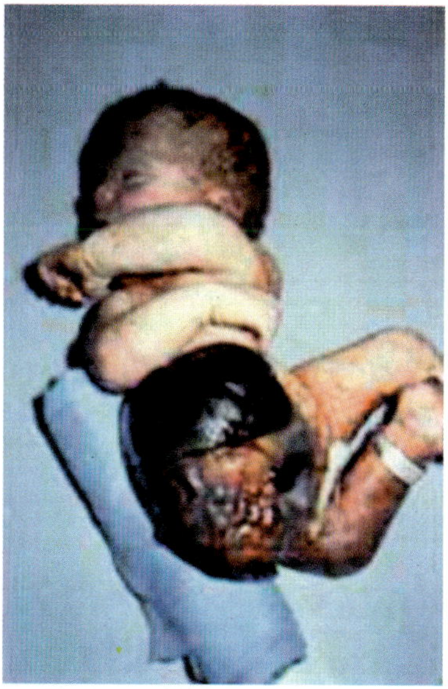

图 59 脐疝在出生后
Exomphalos after birth

肾管畸形

Potter 序列

发病率
3000 例活胎出生中有 1 例。

病因学
由产生羊水过少的情况引起（比如肾发育不全引起的原发 Potter 综合征）、发育异常的肾、多囊肾、泌尿系梗阻以及慢性羊水渗漏。

临床特征
羊水过少、胎儿生长受限以及胎儿畸形。低置的耳朵 (图 60)、伴肢体屈曲挛缩的压缩畸形以及肺发育不全。由泌尿生殖原因引起的肾衰。

预后
死亡通常是由于出生后很快发生的呼吸衰竭（肺发育不全）。

泌尿道梗阻

病因学
可能发生在盆腔输尿管水平或者膀胱输尿管连接处，或者尿道（通常在男性：后尿道瓣膜）。

特征
可以引起肾积水（图 61）或肾发育异常。严重的两侧疾病将会引起羊水过少和肺发育不全。严重膨大的膀胱可能伴发后尿道瓣膜（图 62）。

处理
正常的液体体积提示着某种程度的肾功能。密切的出生后的随访是重要的，然而结局并不与出生前检查结果密切相关。伴有严重羊水过少的妊娠经常被终止。在经过认真地病例选择后，通过膀胱－羊膜导管插入的方法在子宫里可以治疗后尿道瓣膜。

异位膀胱

特征
耻骨联合明显分离，膀胱腹壁疝出，膀胱粘膜暴露 (图 63)。外科整形是可能的，但是尿失禁常见。

Renal tract anomalies

Potter sequence

Incidence

1 in 3000 live births.

Aetiology

Caused by conditions producing oligohydramnios (e.g. renal agenesis-cause of original Potter syndrome), dysplastic kidneys, polycystic kidneys, urinary obstruction and chronic leakage of amniotic fluid.

Clinical features

Oligohydramnios, fetal growth restriction and fetal deformation. Low-set ears (Fig 60), compression abnormalities with limb flexion contractures, and hypoplastic lungs. Renal failure with urogenital causes.

Prognosis

Death is normally due to respiratory failure (pulmonary hypoplasia) soon after birth.

Urinary obstruction

Aetiology

May occur at the level of the pelvi-ureteric or vesico-ureteric junctions or the urethra (usually in males: posterior urethral valves).

Features

Hydronephrosis (Fig 61) or renal dysplasia may result. Severe bilateral disease will cause oligohydramnios and lung hypoplasia. A grossly distended bladder may occur with posterior urethral valves (Fig 62).

Management

Normal liquor volumes indicate some degree of renal function. Close postnatal follow-up is vital, however, and outcome is not well correlated with antenatal scan findings. Pregnancies with severe oligohydramnios are often terminated. Posterior urethral valves can be treated in utero by vesico-amniotic drain insertion, after careful case selection.

Ectopia vesicae

Features

Wide separation of pubic symphysis with ventral herniation of the bladder and exposure of bladder mucosa (Fig 63). Surgical correction is possible but incontinence is common.

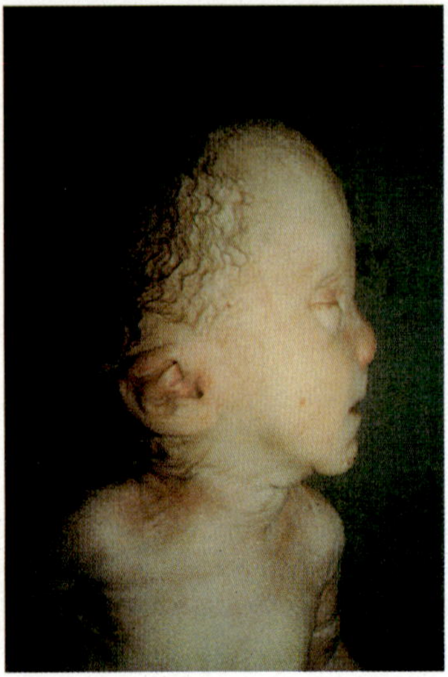

图 60　Potter 面容
Potter facies

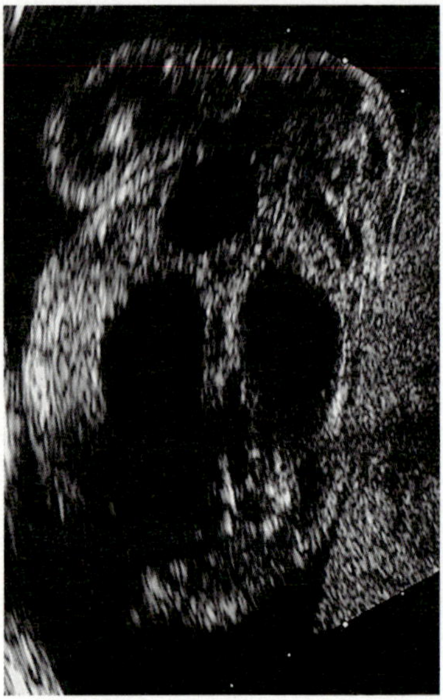

图 61　超声图像显示胎儿肾积水以及扩张的膀胱
Ultrasound image showing fetal hydronephrosis and distended bladder

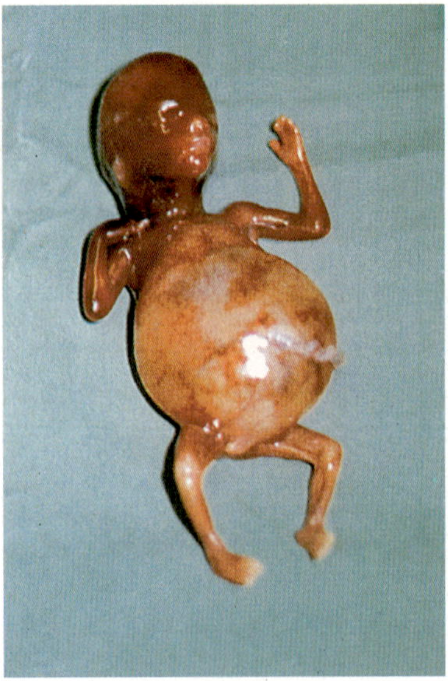

图 62　有后尿道瓣膜及巨大膀胱扩张的胎儿
Fetus with posterior urethral valves and massive bladder distension

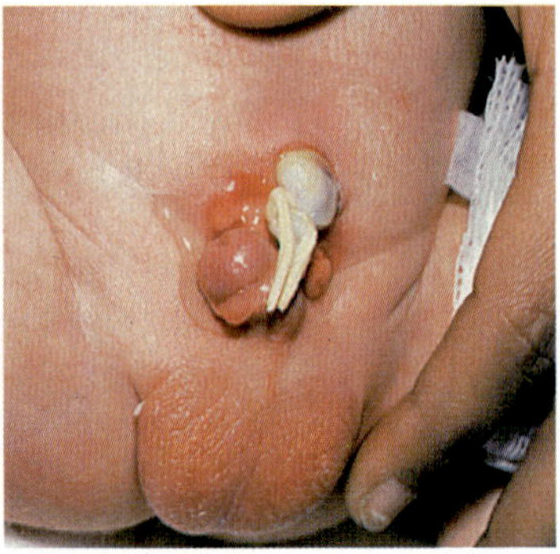

图 63　异位膀胱
Ectopia vesicae

骨骼异常

成骨缺陷

发病率

罕见（50 000 例活胎出生中有 1 例）。

病因

绝大多数是由于 I 型胶原蛋白异常。致命型源于新的显性突变。在不太严重型证实了显性遗传。

特征

类型 I ～Ⅳ。出生前及出生后有严重骨折倾向者能够引起极度的畸形和残废。可能发生异常的牙列和听力丧失。不同的类型预后高度不同。

诊断

在超声下可以看见长骨畸形和变短，矿化很差（如颅骨）伴有多处骨折（图64、65）。累及肋骨可以引起呼吸损害。

短肢侏儒症

发病率

软骨发育不全是最常见的（10 000 例活胎出生中有 10 例）。

病因学

成纤维生长因子受体 -3 基因的新的常染色体显性突变引起大多数的软骨发育不全以及更严重的致死性侏儒（图66）。畸形发育不全的硫酸盐转移基因的突变引起软骨成长不全和畸形发育不全。Campomelic 发育不全是由于 SOX-9 的突变。

特征

每个病例都有其畸形的类型，但是可能包括肢体短小、大头、突出的前额、窄胸、骨化差、多指 / 趾畸形、面裂。预后不同，表现从好（软骨发育不全）到致死性（比如致死性发育不良）。

短肢畸形

病因包括遗传综合征、早于 10 周的绒毛膜绒毛采样、环境的毒素（比如反应停）以及羊膜带（图67），在这些情况下裂口、脑膨出和腹裂都有可能发生。

Skeletal abnormalities

Osteogenesis imperfecta

Incidence
Rare (1 in 50 000 live births).

Aetiology
Mostly due to type I collagen abnormalities. Lethal forms result from new dominant mutations. Dominant inheritance is demonstrated in less severe forms.

Features
Types I-IV. Excessive tendency to antenatal and postnatal fractures which can be extremely deforming and disabling. Abnormal dentition and hearing loss may occur. Highly variable prognosis depending on type.

Diagnosis
The long bones are seen to be deformed and shortened on ultrasound and are poorly mineralized (as is the skull) with multiple fractures (Figs 64, 65). Rib involvement may cause respiratory compromise.

Short-limbed dwarfism

Incidence
Achondroplasia is the most common (10 in 10 000 live births).

Aetiology
New autosomal-dominant mutations in the fibroblast growth factor receptor-3 gene are responsible for most cases of achondroplasia and the more severe thanatophoric dwarfism (Fig 66). Mutations in the diastrophic dysplasia sulphate transporter gene cause achondrogenesis and diastrophic dysplasia. Campomelic dysplasia results from SOX-9 mutations.

Features
Each has its own pattern of abnormalities, but may include short limbs, large head, prominent forehead, narrow chest, poor ossification, polydactyly and facial clefting. Prognosis varies from good (achondroplasia) to lethal (e.g. thanatophoric dysplasia).

Limb reduction deformities
Causes include genetic syndromes, chorionic villus sampling earlier than 10 weeks, environmental toxins (e.g.thalidomide) and amniotic bands (Fig 67), in which clefting, encephalocele and gastroschisis may also occur.

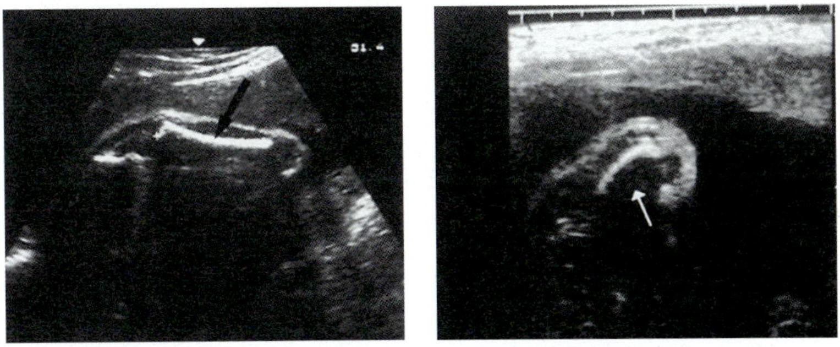

图 64　超声图像　（a）正常胎儿的股骨；（b）异常的股骨（变短和变成弓形）（箭头）

Ultrasound images of (a) a normal fetal femur; (b) an abnormal femur (shortening and bowing) (arrowed)

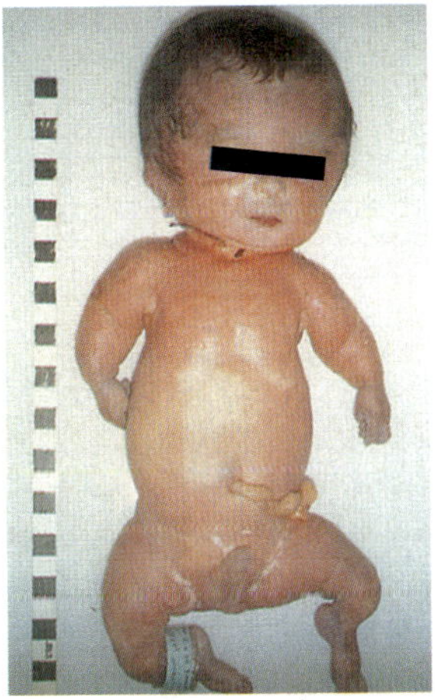

图 65　骨化作用异常

Osteogenesisimperfecta

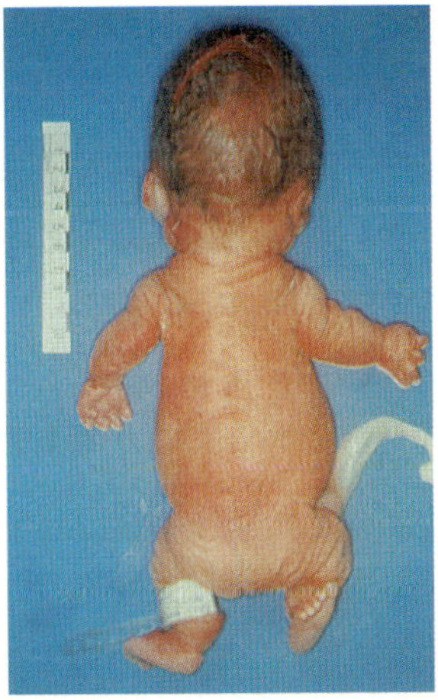

图 66　致死性发育不良

Thanatophoric dysplasia

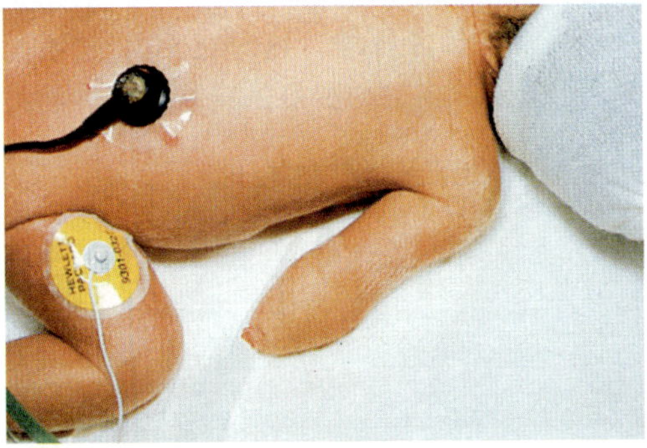

图 67　由羊膜带引起的远端肢体切断

Distal limb amputation caused by amniotic bands

胃肠道异常

膈疝

发病率

在 1500 例活胎分娩中有 1 例。

病因学

横膈的前叶和后叶的融合或者肌化失败引起腹腔内容物凸入胸腔（图68）。通常与非整倍体、多畸形综合征、心脏缺陷相关。

诊断

超声通常会证实腹腔内容物（肝或肠管）出现在胸腔，伴有心脏的移位（图69）。应提供核型分析以及寻找其他的异常。

预后

结局由肺发育不良的程度以及其他异常的出现来决定。整体的存活率是 70%。

气管 - 食管瘘

发病率

3000 例活胎分娩中有 1 例。

病因学

食管的末端为有不同程度的一个盲端囊。发现了气管、支气管或者更低段的食管间病理性交通。在60%的病例与其他的异常相关。

特征

60% 的病例有羊水过多。在超声发现胃泡缺失是一个不可靠的诊断征象，这时在 90% 的情况下出现瘘。婴儿在通过胃管检测到胃酸之前不应该喂食。

肠梗阻

羊水过多常与小肠梗阻同在。有十二指肠闭锁时在超声可能显示“双泡征”（图 70）（第一个泡是胃，第二个泡是扩张的近段十二指肠—— 21 三体的标志），空肠闭锁时显示“三泡征”。

Gastrointestinal anomalies

Diaphragmatic hernia

Incidence

1 in 1500 live births.

Aetiology

Failure of fusion or muscularization of the anterior and posterior leaves of the diaphragm allows abdominal contents to protrude into the chest (Fig 68). Often associated with aneuploidy, multiple malformation syndromes and cardiac defects.

Diagnosis

Ultrasound will normally demonstrate abdominal contents (liver or bowel) in the chest with displacement of the heart (Fig 69). Offer karyotyping and look for other anomalies.

Prognosis

The outcome is determined by the degree of pulmonary hypoplasia and the presence of other abnormalities. The overall survival rate is 70%.

Tracheo-oesophageal fistula

Incidence

1 in 3000 live births.

Aetiology

The oesophagus ends as a blind pouch. Varying degrees of pathological communication are found with the trachea, bronchi or lower oesophagus. Associated with other anomalies in 60% of cases.

Features

Polyhydramnios in 60% of cases. Absence of stomach bubble on ultrasound is an unreliable diagnostic sign as a fistula is present in 90%. The baby should not be fed until a gastric tube has been passed to test for gastric acid.

Intestinal obstruction

Polyhydramnios is common with small bowel obstruction. Ultrasound may show a 'double bubble' (Fig 70) with duodenal atresia (the first bubble is the stomach, the second bubble is the distended proximal duodenum-amarker for trisomy 21) and a 'triple bubble' with jejunal atresia.

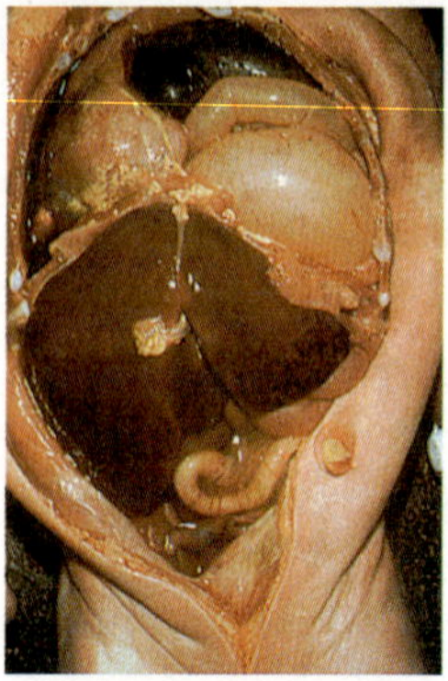

图 68　尸检时膈疝显示肠管在胸部将心脏推向右侧
Postmortem of diaphragmatic hernia showing bowel in chest pushing the heart to the right

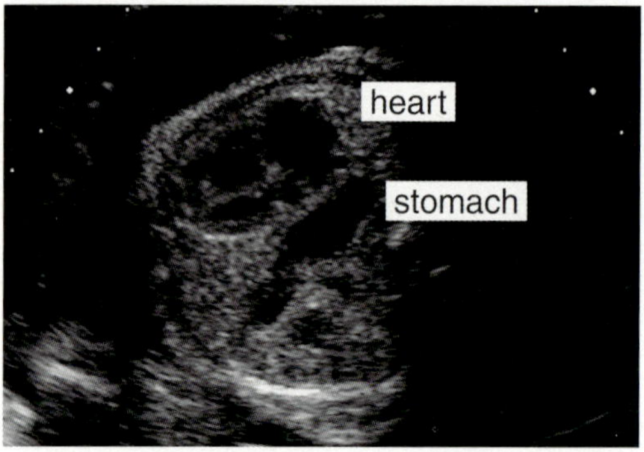

图 69　膈疝的超声图像（胃在胸腔内心脏的一旁）
Ultrasound image of diaphragmatic hernia (stomach lies in the thorax, alongside the heart)

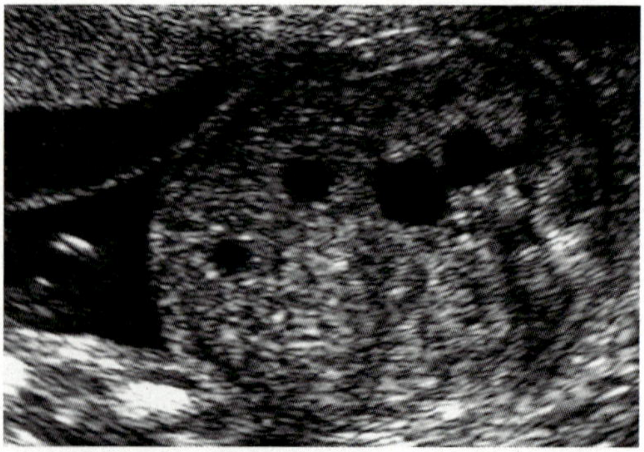

图 70　超声扫描显示十二指肠闭锁的“双泡征”
Ultrasound scan showing ‘double bubble’ of duodenal atresia

Rh 溶血病

病因学

5 个等位基因决定 Rh 型（C、c、D、E、e）。Rh 血型主要由 D 基因决定。当 Rh 阴性的孕妇体内有 Rh 抗体，而胎儿为 Rh 阳性时，可发生 Rh 溶血病。Rh 抗体可通过胎盘，引起胎儿溶血（贫血、黄疸），严重者引起心衰、胎儿水肿（图71）、胎儿死亡。极少数情况下，Kell抗体或Duffy抗体能引起类似的严重疾病。C 或 E 位抗体以及 A 或 B 抗原的抗体引发疾病的严重程度要轻一些。

致敏

当Rh阳性胎儿/婴儿的红细胞进入Rh阴性孕妇的血液循环时（分娩、流产、胎盘出血、羊膜腔穿刺术、绒毛活检、胎头外倒转术或自发倒转时）发生致敏。

预防

当Rh阴性的母亲有潜在的致敏事件时应给予注射抗D免疫球蛋白，或者常规在妊娠28和34周时注射（根据当地政策）。

检测

对未致敏的 Rh 阴性孕妇在妊娠期筛查抗体。

评估

由下列途径判定疾病的严重程度：羊水在 450nm 时的光密度差（图 72）、采胎儿血样测胎儿血红蛋白，或应用测量大脑中动脉血流速度的非侵袭性方法（图 73）。超声下见到的胎儿水肿是晚期征象。

干预

轻、中度溶血病不需频繁化验，可以足月分娩。重者需行侵袭性检查和宫内输血，通常是每 2 ~ 3 周一次。在妊娠期过早而不适宜胎儿输血的严重病例，可用免疫球蛋白静脉给药。

产后护理

采脐带血查血红蛋白、做 Coombs 试验、胆红素水平。黄疸在轻型病例中可行光线疗法，严重者行换血疗法以预防核黄疸。

Rhesus disease

Aetiology

Five allelic pairs of genes determine rhesus groups (C, c, D, E, e). The principal rhesus blood group is determined by the D locus. Rhesus (Rh) disease occurs when a Rh-negative mother has Rh antibodies and a Rh-positive baby. The antibodies cross the placenta and cause fetal haemolysis (anaemia, jaundice) and, in the extreme, cardiac failure and hydrops fetalis (Fig 71) and death. Rarely, Kell or Duffy antibodies can produce a similar severe disease. Less severe disease can be produced by antibodies to the C or E loci, A or B antigens.

Sensitization

Occurs when red blood cells from a Rh-positive fetus/baby enter the circulation of a Rh-negative woman (at delivery, abortion, placental bleeding, amniocentesis, chorionic villus sampling, external cephalic version or spontaneously).

Prevention

By administration of anti-D immunoglobulin to Rh-negative mothers at potentially sensitizing events, or routinely at 28 and 34 weeks (depending on local policy).

Detection

Unsensitized Rh-negative women are screened for antibodies during pregnancy.

Assessment

The severity of disease may be assessed by amniotic fluid optical density difference at 450 nm (Fig 72), fetal blood sampling for fetal haemoglobin or non-invasively by measuring middle cerebral artery blood flow velocities (Fig 73). Hydrops on ultrasound is a late feature.

Intervention

Mild or moderate disease demands less frequent testing and delivery at term. More severe disease necessitates invasive testing and intrauterine transfusion of blood, often every 2-3 weeks. Intravenous immunoglobulins have been tried for severe disease at gestations too early for fetal blood transfusion.

Postnatal care

Cord blood is taken for haemoglobin, Coombs' test and bilirubin levels. Jaundice should be treated by phototherapy in mild cases and exchange transfusions in the more severe, to prevent kernicterus.

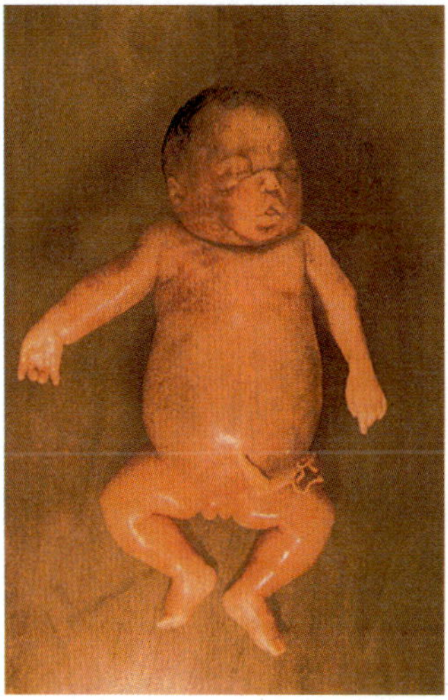

图 71　Rh 溶血病导致的胎儿水肿
Hydrops fetalis secondary to rhesus disease

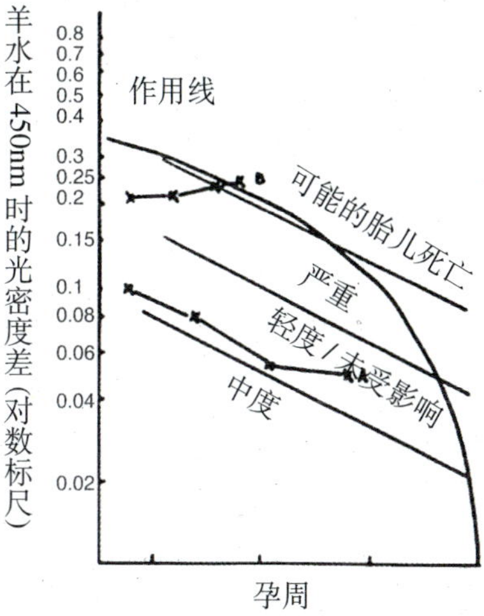

图 72　中度（a）和重度（b）溶血病的 Liley 曲线
Liley curve with examples of moderate (a) and severe (b) disease

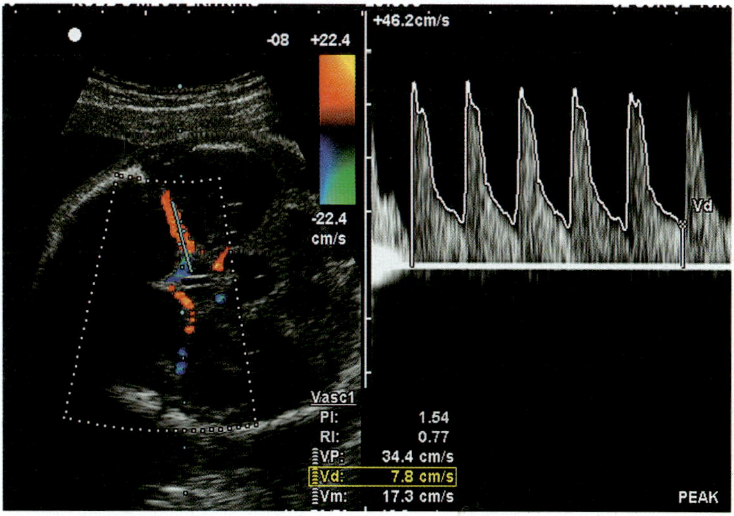

图 73　大脑中动脉多普勒超声图
Doppler ultrasound of the middle cerebral artery

诊断

由除红细胞抗原同种免疫之外的原因引起，液体积聚于皮肤（水肿）（图 74）、腹部（腹水）（图 75）或胸腔（胸腔积液或心包积液）（图 76）。

病因学

- 贫血：溶血（红细胞酶缺陷、纯合型α地中海贫血）、出血（双胎输血综合征、胎儿向母体出血）、骨髓浸润（Gaucher病）或细小病毒（B19）感染。
- 心衰：心律失常、心脏畸形、心脏肿瘤或动静脉分流（胎儿或胎盘的）。
- 低蛋白血症：先天肾病综合征、肝酶缺陷。
- 静脉回流受阻：神经母细胞瘤、肺部囊腺瘤畸形、卵巢囊肿、腹膜后纤维变性。
- 混杂因素：先天感染（细小病毒B19、巨细胞病毒、梅毒）、染色体异常（如Turner综合征）、骨骼发育不良、乳糜胸/胸腔积液、先天代谢病、神经系统疾病。

处理

一旦发现胎儿水肿，应确定病因，如果可能的话，可联合进行超声检、孕妇血化验、胎儿侵袭性检查。即使发现病因（80%），可能也无法治疗。可治疗的病因包括：胎儿贫血（可行宫内输血）、胎儿心律失常（给予孕妇地高辛或氟卡尼）、胸腔积液（插入胸膜羊膜分流器），这些通常是引起更加泛发水肿的原因。总体存活率约 25%。

临床特征

在可能的情况下于产前纠正水肿可改善预后。分娩时，隐性水肿的新生儿表现为苍白，由于肺水肿或肺发育不良合并胸腔积液而引起先天性心脏衰竭或严重的呼吸窘迫。

Non-immune hydrops fetalis

Diagnosis

Fluid accumulation in skin (oedema) (Fig 74), abdomen (ascites) (Fig 75) or chest (pleural or pericardial effusions) (Fig 76), secondary to causes other than isoimmunization against red blood cell antigens.

Aetiology

- Anaemia: by haemolysis (red cell enzyme defects, homozygous α -thalassaemia), haemorrhage (twin-twin transfusion, fetomaternal haemorrhage), marrow infiltration (Gaucher disease) or parvovirus (B19) disease.
- Cardiac failure: arrhythmias, cardiac anomalies, cardiac tumour, or arteriovenous shunts (fetal or placental).
- Hypoproteinaemia: congenital nephrotic syndrome, hepatic enzyme defects.
- Obstructed venous return: neuroblastoma, cystic adenomatous malformation of lung, ovarian cysts, retroperitoneal fibrosis.
- Miscellaneous: congenital infection (parvovirus B19, cytomegalovirus, syphilis), chromosomal anomaly (e.g. Turner syndrome), skeletal dysplasias, chylo/hydrothorax, inborn errors of metabolism, neurological disorders.

Management

Once fetal hydrops has been noted, the cause should be identified, if possible, by a combination of ultrasound, maternal blood tests and fetal invasive testing. Even if a cause is found (80%), treatment may not be possible. Treatable causes include fetal anaemia (with intrauterine transfusion), fetal cardiac arrhythmia (with maternal administration of digoxin or flecainide) and pleural effusions (with insertion of pleuroamniotic shunts), which are occasionally the cause of more widespread oedema. Overall survival is about 25%.

Clinical features

The prognosis is improved by correction of the hydrops antenatally where possible. At delivery, a baby born with unresolved hydrops may be pale and suffer from congestive heart failure or severe respiratory distress due to pulmonary oedema or pulmonary hypoplasia with pleural effusions (Fig 77).

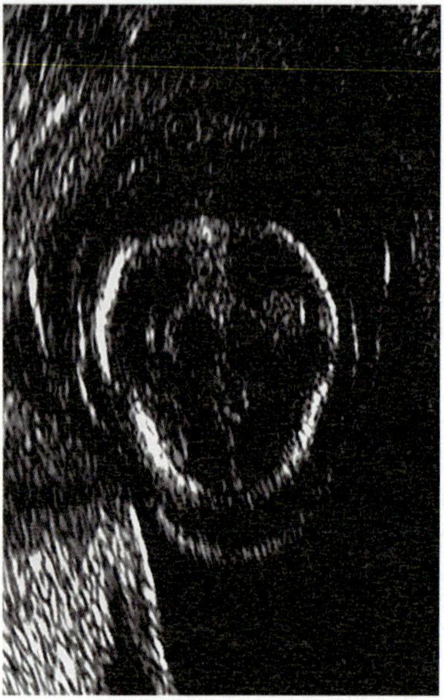

图 74　超声图像示皮肤水肿
Ultrasound image showing skin oedema

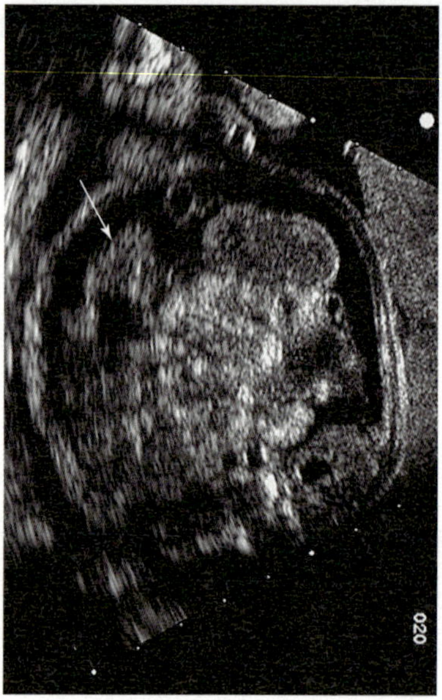

图 75　超声图像示胎儿腹水
Ultrasound image showing fetal ascites

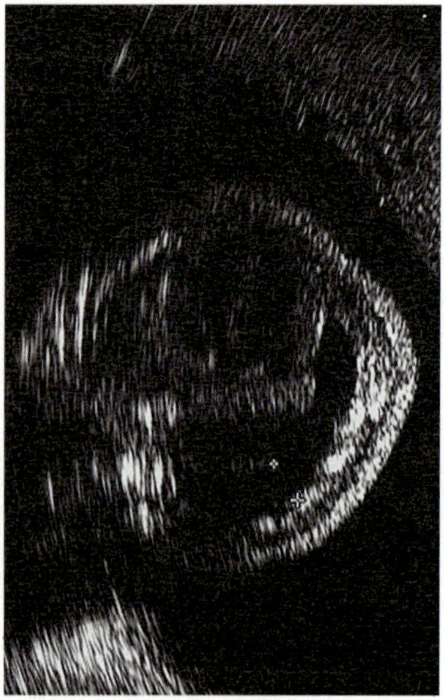

图 76　超声示胎儿胸腔积液
Ultrasound image showing a fetal pleural effusion

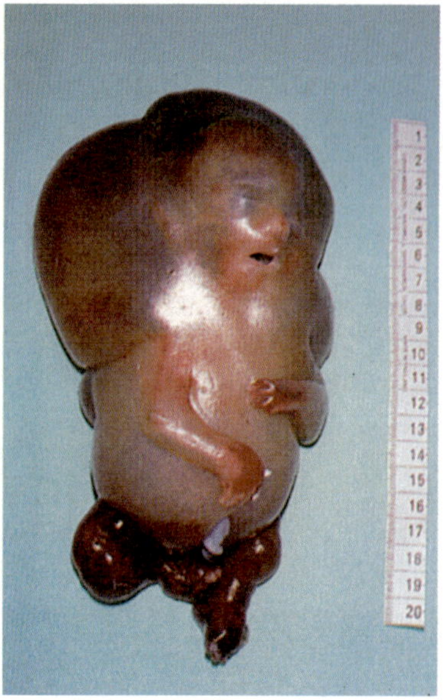

图 77　死亡的水肿的婴儿
Dead hydropic baby

贫血

定义

血红蛋白浓度随妊娠改变。在妊娠早期血红蛋白的正常低值为11g/dl。妊娠28周后正常低值降至10.5 g/dl。

病因学

生理性的（由于血液稀释）（图78）、缺铁（低色素性贫血、小细胞性、血清铁蛋白降低）（图79）或叶酸缺乏（大细胞深染性、低红细胞叶酸）（图80）。维生素 B_{12} 缺乏、感染、血红蛋白病及其他原因不常见。

预防

有些妇女的饮食不能满足每日铁需要量。对这些孕妇推荐补充铁剂（元素铁每日100mg），同时加用叶酸（每日300mg）。对所有孕妇补充叶酸和铁以预防贫血的方法尚有争议。然而每日摄入400 μg叶酸在理论上可预防神经管缺陷（见第8章）。

检查

一旦确诊，还应进行其他的检查，检查红细胞指数（平均红细胞体积、平均红细胞血红蛋白浓度）、网织红细胞计数、血涂片、血清铁蛋白、红细胞叶酸及血清维生素 B_{12} 浓度，如疑有血红蛋白病应行电泳。

治疗

根据病因决定治疗方案。轻度的生理性贫血无需治疗。缺乏叶酸和/或铁者可给予铁和叶酸共同口服，虽然口服铁剂通常不耐受（胃肠道紊乱）。胃肠外铁剂可引起过敏反应（皮疹、关节痛、血管神经性水肿），只在不能口服铁剂时使用，且必须入院使用。应同胃肠外铁剂时口服叶酸，以促进造血。妊娠期输血应该是一种少见的情况（比如有症状的严重贫血）。

Anaemia

Definition

The haemoglobin concentration varies with gestation. The lower limit of normal is 11 g/dL in the first trimester and 10.5 g/dL after 28 weeks.

Aetiology

Physiological (due to haemodilution) (Fig 78), iron deficiency (hypochromic, microcytic, low serum ferritin) (Fig 79) or folate deficiency (hyperchromic macrocytic, low red cell folate) (Fig 80). Vitamin B_{12} deficiency, infection, haemoglobinopathies and other causes are uncommon.

Prophylaxis

In some women, the daily iron requirement cannot be met by the diet. For such mothers, supplementation with iron (100 mg elemental iron per day), often with folic acid (300 mg/day), is recommended. The use of iron and folate supplements for all mothers is controversial in the prevention of anaemia; however, daily intake of folic acid of 400 μg periconceptually is recommended to prevent neural tube defects (see Ch 8).

Investigations

Once the diagnosis has been made, other investigations include red cell indices (mean corpuscular volume, mean corpuscular haemoglobin concentration), reticulocyte count, film, serum ferritin, red cell folate and serum vitamin B_{12} concentrations, and electrophoresis if a haemoglobinopathy is suspected.

Treatment

Depends on the cause. Mild physiological anaemia requires no treatment. Iron and/or folate deficiency can be treated with oral iron and folic acid together, although oral iron is often poorly tolerated (gastrointestinal disturbance). Parenteral iron can cause anaphylaxis (rashes, arthralgia, angioneurotic oedema) and should only be given when all oral preparations have been unsuccessful, and in hospital. Oral folic acid should be given with parenteral iron because of the stimulus to haemopoiesis. Blood transfusion in pregnancy should be a rare event (e.g. with symptomatic severe anemia).

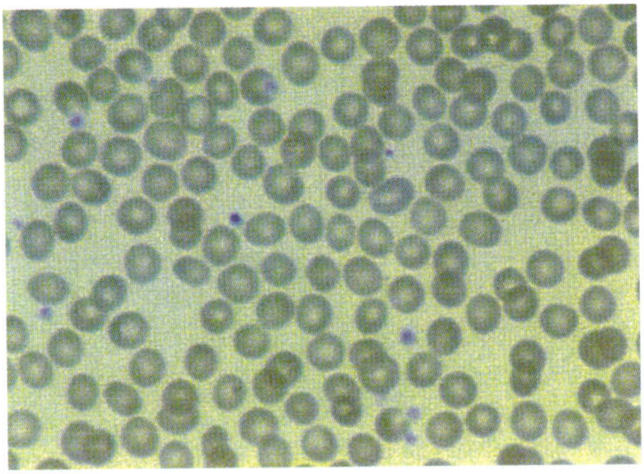

图 78　正常血涂片
Normal blood film

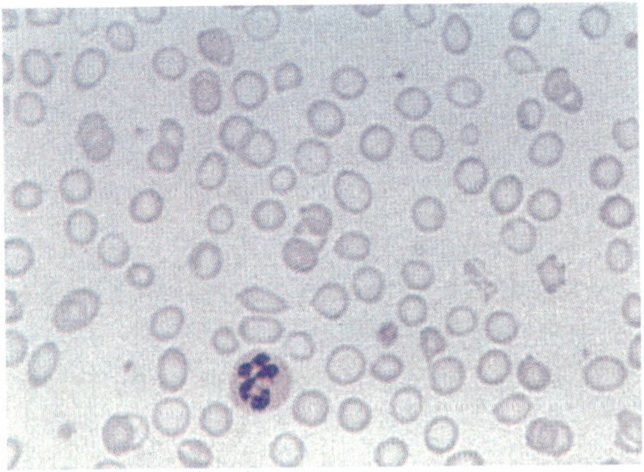

图 79　血涂片显示缺铁（低色素和小细胞）
Blood film showing iron deficiency
(hypochromia and microcytosis)

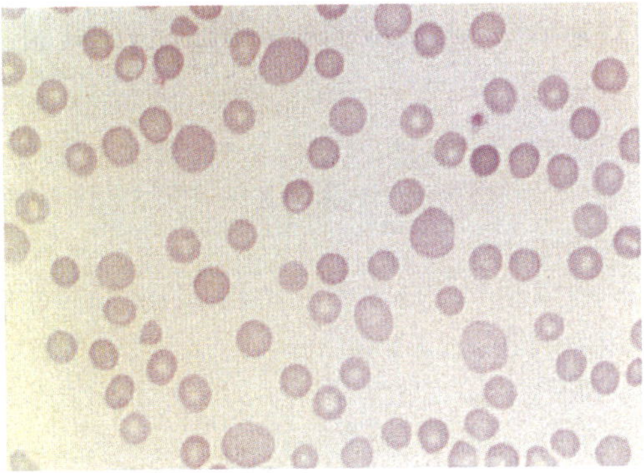

图 80　血涂片显示叶酸缺乏（巨红细胞症）
Blood film showing folate deficiency
(macrocytosis)

高血压

定义

4 小时内有一次以上的血压持续高值，收缩压达140mmHg或舒张压达90mmHg。另外一种定义是收缩压超过基础血压30mmHg，和/或舒张压超过基础血压15mmHg。第二种定义与围生期发病率相关性小。由于妊娠引起的高血压通常发生在妊娠20周后。

检查

孕妇安静状态下于半卧位/坐位，上臂、心脏及血压计处于同一水平（图81）（肥胖孕妇使用大号袖带）（图82）。脉搏搏动消失时（Korotkoff V期）为舒张压读数，Korotkoff V期比Ⅳ期更接近动脉内压（Ⅳ期为脉搏搏动变低沉时）。不同血压计测量可能产生明显不同的数值（图83）。

分类

- 妊娠引起的单纯高血压。
- 妊娠引起的高血压合并蛋白尿（先兆子痫）。
- 原先存在的高血压。
- 原先存在的高血压合并先兆子痫。

原先存在的高血压

病因学

大多为原发性高血压，其他诊断包括肾病（多囊肾、肾动脉狭窄）、内分泌疾病（Cushing综合征、Conn综合征、嗜铬细胞瘤）、结缔组织病、主动脉缩窄、药物（口服避孕药、类固醇）。

处理

调换不适宜的抗高血压药（如阿替洛尔、利尿剂、ACEI类）。使用妊娠期安全的药物（拉贝洛尔、甲基多巴、硝苯地平）。

连续超声扫描寻找胎盘疾病的证据。对反复先兆子痫孕妇进行监护。

伴有中度-重度高血压的妊娠通常在妊娠38周进行引产，如果不是更早的话。

Hypertension

Definition

A sustained absolute systolic BP of 140 mmHg or a diastolic BP of 90 mm Hg on more than one occasion at least 4 h apart. An alternative definition is a sustained rise of systolic BP by 30 mmHg and/or diastolic BP by 15 mmHg over booking values. This latter definition correlates less well with perinatal morbidity. Hypertension caused by pregnancy does not usually occur until after 20 weeks.

Examination

Semirecumbent/sitting relaxed mother, upper arm level with heart (Fig 81) and sphygmomanometer (larger cuff with obese women) (Fig 82). Diastolic BP is taken as the point at which the pulse can no longer be heard (Korotkoff phase V) and is more closely related to intra-arterial pressure than Korotkoff phase IV (muffling of the pulse). Different equipment (Fig 83) may produce significantly different values.

Classification

- Pregnancy-induced hypertension alone.
- Pregnancy-induced hypertension with proteinuria (pre-eclampsia).
- Pre-existing hypertension.
- Pre-existing hypertension with added pre-eclampsia.

Pre-existing hypertension

Aetiology

Mostly essential hypertension. Other diagnoses include renal pathology (multicystic/polycystic kidney disease, renal artery stenosis), endocrinopathies (Cushing syndrome/disease, Conn syndrome, phaeochromocytoma), connective tissue disorders, aortic coarctation, drugs (oral contraceptives, steroids).

Management

Change unsuitable antihypertensives (e.g. atenolol, diuretics and ACE inhibitors) where possible to medications safe for use in pregnancy (labetalol, methyldopa, nifedipine).

Serial scanning for evidence of placental disease and maternal monitoring for superimposed pre-eclampsia.

Pregnancies complicated by moderate-to-severe hypertension are usually induced at 38 weeks, if not sooner.

Pregnancy-

Management

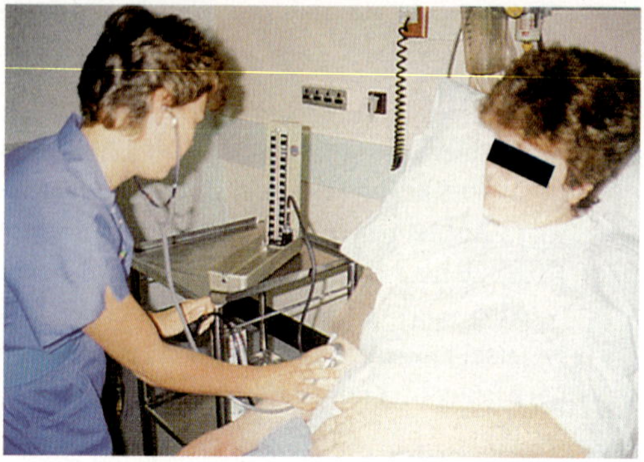

图 81　测量血压
Measuring blood pressure

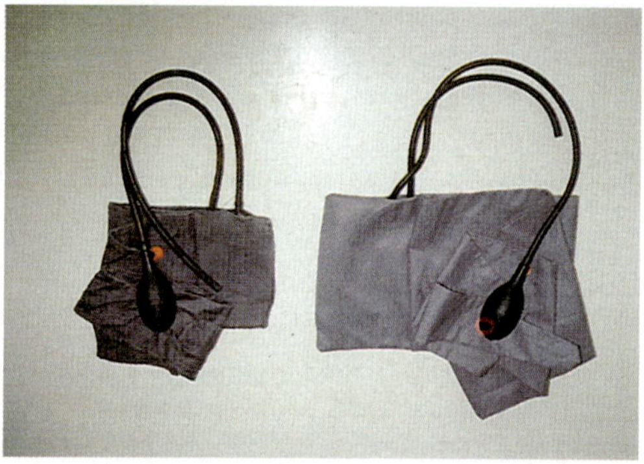

图 82　不同大小的袖带
Cuff size variation

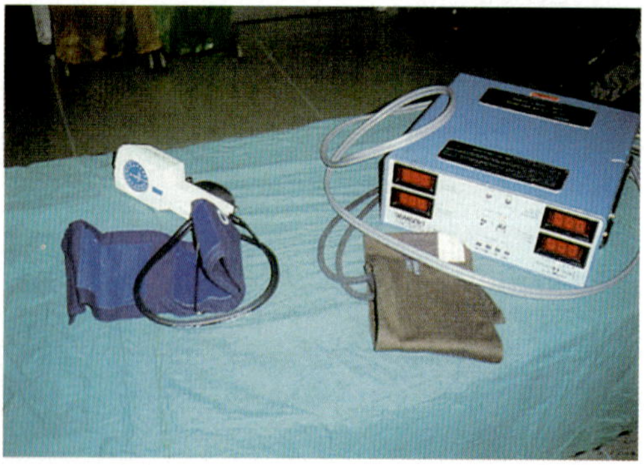

图 83　不同血压仪
Equipment variation

妊娠引起的高血压（不伴有蛋白尿）

处理

密切监护胎儿及孕妇，及时发现子痫前期或胎盘功能不良。单纯轻度高血压（< 160/100mmHg）无需过早引产。一般不会并发胎儿生长受限，产妇/围产期发病率、死亡率不会增加。

先兆子痫

定义

高血压伴有大量蛋白尿（24 h尿蛋白定量> 0.3g），需排除泌尿系统感染。

病因学

是孕妇特有的具体病因不详的疾病，与多系统内皮损伤和胎盘血流灌注不足有关。其发生占所有妊娠的5%。高危因素有：初产妇、既往先兆子痫病史、家族史、原有高血压、偏头痛、糖尿病、结缔组织病、抗磷脂综合征、与胎盘过大有关的任何情况（多胎妊娠、葡萄胎、水肿）。

临床特征

表现为高血压、蛋白尿、肾损害、液体潴留及胎儿生长受限。急性并发症包括：子痫（继发于脑水肿、脑血管痉挛）（图84）、弥漫性血管内凝血（图85）、肝包膜膨胀（图 86）、肺水肿（图 87）及胎盘早剥（图 127）。

症状有：头痛、视物模糊、上腹部疼痛。查体可发现明显水肿、反射亢进、抽搐及上腹部压痛。

处理

解决先兆子痫的唯一方法是分娩。如为非常早期的早产（妊娠<34周），应入院密切监测胎儿及产妇。如有早产，需给母体使用糖皮质激素。应该考虑应用抗高血压药和解痉药（硫酸镁）。

induced hypertension (without proteinuria)

Close fetal and maternal surveillance for evidence of pre-eclampsia or placental insufficiency. When the isolated hypertension is mild (<160/100 mmHg), early induction is not usually necessary. These pregnancies are not usually complicated by fetal growth restriction or increased maternal/perinatal morbidity or mortality.

Pre-eclampsia

Definition

Hypertension associated with significant proteinuria (>0.3 g per 24-h urine collection) in the absence of a urinary tract infection.

Aetiology

Condition peculiar to pregnancy of unknown aetiology, associated with multisystem endothelial damage and placental hypoperfusion. Occurs in 5% of all pregnancies. Risk factors: primigravidity, previous pre-eclampsia, family history, pre-existing hypertension, migraine, diabetes, connective tissue disorders, antiphospholipid syndrome, any condition associated with a large placenta (multiple pregnancy, hydatidiform mole, hydrops).

Clinical features

Characterized by hypertension, proteinuria, renal impairment, fluid retention and fetal growth restriction. Acute complications include eclampsia (secondary to cerebral oedema and vasospasm) (Fig 84), disseminated intravascular coagulation (Fig 85), liver capsule distension (Fig 86), pulmonary oedema (Fig 87) and abruption (Fig 127).

Symptoms include headache, visual disturbances and epigastric pain. Marked oedema, brisk reflexes, clonus and upper abdominal tenderness may be found on examination.

Management

Resolution of pre-eclampsia comes only with delivery. If very preterm (less than 34 weeks), close fetal and maternal monitoring as an inpatient is indicated. Maternal steroids should be given as preterm delivery may be necessary. Antihypertensives and anticonvulsants (magnesium sulphate) should be considered.

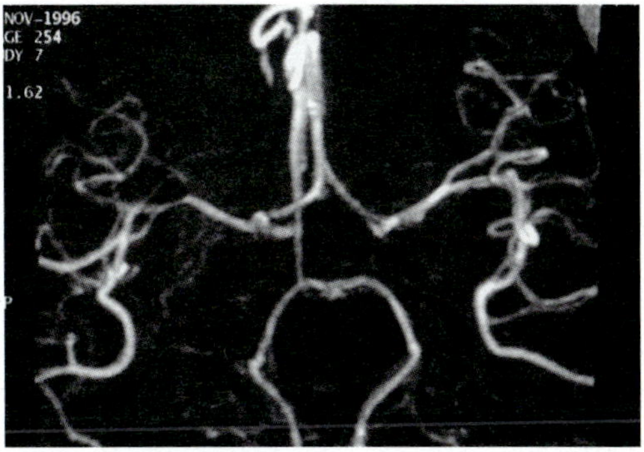

图 84　先兆子痫脑 MRI
MRI of pre-eclamptic brain

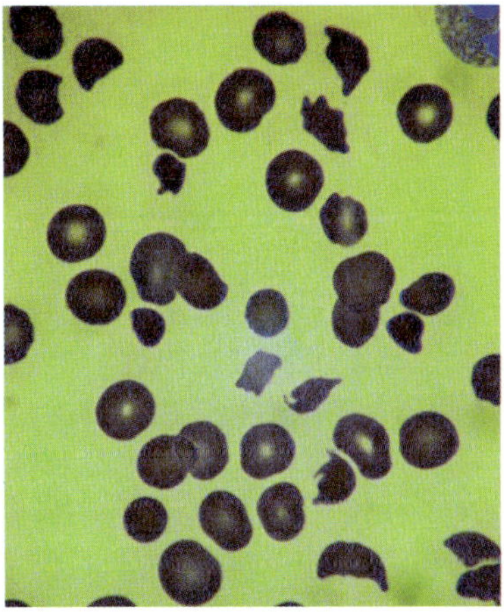

图 85　血涂片显示溶血
Blood film showing haemolysis

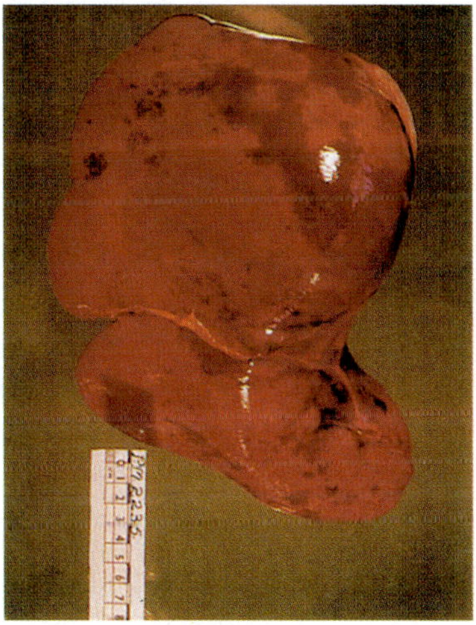

图 86　肝包膜下出血
Subcapsular hepatic haemorrhage

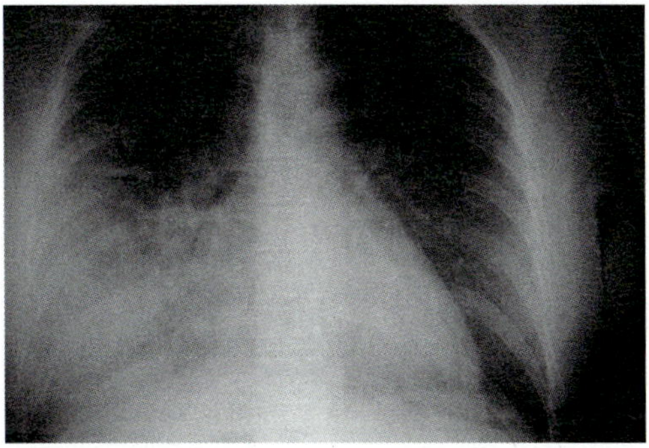

图 87　胸部 X 线显示肺水肿
Chest X-ray showing pulmonary oedema

糖尿病（diabetes mellitus，DM）

定义

是由于胰岛素生成缺乏（Ⅰ型）或胰岛素抵抗（Ⅱ型及妊娠期糖尿病）导致的血糖控制不良。口服葡萄糖耐量试验（OGTT）可确诊。

原有糖尿病

对孕妇影响：胰岛素需求量增加、低血糖发作、视网膜病变恶化、先兆子痫、产伤/剖宫产。

对胎儿影响：先天畸形的危险增加（特别是心脏、肌肉骨骼、神经管缺陷）（图88）、巨大儿（图89）、羊水过多、死胎、产伤（如肩难产、Erb麻痹）（图90）、呼吸窘迫、低血糖及黄疸。

治疗

孕前期：应用大剂量叶酸、合理控制血糖可减少先天畸形的风险。

产前：严格控制血糖（图91）。目标定在餐前血糖≤6mmol/L，餐后2小时血糖≤9mmol/L。应用胰岛素代替口服降糖药。定期检查血压和眼底。妊娠11～13周（颈部半透明度）和20周时进行超声检查监测胎儿。此后定期超声扫描检查胎儿生长和健康状态。妊娠38～40周分娩。对巨大儿考虑选择性剖宫产。分娩后胰岛素需求量下降。

妊娠期糖尿病

随机血糖和口服葡萄糖耐量试验可确诊。适用于所有孕妇或仅针对有高危因素的孕妇（糖尿、糖尿病家族史、原因不明的死产、既往巨大儿史、孕妇肥胖、羊水过多）。

妊娠期糖尿病可单纯通过饮食控制。经常需用胰岛素。妊娠期糖尿病通常发生于妊娠24周后，主要危险是巨大儿及其并发症。

Diabetes mellitus (DM)

Definition

Inadequate blood sugar control due either to a deficiency in production of insulin (type I) or to a state of insulin resistance (type II and gestational diabetes mellitus). Diagnosed by an oral glucose tolerance test (OGTT).

Pre-existing DM

Maternal risks Increased insulin requirement, hypoglycaemic episodes, deterioration of retinopathy, pre-eclampsia and traumatic labour/caesarean section.

Fetal risks Increased risk of congenital malformations (especially cardiac, musculoskeletal, neural tube defect) (Fig 88), macrosomia (Fig 89), polyhydramnios, fetal death, traumatic delivery (e.g. shoulder dystocia and Erb's palsy) (Fig 90), respiratory distress, hypoglycaemia and jaundice.

Management

Prepregnancy High-dose folic acid and improved blood glucose control reduce the risk of congenital anomalies.

Antenatal Close control of blood glucose (Fig 91). Aim for preprandial values of less than 6 mmol/L, and 2-h postprandial values less than 9.0 mmol/L. Insulin is substituted for oral hypoglycaemic agents. Regular checks of BP and optic fundi. Fetal screening for normality by ultrasound at 11-13 weeks (nuchal translucency) and 20 weeks. Later, regular scans for growth and well-being. Delivery at 38-40 weeks. Consider elective caesarean section for macrosomic babies. After delivery, insulin requirements fall.

Gestational DM

Diagnosis follows screening with random blood sugars and OGTT. This may be universal or include only those pregnant women with risk factors (glycosuria, family history of diabetes, unexplained stillbirth, previous macrosomia, maternal obesity, polyhydramnios).
Gestational DM may be managed by dietary changes alone. Insulin often required. Onset is usually after 24 weeks. Main risk is macrosomia and its complications.

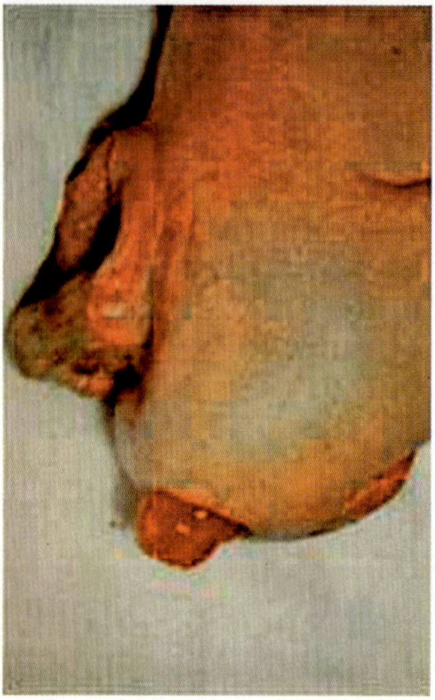

图 88　神经管缺陷
Neural tube defect

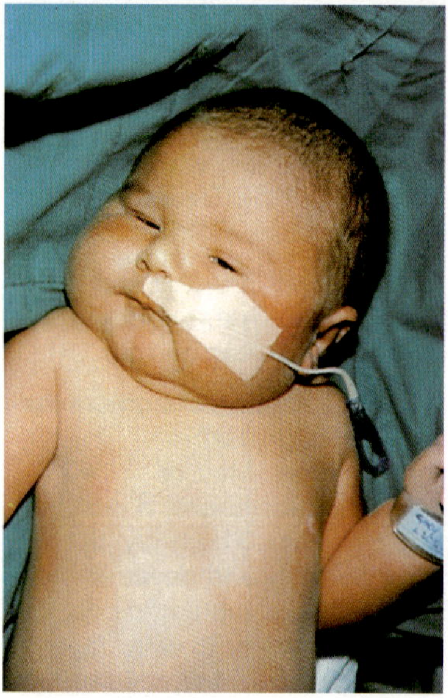

图 89　巨大儿
Macrosomia

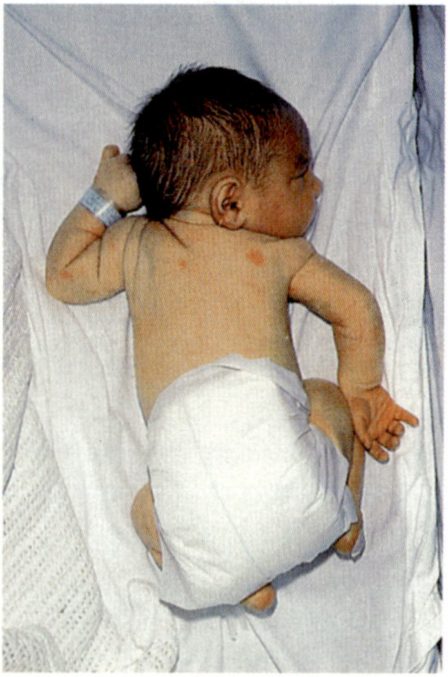

图 90　Erb 麻痹
Erb's palsy

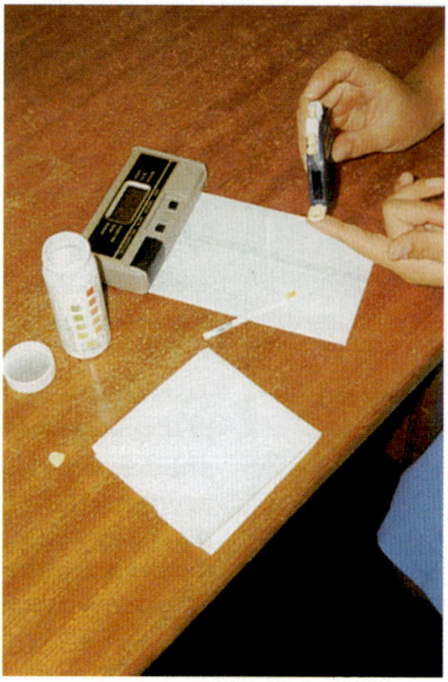

图 91　频繁的血糖检测以改善对血糖的控制
Frequent glucose testing to improve control

静脉血栓栓塞性疾病

发病率

每1500例妊娠发生1例。在英国，该病为孕妇致死的最重要原因。

病因学

由于妊娠时凝血因子增多、纤溶减少及内源性抗凝血因子水平降低，故妊娠本身就是高危因素，这些改变尤以产褥期显著。其他危险因素包括：肥胖、不活动、年龄（>35岁）、脱水、先兆子痫、遗传性血栓形成倾向（如抗凝血酶Ⅲ缺乏）、获得性血栓形成倾向（如原发性/继发性抗磷脂综合征）及手术分娩。

临床特征

可能表现为深静脉血栓形成（DVT，肿胀、疼痛、大腿和小腿皮温增高）（图92）、肺栓塞（胸痛、咯血、气短、心动过速、虚脱），或者更罕见的大脑静脉窦血栓形成（头痛、呕吐、意识障碍）。

诊断

DVT通常可以通过下肢静脉多普勒检查诊断。肺栓塞诊断靠通气/血流扫描（图93）或血管造影。MRI在诊断妊娠期各种形式的血栓栓塞性疾病被证实有越来越重要的意义（图94）。

治疗

目前用低分子量肝素皮下注射代替传统的未分馏肝素给药治疗DVT及肺栓塞。在个别病例，可通过在下腔静脉中插入滤过器的方法预防DVT发生多发性肺栓塞（图95）。妊娠期抗凝会增加产前和产后出血的危险。

预防

认识血栓栓塞性疾病的高危因素很重要。产后特别是剖宫产术后的预防尤为重要。经常建议在产前及分娩后6周内使用低分子量肝素预防。

Venous thromboembolic disease

Incidence

1 in 1500 pregnancies. It remains the leading cause of maternal mortality in the UK.

Aetiology

Pregnancy itself is a risk factor because of raised coagulation factors, reduced fibrinolysis and decreased levels of endogenous anticoagulants. These changes are most marked in the puerperium. Other risk factors include obesity, immobility, age (older than 35 years), dehydration, pre-eclampsia, inherited thrombophilias (e.g. antithrombin III deficiency), acquired thrombophilias (e.g. primary/secondary antiphospholipid syndrome) and operative delivery.

Clinical features

May present as a deep vein thrombosis (DVT; swollen, painful, warm lower leg and thigh) (Fig 92), pulmonary embolism (chest pain, haemoptysis, shortness of breath, tachycardia, collapse) or more rarely cerebral venous sinus thrombosis (headache, vomiting and reduced level of consciousness).

Diagnosis

A DVT is usually diagnosed by venous Doppler of the lower limbs. Pulmonary emboli are diagnosed by ventilation/perfusion scanning (Fig 93) or angiography. MRI is proving increasingly valuable in the diagnosis of all forms of thromboembolic disease in pregnancy (Fig 94).

Treatment

Traditional treatment of DVT and pulmonary embolism with intravenous unfractionated heparin is being replaced by subcutaneous injections of low molecular weight heparin. In rare cases, multiple pulmonary embolisms arising from a DVT can be prevented by insertion of a filter in the inferior vena cava (Fig 95). Anticoagulation during pregnancy increases the risks of antepartum and postpartum haemorrhage.

Prevention

Recognition of risk factors for thromboembolic disease is vital. Prophylaxis in the postpartum period, especially after caesarean section, is particularly important. Prophylaxis with low molecular weight heparin is often commenced antenatally and continued 6 weeks after delivery.

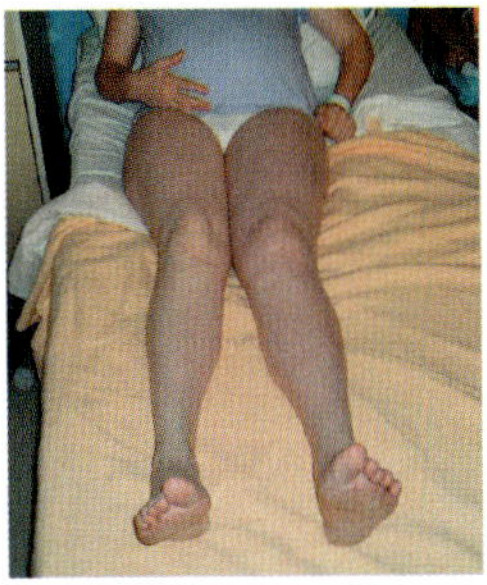

图 92　左下肢深静脉血栓
Left deep vein thrombosis

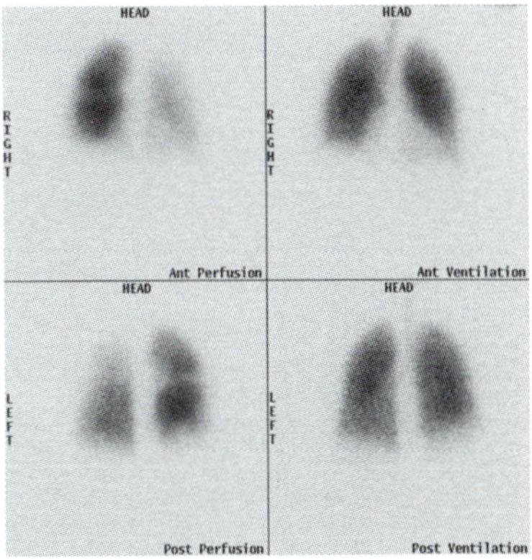

图 93　扫描显示由于肺栓塞导致的通气 / 血流比例失调
Scan showing ventilation/ perfusion mismatch due to pulmonary emboli

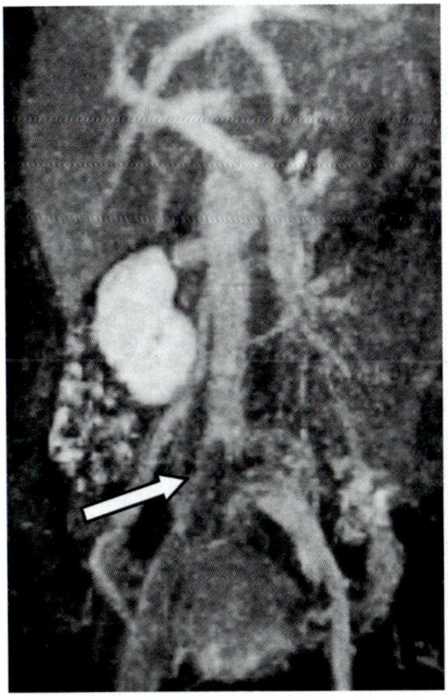

图 94　左侧回肠股骨血管血栓形成的 MRI 图像
MRI of left ileofemoral thrombosis

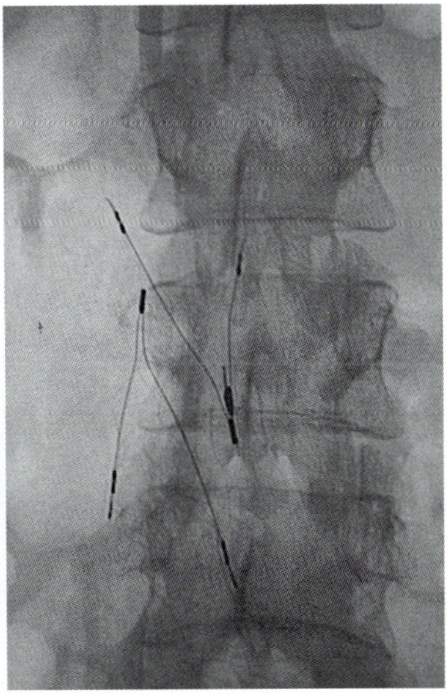

图 95　下腔静脉内过滤器的 X 线片
X-ray of inferior vena cava filter

性传播感染疾病

人类免疫缺陷病毒（HIV）

高危因素包括静脉药物滥用、来自非洲、高危性伴侣（如双性恋、无防护性交）。对所有孕妇提供HIV检测。

高危因素

如不进行干预，则有15%～25%的病例可发生HIV由孕妇传播给胎儿。妊娠期使用抗逆转录病毒药物、选择性剖宫产、避免母乳喂养可使其发生减少至低于2%。在无AIDS疾病的情况下，HIV对妊娠的结局没有不利影响（图96）。

治疗

与HIV内科医生合作。抗逆转录病毒药物应该持续应用，或者对尚未使用的孕妇建议用药。生殖器感染的筛查和治疗、选择性剖宫产、人工喂养有助于减少传播。定期检查CD4计数。谨慎处理HIV感染者的体液。

生殖器疱疹

原发性疱疹感染者（图97）应口服阿昔洛韦5天。建议妊娠晚期使用阿昔洛韦以预防复发。妊娠30周以后发生疱疹的孕妇应行剖宫产，以预防新生儿感染。再发患者感染新生儿的危险很小（由于被动免疫）。

B族链球菌

B族链球菌是新生儿败血症早期发病的最常见原因，在英国每年约有40例新生儿死于此病。20%～30%产妇阴道内有B族链球菌寄居（图98）。既往有新生儿感染史的产妇在产时应预防性应用抗生素青霉素。无既往新生儿感染史的携带者产妇在产时也应使用抗生素。

其他

淋病奈瑟菌及沙眼衣原体长期潜伏于宫颈。产时感染可引起结膜炎（图99）、关节炎、脑膜炎或全身性败血症。妊娠期间的这些病原菌感染分别使用青霉素和红霉素治疗。

Sexually transmitted infections

Human immunodeficiency virus

Risk factors include intravenous substance abuse, African origin, partners with high-risk behaviours (e.g. bisexuality and unprotected intercourse). All pregnant women are offered HIV testing.

Risks

Without interventions, HIV is transmitted from mother to fetus in 15-25% of cases. Use of antiretroviral drugs through pregnancy, elective caesarean section and avoidance of breast feeding reduce this to less than 2%. HIV does not adversely affect pregnancy outcome in the absence of AIDS-defining illnesses (Fig 96).

Management

Jointly with an HIV physician. Antiretroviral drugs should be continued or commenced in those women not yet taking them. Screening and treatment of genital infections helps to reduce transmission, as does elective caesarean section and bottle-feeding. Regular CD4 counts. Extreme care in handling body fluids.

Genital herpes

Primary herpes infections (Fig 97) should be treated with 5 days of oral aciclovir; this should be recommenced in the late third trimester to prevent recurrences. Those presenting after 30 weeks' gestation should be delivered by caesarean section to prevent neonatal infection. The risk of this is almost negligible with secondary recurrences (due to passive immunity).

Group B streptococcus (GBS)

The most frequent cause of early onset neonatal sepsis, accounting for approximately 40 deaths per year in the UK. 20-30% of women have vaginal colonization (Fig 98). Those with previous neonatal infection should receive intrapartum antibiotic prophylaxis with penicillin. It is common practice for carriers without such a history to receive intrapartum antibiotics.

Others

Neisseria gonorrhoeae and Chlamydia trachomatis reside in the cervix. Intrapartum infection may cause conjunctivitis (Fig 99), arthritis, meningitis or generalized septicaemia. During pregnancy these infections are treated with penicillin and erythromycin, respectively.

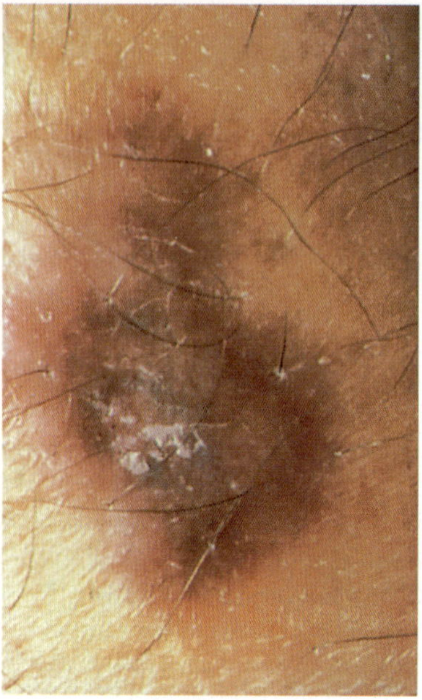

图 96　卡波齐肉瘤
Kaposi's sarcoma

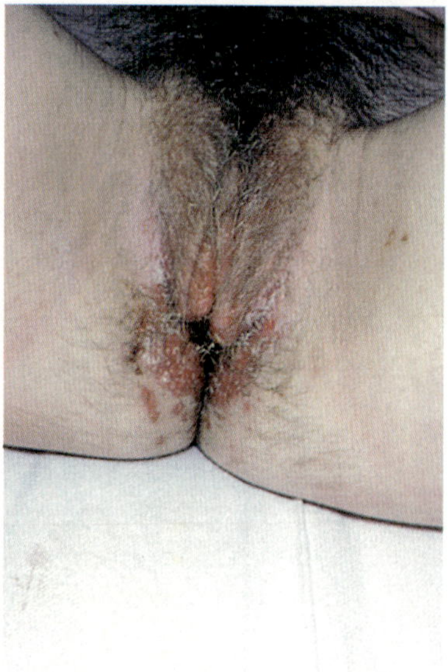

图 97　单纯性感染生殖器的疱疹
Herpes simplex infection of the genitalia

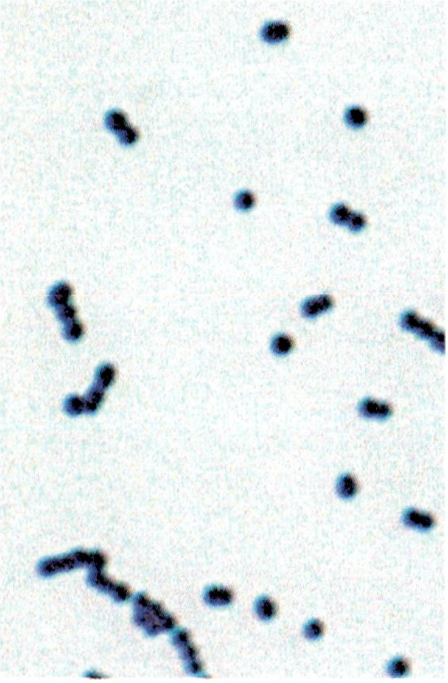

图 98　B 族链球菌的革兰染色
Gram stain of group B streptococcus

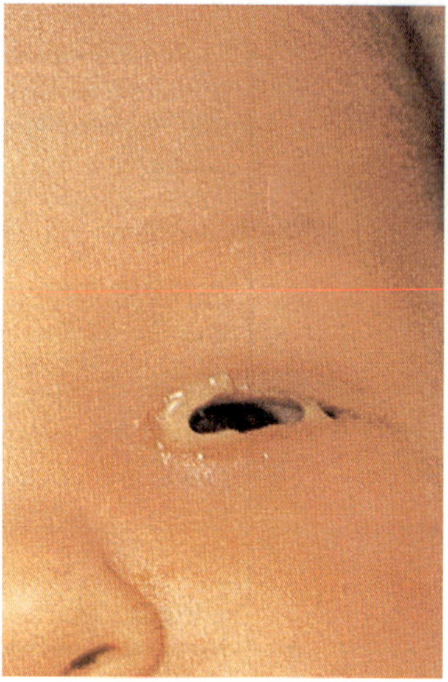

图 99　新生儿眼炎
Ophthalmia neonatorum

皮肤病

妊娠前即患皮肤病

系统性红斑狼疮（systemic lupus erythematosus，SLE）、皮肌炎、系统性硬化病的皮肤损害表现可发生在妊娠期，需口服皮质类固醇激素。这三种疾病中常见发生胎儿生长受限、胎死宫内的风险。

湿疹和牛皮癣可在妊娠期加重或好转。

妊娠期间皮肤病的治疗大多数是安全的。但是类视黄醇（牛皮癣、痤疮）、甲氨蝶呤（牛皮癣）、鬼臼树脂（生殖器疣）及灰黄霉素（皮肤真菌感染）应避免使用。

妊娠期特殊的皮肤病

妊娠期特殊的皮肤病包括：多形性疹（图 100）（发病率0.75%，水肿性红斑丘疹）、瘙痒性毛囊炎（图101）（瘙痒性小红泡丘疹）、痒疹（图 102）（发生率 0.3%，脱皮性痒疹）及妊娠性类大疱疹（图 103）（发生率 1∶50 000，再发与其自身免疫情况、瘙痒性丘疹、小泡及大疱有关）。主要分布于腹部和大腿。口服抗组胺药、1%氢化可的松局部上药通常有效。但妊娠性类天疱疹通常需口服皮质类固醇激素。

妊娠期胆汁淤积症

产科的胆汁淤积症继发于妊娠相关性肝内胆汁淤积症（发生于 0.2% 的妊娠），表现为瘙痒。复发率为 40%。典型表现为妊娠晚期手掌和足底瘙痒，无皮疹，但可见表皮脱落痕迹。妊娠期胆汁淤积症可增加早产和死产的危险。血清胆汁酸和肝转氨酶升高可诊断胆汁淤积症。有时使用熊去氧胆酸可控制皮肤瘙痒。分娩方可治愈此病（通常选择在妊娠 37 ～ 38 周）。

Dermatological problems

Pre-existing conditions

The skin manifestations of systemic lupus erythematosus (SLE), dermatomyositis and systemic sclerosis can recur in pregnancy, requiring treatment with oral steroids. Risk of fetal growth retardation and death is more common with all three conditions.

Eczema and psoriasis can worsen or improve in pregnancy.

Most dermatological treatments are safe during pregnancy, but the retinoids (psoriasis and acne), methotrexate (psoriasis), podophyllin (genital warts) and griseofulvin (fungal skin infections) should all be avoided.

Pregnancy-specific dermatoses

Specific dermatoses of pregnancy include polymorphic eruption (Fig 100) (0.75% incidence, erythematous edematous papules), pruritic folliculitis (Fig 101) (pruritic erythematous follicular papules), prurigo (Fig 102) (0.3% incidence, itchy excoriated papules) and pemphigoid ('herpes') gestationis (Fig 103) (1 : 50 000 incidence, recurrent condition associated with autoimmune conditions, pruritic urticarial papules, vesicles and bullae). The distribution is especially over abdomen and thighs. Treatment with oral antihistamines and topical 1% hydrocortisone is usually effective, although oral steroids may be required for pemphigoid gestationis.

Cholestasis of pregnancy

Obstetric cholestasis is itching secondary to pregnancy-related intrahepatic cholestasis (0.2% of pregnancies). There is a 40% recurrence risk. Typically presents in the third trimester with itching of palms of hands and soles of feet. There is no skin rash but excoriation marks may be present. Associated with an increased risk of prematurity and stillbirth. Diagnosis is by elevated serum bile acids and liver transaminases. The itching can sometimes be controlled with ursodeoxycholic acid. Delivery is the cure (normally electively at 37-38 weeks' gestation).

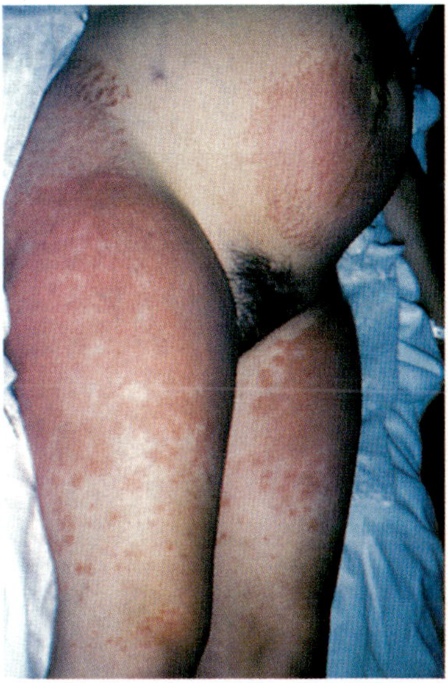

图 100　妊娠期多形性疹
Polymorphic eruption of pregnancy

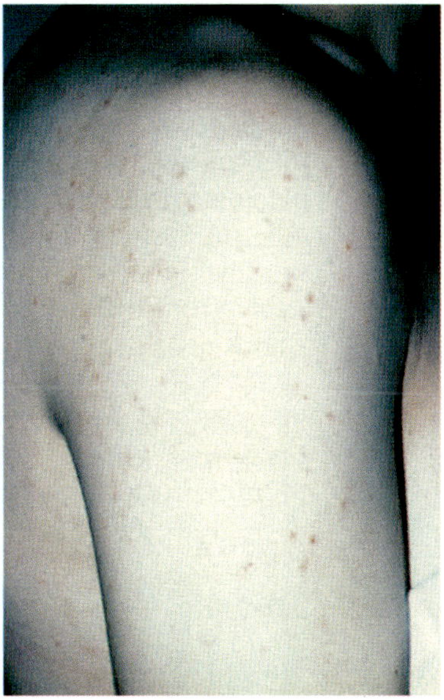

图 101　妊娠期瘙痒性毛囊炎
Pruritic folliculitis of pregnancy

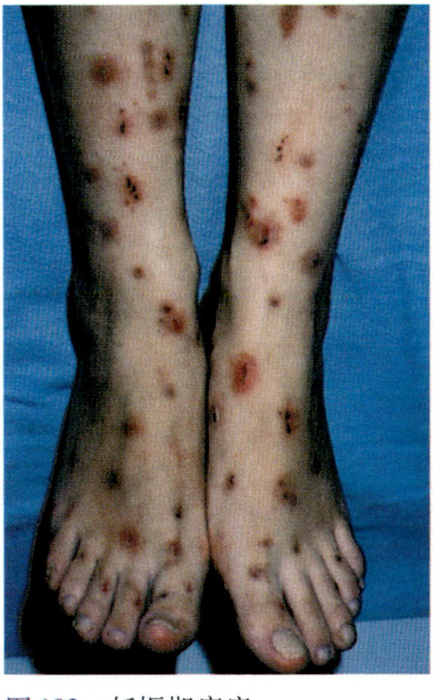

图 102　妊娠期痒疹
Prurigo of pregnancy

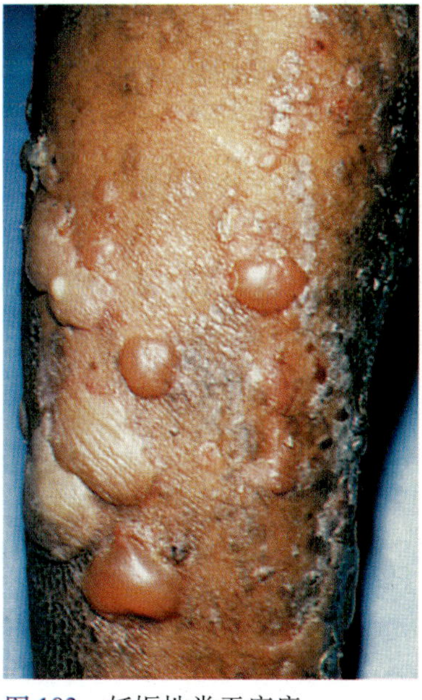

图 103　妊娠性类天疱疹
Pemphigoid gestationis

药物和物质滥用

处方药物

大多数药物可通过胎盘和在乳汁分泌，但只有少数药物被确认有致畸作用（如丙戊酸盐、华法林、甲氨蝶呤）。但妊娠最初三个月期间应尽可能避免使用药物治疗。胎儿以后的生长与发育能受影响：如四环素引起的胎儿牙齿染色（图104），抗甲状腺药物可导致胎儿甲状腺肿（图105）。妊娠后期用药可能影响新生儿（如麻醉药止痛可引起新生儿窘迫）。只有当使用药物有明确用药指征或利大于弊时方可使用。

吸烟

孕妇吸烟可使新生儿平均出生体重减低200 ~ 300g。妊娠后半期戒烟可使胎儿生长受限受到限制。孕妇吸烟也会增加早产、胎膜早破、胎盘早剥、胎儿突然死亡的危险。

酒精

每周酒精摄入超过20单位可导致智力损害、酒精相关性出生缺陷及胎儿酒精综合征（智力低下，生长受限，短眼裂、鼻唇间纵沟发育不良、小颌的特征面容）（图106）。

物质滥用

妊娠期滥用药物的孕妇常见并发症包括：贫血、胎膜早破、产前出血、早产、胎儿生长受限、新生儿窒息及围生期死亡。同时也有感染HBV和HIV的危险。可能发生新生儿戒断症状，其发生时间取决于药物及其半衰期。

Drugs and substance abuse

Prescribed drugs

Most drugs cross the placenta and are excreted in breast milk, but teratogenic effects have been confirmed for only a few (e. g. valproate, warfarin, methotrexate). However, drug therapy in the first trimester should be avoided if possible. Fetal growth and development can be affected later:
e.g. tetracycline-induced staining of fetal teeth (Fig 104), antithyroid drugs producing fetal goitre (Fig 105). Drugs used in the third trimester may affect the newborn
(e.g. narcotic analgesia causing neonatal depression). Drugs should only be prescribed when there are clear indications and benefits outweigh the risks.

Smoking

Maternal smoking reduces the mean birth weight by 200-300g. Fetal growth restriction is limited by stopping smoking in the second half of pregnancy. Maternal smoking during pregnancy also increases the risk of preterm labour, preterm rupture of membranes, abruption and sudden infant death.

Alcohol

Consumption of more than 20 units of alcohol per week has been associated with intellectual impairment, alcohol-related birth defects and the fetal alcohol syndrome (mental retardation, growth retardation, characteristic facies with short palpebral fissures, hypoplastic nasal philtrum, and micrognathia) (Fig 106).

Substance abuse

Complications more common in women who abuse drugs during pregnancy include anaemia, premature membrane rupture, antepartum haemorrhage, preterm delivery, fetal growth restriction, birth asphyxia and perinatal death. They are also at risk of hepatitis B and HIV infection. Neonatal withdrawal symptoms may occur, the timing depending on the drug and its half-life.

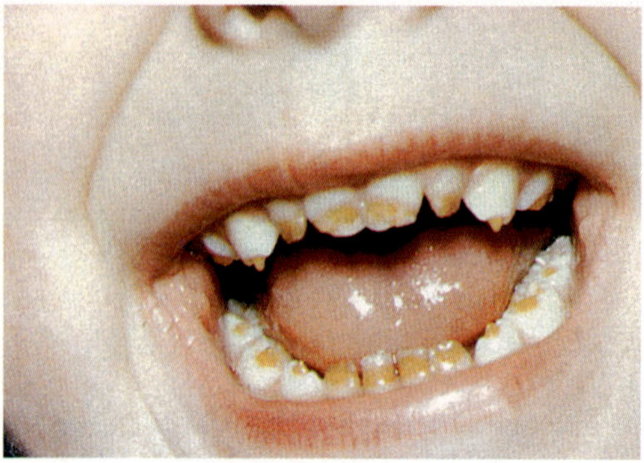

图 104　四环素牙
Tetracycline teeth

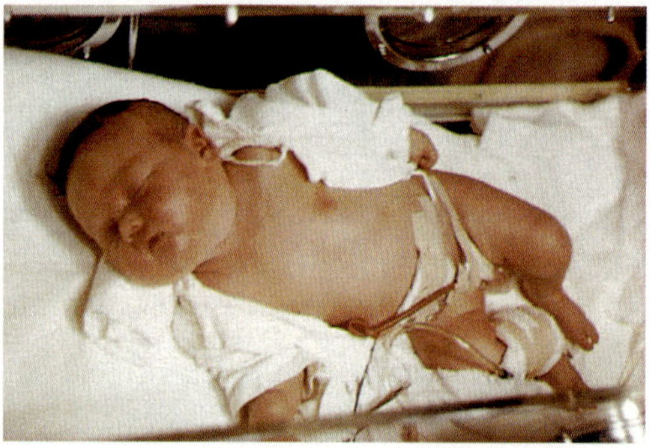

图 105　由于孕妇使用抗甲状腺药物导致的新生儿甲状腺肿
Neonatal goitre secondary to maternal antithyroid treatment

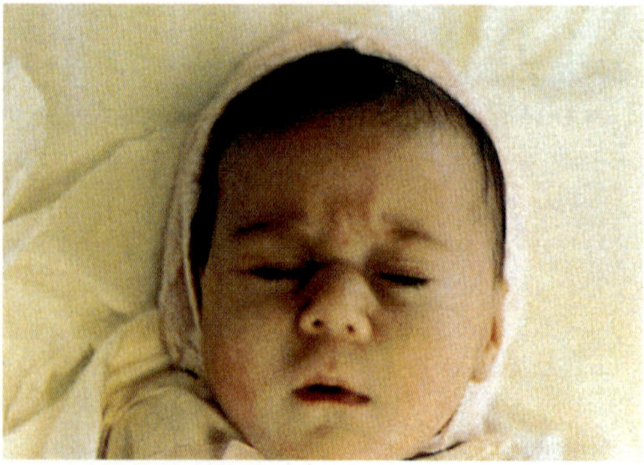

图 106　胎儿酒精综合征
Fetal alcohol syndrome

发病率

约占出生活婴的10%，30%体重小于2.5kg的胎儿患有宫内生长受限（intrauterine growth restriction, IUGR）。其围生期死亡率、发病率及往后的发育问题显著增加。

定义

IUGR 的定义为“胎儿不能获得其遗传上的生长潜能”(图107) 。但实际上由于种族和地域差异通常不易做出诊断。产前确诊主要依赖于超声：胎头双顶径低于正常群体范围的百分位点，或头围（图108）与腹围（图109）显著不匀称。但应注意到如此诊断时胎儿大小并没有落在正常范围值之外。

在正常生长中，胎儿线性生长的最大速率发生在妊娠20周，胎儿体重增长的最大速率在妊娠34周。妊娠末期由于身体限制使胎儿生长变得缓慢。遗传因素、激素及营养补充可影响体重。

病因

- 内因：畸形，包括染色体异常（5%～10%）和病毒感染（2%）。
- 外因：子宫胎盘血管功能不良（如先兆子痫）、紫绀型心脏病、严重的孕妇营养不良、吸烟、酗酒、可卡因、药物（如阿替洛尔）及先天性原因（30%）。

高危因素

身材矮小、既往分娩低体重儿史、孕妇低体重（<45kg）和低身体质量指数、体重增长不良、多胎妊娠、吸烟、酗酒、甲胎蛋白升高及其他情况（参见以上原因）。

12 Fetal growth restriction

Incidence

Approximately 10% of all live-born babies and 30% of those weighing less than 2.5 kg suffer from intrauterine growth restriction (IUGR). They experience greater perinatal mortality and morbidity and have more developmental problems later in life.

Definition

IUGR is defined as 'failure of a fetus to achieve its genetic growth potential' (Fig 107). In practice, however, the diagnosis is not always easy as there are ethnic and geographical variations. Antenatal identification is usually based on ultrasound: failure of fetal biometric measurements to progress along an earlier centile within the normal population range, or marked asymmetry between the head circumference (Fig 108) and abdominal circumference (Fig 109). It is important to note that fetal size does not have to fall outside the normal range for this diagnosis to be made.

In normal growth, maximum velocity of linear growth occurs at 20 weeks, and of body weight at 34 weeks. At the end of pregnancy, physical constraints probably slow fetal growth. Control is influenced by genetic and hormonal factors and nutrient supply.

Causes

- *Intrinsic causes*: malformations, including chromosomal abnormalities (5-10%) and viral infections (2%).
- *Extrinsic causes*: uteroplacental vascular insufficiency (e.g. pre-eclampsia), cyanotic heart disease, maternal malnutrition if severe, smoking, alcohol, cocaine, medications (e.g. atenolol) and idiopathic causes (30%).

Risk factors

Short stature, previous small baby, low maternal weight (<45 kg) and body mass index, poor weight gain, multiple pregnancy, smoking, alcohol, raised a-fetoprotein and other conditions (see causes above).

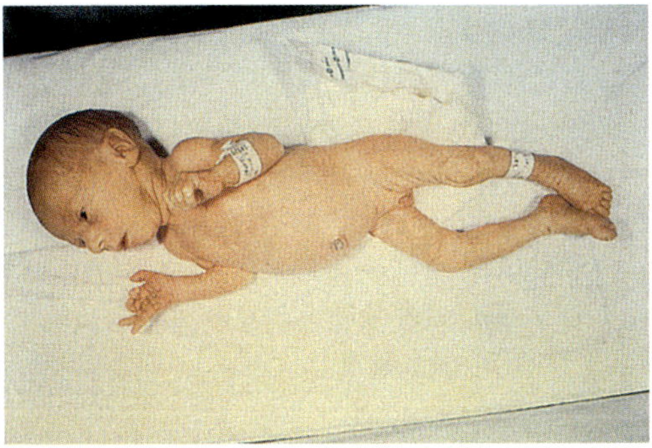

图 107　生长受限的新生儿
Growth-restricted newborn infant

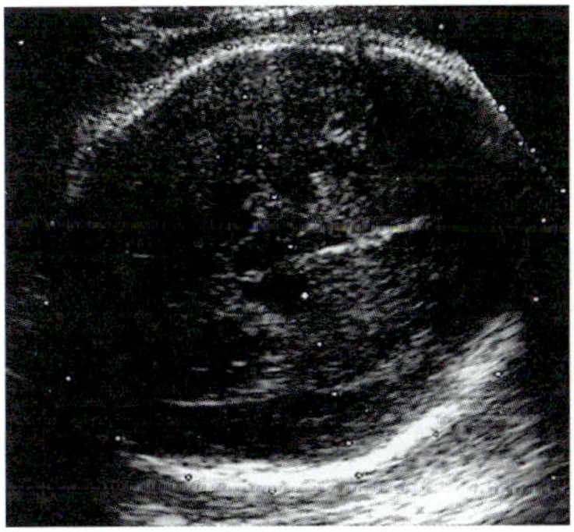

图 108　超声下测量头围
Head circumference measure -ment at ultrasound.

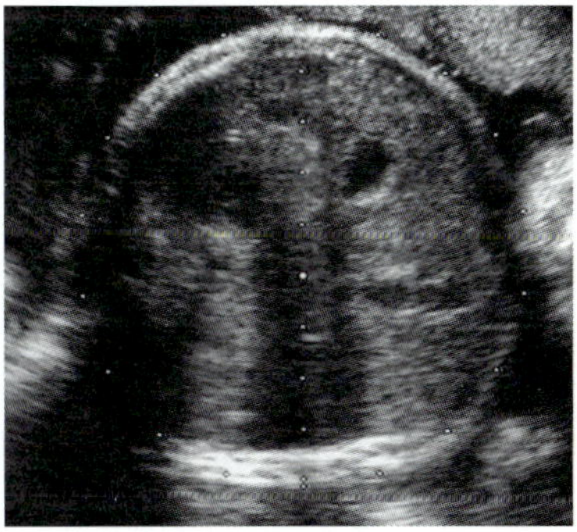

图 109　超声下测量腹围
Abdominal circumference measurement at ultrasound

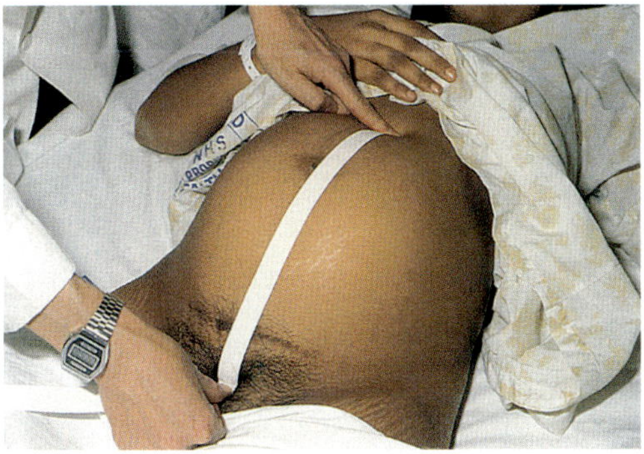

图 110　测量宫高
Fundal height measurement

诊断

尽管根据高危因素可在临床上高度怀疑IUGR，但仍有30%～50%生长受限胎儿无法通过临床检查查出。连续记录耻骨上宫高有助于增加检查的敏感性，但仍是不完善的(图110)。多胎妊娠、羊水过多、横位、肥胖孕妇可降低临床检测率。使用超声连续测量头围和腹围是诊断病理性胎儿生长的最佳方法。

IUGR 可分为两类：

- *匀称型/早期*：通常由内因引起（如先天畸形、病毒感染）。超声下测量出的头围、腹围均低于预计生长轨迹（图 111）。
- *非匀称型/晚期*：通常由外因引起（如先兆子痫、多胎妊娠）。超声下测量的腹围低于预计生长轨迹，而头围增长大多正常。

处理

生长受限胎儿应检查有无先天畸形。对于早期出现IUGR或匀称型IUGR，应行羊膜腔穿刺、绒毛活检进行染色体核型分析及病毒检测。必须对胎儿健康进行持续监测。选择性分娩的时间选择取决于妊娠及胎儿健康评估。早产病例应考虑给予糖皮质激素。脐动脉血流多普勒分析可用于鉴别是正常生长的小样儿还是由于子宫胎盘疾病导致的病理性生长。

新生儿并发症

围生期窒息、胎粪吸入、肺出血、低体温、低血糖、红细胞增多症、可能的早产及先天畸形。

Diagnosis

Even with a high degree of clinical suspicion based on risk factors, 30-50% of growth-restricted fetuses remain undetected by clinical examination. Serial recording of symphysiofundal height improves the sensitivity of detection but is nevertheless poor (Fig 110). Multiple pregnancy, polyhydramnios, transverse lie and maternal obesity further reduce clinical detection rates. Ultrasound is the best method of diagnosing pathological fetal growth using serial measurements of head (HC) and abdominal (AC) circumferences.

Two patterns of IUGR are recognized:

- *Symmetrical/early*: usually due to intrinsic problems (e.g. congenital abnormality, viral infection). On ultrasound, both HC and AC measurements fall away from expected growth trajectories (Fig 111).
- *Asymmetrical/late*: usually due to extrinsic problems (e.g. pre-eclampsia, multiple pregnancy). On ultrasound, AC values fall away from expected growth trajectories but HC growth is mostly maintained (Fig 112).

Management

The growth-restricted fetus should be scanned for congenital abnormalities. Karyotyping by amniocentesis or chorionic villus sampling and viral studies should be considered in early-onset or symmetrical cases. Serial monitoring of fetal health is mandatory. The timing of elective delivery is determined by gestation and fetal health assessment. Consideration should be given to administering steroids in preterm cases. Doppler analysis of umbilical artery blood flow may be used to differentiate the normally grown small fetus from one with pathological growth due to uteroplacental disease.

Neonatal complications

Perinatal asphyxia, meconium aspiration, pulmonary haemorrhage, hypothermia, hypoglycaemia, polycythaemia and possibly prematurity and congenital abnormalities.

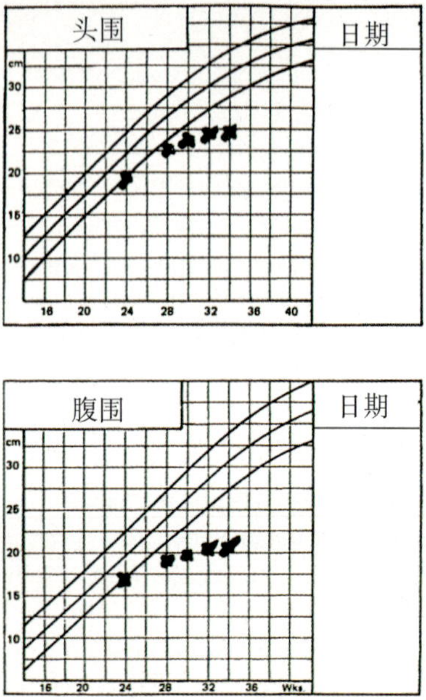

图 111　匀称型 / 早期胎儿生长受限
Symmetrical/early fetal growth restriction

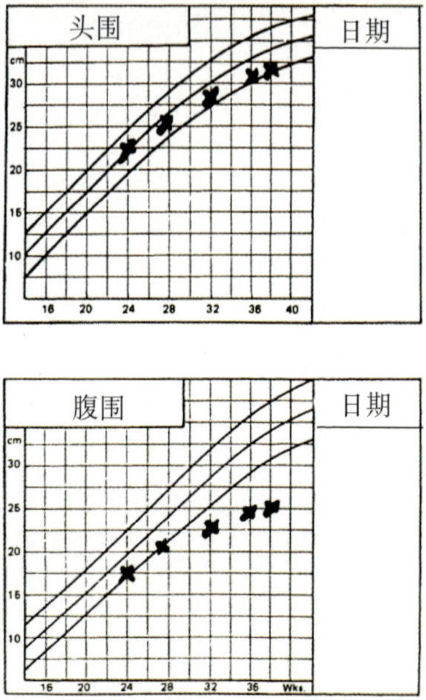

图 112　非匀称型 / 晚期胎儿生长受限
Asymmetrical/late fetal growth restriction

常规检查

在低危妊娠中，常规检查限于胎儿生长的临床评估和孕妇自觉胎动。一般使用皮氏听诊器(图113)或简易的手持多普勒超声仪(图114)常规记录胎心。这种记录胎心的方式对胎儿健康的评估是有限的。它只能证实某一时刻胎心是否存在以及胎心率是否正常。

高危妊娠

既往有内科/产科病史（如母亲患系统性红斑狼疮、既往死产史）或妊娠期有事故发生（如血清甲胎蛋白升高、反复的产前出血、妊娠期高血压疾病、超声诊断的胎儿生长受限）的妊娠被认为是高危妊娠。高危妊娠应连续进行超声检查胎儿双顶径、羊水量以及胎儿生物物理检查和脐动脉多普勒检查。无应激试验检测在胎儿产前评估中也起作用（图 115)。但这些监测方法对某些疾病（如糖尿病、妊娠胆汁淤积症）的意义尚未被证实。

生物物理方法

根本的原则是当胎儿暴露于慢性刺激中时（特别是缺氧）其中枢神经系统（胎心率变异、胎动、肌张力、胎儿呼吸运动均减少）将受到抑制。更严重者可抑制胎儿肾功能（导致羊水过少)。采用的检查包括胎动表(每日记录母体的自觉胎动)、无应激胎心率记录及生物物理图（见下)。

胎心产力描述图

异常胎心率与胎儿急性窘迫有密切联系。足月时正常的胎心率取决于胎儿状况。一个成熟胎儿有 30%的时间安静（表现为基线摆动幅度小，无胎心加速)，70%的时间活跃（基线幅度摆动大，有胎心加速，胎心率加速>15次/分，持续至少15秒）(图116)。有胎心加速、胎心基线在 110 ~ 160 次/分之间、没有胎心减速的胎心产力描述图为正常的胎心图，又称“反应型”。胎心图只可确保排除即刻的胎儿窘

13 Antepartum fetal health assessment

Routine screening

In low-risk pregnancies this is limited to clinical assessment of fetal growth and the maternal perception of fetal movements/activity. The fetal heart is recorded routinely either by auscultation with a Pinard stethoscope (Fig 113) or with simple hand-held Doppler ultrasound (Fig 114). Recording of the fetal heart in this way is a limited assessment of fetal well-being. It is able to detect only whether the fetal heart is present, and whether the rate is normal at any given moment.

Pregnancies at risk

A pregnancy may be deemed 'high-risk' as a result of previous medical/obstetric history (e.g. maternal systemic lupus erythematosus, previous stillbirth) or because of events occurring during pregnancy (e.g. raised serum α-fetoprotein, recurrent antepartum haemorrhage, pregnancy-induced hypertension, ultrasonically diagnosed intrauterine growth restriction-IUGR). Serial ultrasound should be performed in such pregnancies for biometric parameters, estimation of liquor volume, fetal biophysical testing and possibly umbilical artery Doppler measurement. Non-stress fetal heart rate (FHR) monitoring also has a role in fetal antenatal assessment (Fig 115). The value of these monitoring techniques has not been established for certain conditions (e.g. diabetes, obstetric cholestasis).

Biophysical methods

The underlying principle is that the fetus exposed to a chronic insult (especially hypoxia) will have a depressed central nervous system (reduced heart-rate variability, movements, tone and breathing movements) and, if severe, depressed renal function (oligohydramnios). The tests used are the kick chart (daily record of maternally perceived movements), non-stress FHR recording and the biophysical profile (see below).

Cardiotocography

There is a close association between an abnormal FHR pattern and an acutely asphyxiated fetus. The normal FHR trace at term is dependent on the state of the fetus. A mature fetus will be quiet for about 30% of the time

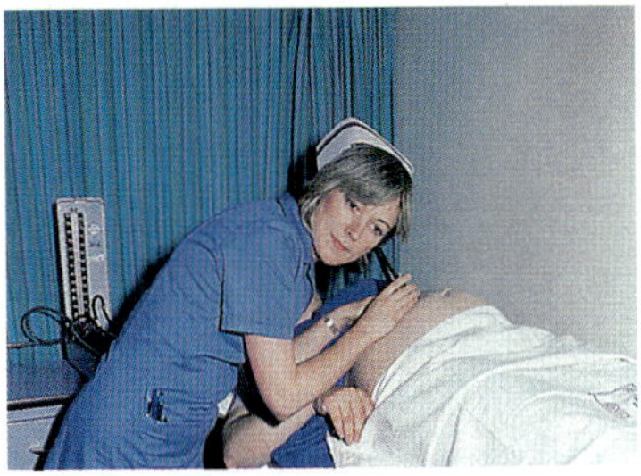

图 113　使用皮式听诊器听胎心
Fetal heart auscultation with a Pinard stethoscope

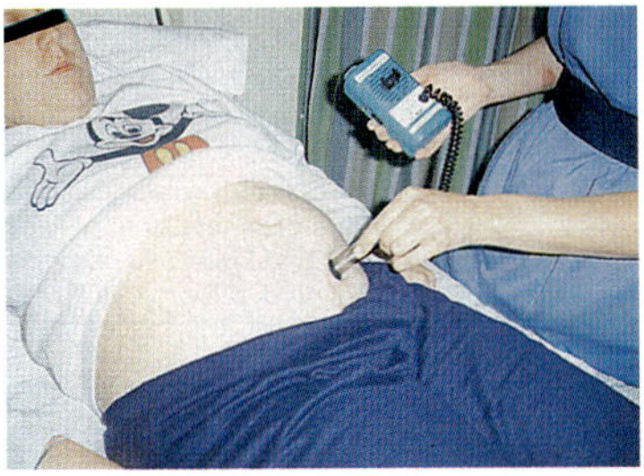

图 114　使用手持式多普勒仪听胎心
Fetal heart auscultation with hand-held Doppler

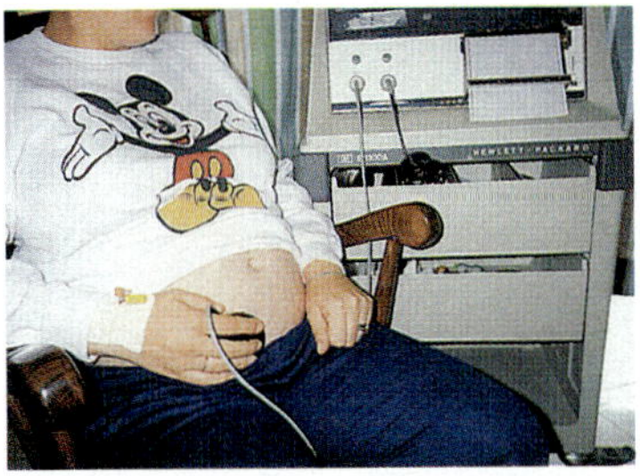

图 115　使用胎心图记录胎心图
Fetal heart rate recording with cardiotocography

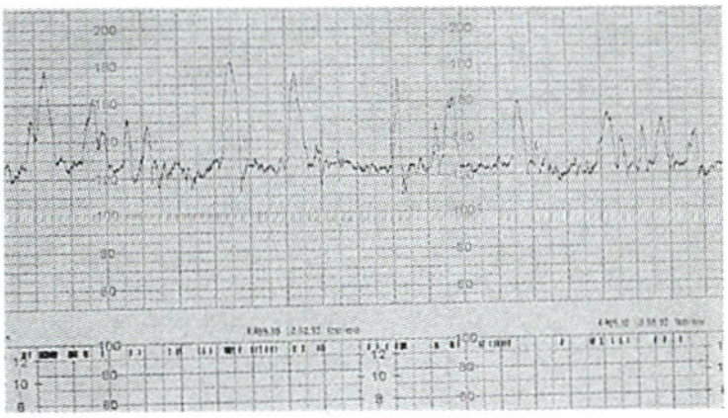

图 116　足月儿反应型胎心图
Reactive fetal heart rate recording at term

迫，但对远期的胎儿缺氧缺乏保证。对已知有胎儿窘迫的产妇进行胎儿监护以及分娩过程中对胎儿进行监护有重要意义。

胎儿生物物理评分(biophysical profile scoring, BPS)

BPS 是一种更能综合评估胎儿窘迫危险的方法。它可记录5种生物物理参数：胎心率模式（前面提到的无应激试验）、胎动、胎儿肌张力、胎儿呼吸运动以及羊水量。如果记录30分钟内存在以上参数中的4～5 个参数，那么胎儿晚期窒息的危险性是低的。

羊水量(amniotic fluid volume, AFV)

超声检测羊水量有两种指标：最大羊水池径线（maximum pool diameter, MPD）（正常范围 20 ～ 80mm）或羊水指数（amniotic fluid index，AFI；子宫内四个象限的羊水暗区垂直深径相加之和）（图117）。

- *羊水过少*（MPD ＜ 20mm 或 AFI ＜第 3 百分位数）：可由破膜、胎儿肾畸形或胎儿疾病（如严重 的胎儿宫内生长受限）引起。
- *羊水过多*（MPD ＞ 80mm 或 AFI ＞第 97 百分位数）：可由胎儿吞咽不能（如气管 - 食管闭锁）、胎儿多尿（如母亲患糖尿病的胎儿）或双胎输血综合征引起。

脐动脉血流多普勒记录

小于相应孕龄胎儿的脐动脉舒张期缺乏向前的血流（图118），甚至出现反向血流，与下列情况相关：围生期死亡率增加、胎儿出生时窒息、需要提前终止妊娠或坏死性小肠结肠炎。这是经随机实验证实了的检测胎儿健康的唯一方法。胎儿其他血管中血流图形改变，如胎儿静脉导管（图119）或大脑中动脉（图73），有助于对严重早发的有宫内生长受限的产妇的分娩时间做出决定。

(associated with little oscillation of the baseline and no accelerations) and active for about 70% of the time (wide oscillations of the baseline and many accelerations, i.e. rises in the FHR of 15 beats/min above the baseline lasting for at least 15 s) (Fig 116). A cardiotocogram (CTG) with accelerations, a baseline rate of between 110 and 160 beats/ min and no decelerations is described as normal or 'reactive'. Cardiotocography is reliable at excluding asphyxia while it is being performed but offers little reassurance in the long term. It is most valuable for monitoring a fetus already known to be compromised and for intrapartum fetal monitoring.

Biophysical profile scoring (BPS)

A more comprehensive assessment of the fetus at risk of asphyxia is provided by the BPS, which records the presence of five biophysical variables: FHR pattern (non-stress test as above), fetal movements, fetal tone, fetal breathing and amniotic fluid volume. If four or five of these parameters are present in up to 30 min of recording, then the risk of terminal fetal asphyxia is low.

Amniotic fluid volume (AFV)

AFV can be measured by ultrasound using either maximum pool diameter (MPD) (range 20-80 mm) or amniotic fluid index (AFI; sum of four vertical pools of amniotic fluid measured in the four quadrants of the uterus) (Fig 117).

- *Oligohydramnios* (MPD <20 mm or AFI <3rd centile): can be due to ruptured membranes, fetal renal abnormality or fetal illness (e.g. severe IUGR).
- *Polyhydramnios* (MPD >80 mm or AFI >97th centile): can be due to a failure of fetal swallowing (e.g.tracheo-oesophageal atresia), excess urine production (e.g. infant of diabetic mother) or the twin-twin transfusion syndrome.

Doppler recording of umbilical artery blood flow

The absence of forward flow in diastole in the umbilical arteries of a small-for-dates fetus (Fig 118), or even reversed flow, is associated with an increased risk of perinatal death, birth asphyxia, need for preterm birth and necrotizing enterocolitis. This is the only test of fetal health with proven benefit from randomized trials. Changes in the blood flow patterns in other fetal blood vessels such as the ductus venosus (Fig 119) or middle cerebral artery (Fig 73) may help optimize decision-making regarding timing of delivery in severe early-onset IUGR.

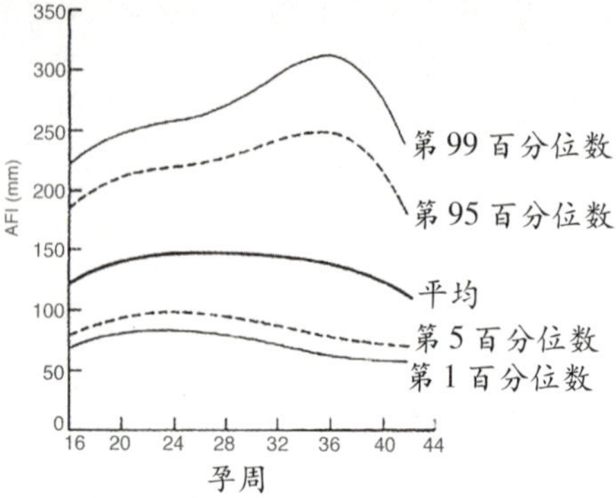

图 117　羊水指数百分位数图
Amniotic fluid index (AFI)
centile chart

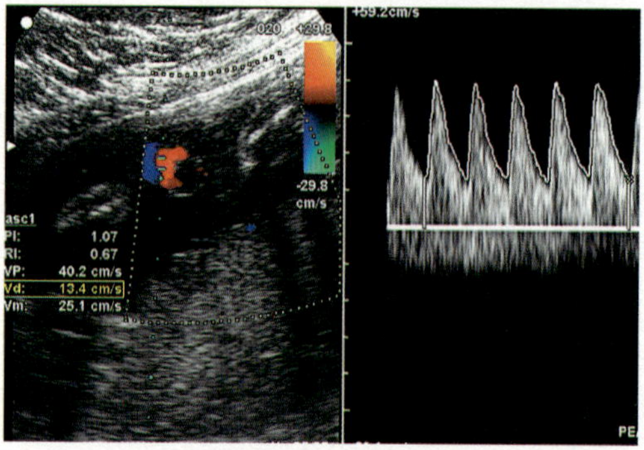

图 118　脐动脉多普勒血流记录
Umbilical artery Doppler
blood flow recording

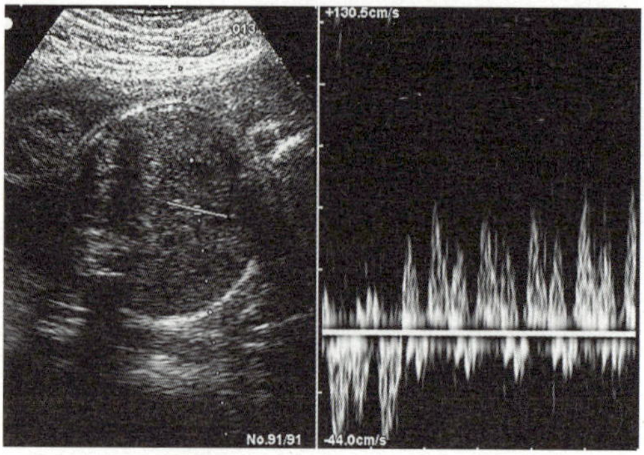

图 119　胎儿静脉导管血流记录
Blood flow recording from the ductus
venosus

早产

定义

妊娠不足 37 周分娩。

发病率

占分娩总数的 5% ~ 8%。

病因

早产的危险因素包括多胎妊娠、产前出血、胎儿畸形、子宫畸形、宫颈内口松弛症、感染、胎膜早破（见下）以及羊水过多。由于先兆子痫、严重的宫内生长受限或孕妇病情恶化，提前终止妊娠可能是必需的。

处理

通过发现宫颈改变及规律宫缩，确定早产的诊断。寻找并处理任何的可逆原因。如无禁忌，应使用保胎药（如阿脱西班、利托君或硝苯地平）。给予地塞米松或倍他米松以减少胎儿呼吸窘迫综合征的发生率（图 120）。

胎膜早破

定义

妊娠不足37周在子宫收缩前发生胎膜破裂。30%早产发生于胎膜早破后。

诊断

阴道口有液体或者窥器检查发现阴道内有液体（图 121），如羊水间断排出则较难做出诊断。已经设计出了专门用于诊断的生化拭子实验（图 122）。超声检查对此病不敏感。

结局

早产、绒毛膜羊膜炎、产后子宫内膜炎以及新生儿败血症。妊娠早期发生的持续性胎膜早破可导致胎儿肺发育不良、脐带受压及体位畸形。

14 Prematurity

Preterm birth

Definition

Delivery at less than 37 weeks' gestation.

Incidence

5-8% of all deliveries.

Causes

Risk factors for preterm labour include multiple gestation, antepartum haemorrhage, fetal abnormality, uterine abnormality, incompetent cervix, infection, preterm rupture of membranes (see below) and polyhydramnios. Preterm birth may be necessary because of pre-eclampsia, severe intrauterine growth restriction (IUGR), or deteriorating maternal health.

Management

Confirm the diagnosis of preterm labour by finding cervical change in association with regular uterine activity. Look for and treat any reversible causes. Use tocolysis (e.g. atosiban, ritodrine or nifedipine) if there are no contraindications. Give dexamethasone or betamethasone to reduce the incidence of respiratory distress syndrome (Fig 120).

Preterm rupture of membranes

Definition

Membrane rupture before uterine contractions at less than 37 weeks' gestation. 30% of preterm deliveries are preceded by preterm membrane rupture.

Diagnosis

Liquor at the introitus or in the vagina on speculum examination (Fig 121). The diagnosis can be difficult to make if loss of amniotic fluid is intermittent. Biochemical swab tests have been designed specifically for this purpose (Fig 122). Ultrasound scanning is not a sensitive test for this.

Consequences

Preterm labour and delivery, chorioamnionitis, postpartum endometritis and neonatal sepsis. Prolonged preterm rupture

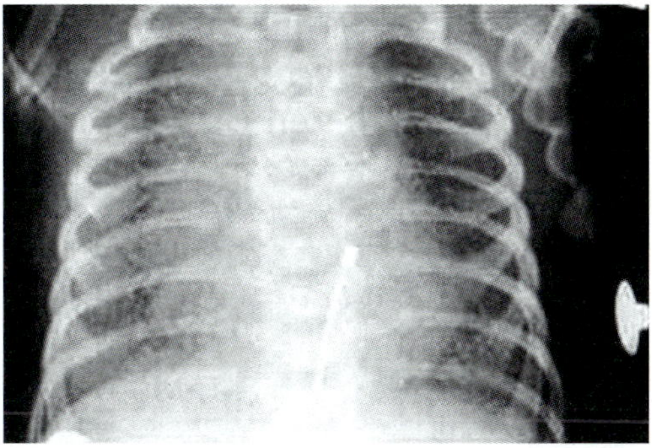

图 120　新生儿胸部 X 线显示呼吸窘迫综合征的“毛玻璃”征
Neonatal chest X-ray showing the ‘ground-glass’ appearance of respiratory distress syndrome

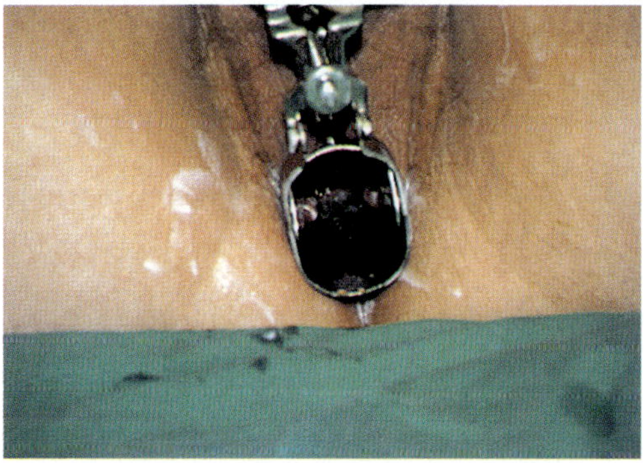

图 121　通过无菌窥器看到阴道内有液体
Liquor in the vagina seen via a sterile speculum

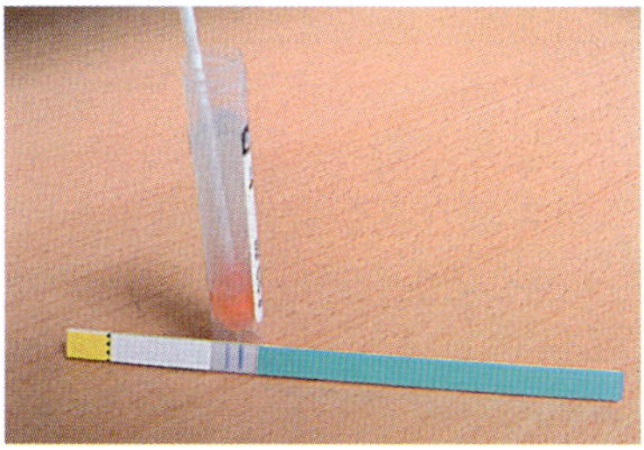

图 122　用于诊断胎膜早破的生化拭子检查
Biochemical swab testing for ruptured membranes

处理

最好入院治疗，但并非必须。高度警惕感染是重要的(疼痛、子宫收缩、子宫压痛、排出物有臭味、孕妇发热、心动过速、C反应蛋白升高、低位阴道拭子阳性)，除非可疑临产，否则应限制阴道内诊。对妊娠24～34周孕妇，经验性使用红霉素可延长妊娠，减少感染发病率。妊娠不足36周者通常给予糖皮质激素，以促进胎肺成熟。

如疑有感染，所有的妊娠均需促进分娩。只有当其发生不足48小时，才试图抑制分娩（假设激素已使用）。对于妊娠延长超过34周者，可在36～38周行引产。

早产结局

早产新生儿并发症包括死亡、呼吸窘迫综合征、心室内出血、室周白质软化（图123)、肺出血、坏死性小肠结肠炎（图124)、败血症、低体温、喂以喂养、黄疸、低血糖。远期并发症包括视网膜病变、慢性肺疾病及神经发育迟缓。

早产的预防

危险评估

风险评估是建立在病史（如既往早产史、锥形活组织检查史)、特异宫颈拭子检测到胎儿纤维连接蛋白、高位阴道拭子行细菌学检查、测量宫颈长度（图125）的基础上。如宫颈长度<2.5cm，特别是宫颈内口呈漏斗状时，早产或胎膜早破的危险显著增加。

处理

有细菌性阴道病及既往早产史的孕妇使用抗生素可能有益。宫颈缩短和/或宫颈呈漏斗状或者既往有宫颈机能不全者缝合宫颈可能有益。

of membranes from a very early gestation results in pulmonary hypoplasia, umbilical cord compression and postural deformities.

Management

Inpatient care is usually preferred but is not mandatory. A high degree of vigilance for infection is vital (pain, contractions, uterine tenderness, offensive discharge, maternal pyrexia, tachycardia, raised C-reactive protein, positive low vaginal swab) and vaginal examinations should be limited unless labour is suspected. For women between 24 and 34 weeks' gestation, empirical treatment with erythromycin prolongs the pregnancy and reduces infectious morbidity. Steroids are usually administered prior to 36 weeks to promote fetal lung maturation.

Delivery should be expedited at all gestations if infection is suspected. Only attempt to stop labour if it occurs within 48 h (provided steroids are given at presentation). For pregnancies extending beyond 34 weeks, an induction is usually organized at 36-38 weeks.

Consequences of preterm birth

Early neonatal complications include death, respiratory distress syndrome, intraventricular haemorrhage, periventricular leukomalacia (Fig 123), pulmonary haemorrhage, necrotizing enterocolitis (Fig 124), sepsis, hypothermia, poor feeding, jaundice, hypoglycaemia. Later complications include retinopathy, chronic lung disease and neurodevelopmental delay.

Prevention of preterm labour

Risk assessment

A risk assessment can be made on the basis of history (e.g. previous preterm birth, history of cone biopsy), specialized cervical swabs that detect fetal fibronectin, high vaginal swabs for bacteriology and cervical length scanning (Fig 125). A cervix shorter than 2.5 cm is significantly associated with an increased risk of preterm labour or rupture of membranes, particularly if cervical funneling is noted at the internal os.

Treatment

Women with bacterial vaginosis and a history of previous preterm birth may benefit from antibiotics. Those with cervical shortening and/or funnelling or with a history of cervical incompetence may benefit from a cervical suture.

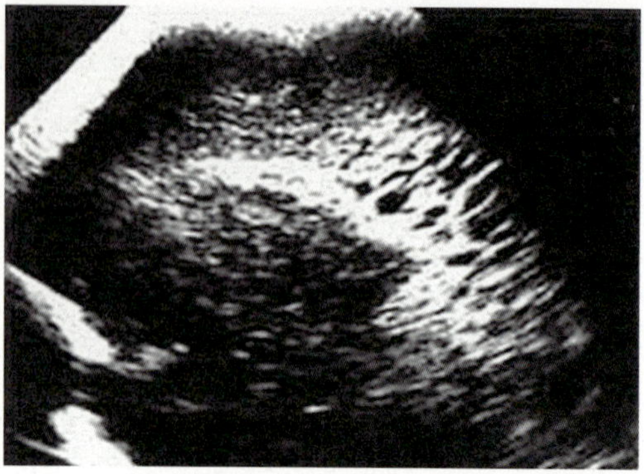

图 123　新生儿脑部超声显示脑室周围白质软化
Ultrasound of neonatal brain showing periventricular leukomalacia

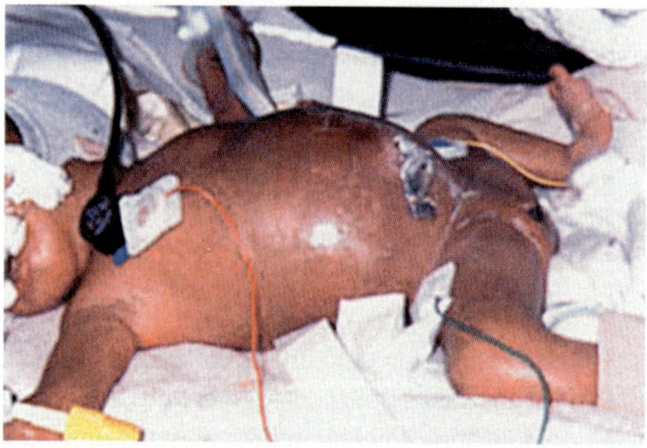

图 124　坏死性小肠结肠炎新生儿
Neonate with necrotizing enterocolitis

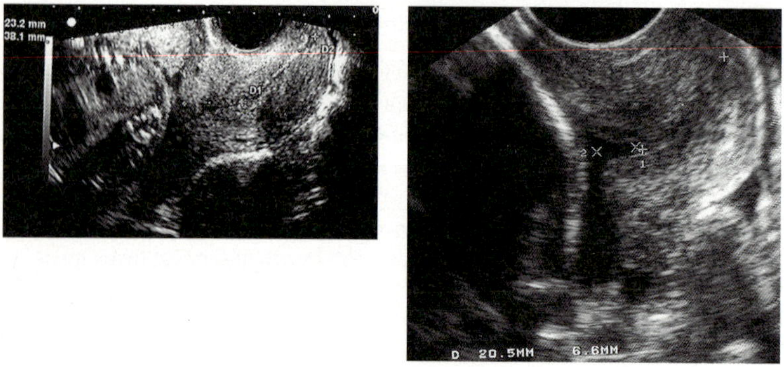

图 125　阴式超声下（a）图示宫颈长（61.3mm）而关闭（b）图示宫颈短（21.5mm）而呈漏斗形
Transvaginal scans showing (a) a long (61.3 mm) closed cervix and (b) a short cervix (21.5 mm) with funnelling

定义

妊娠 24 周后、分娩前发生的生殖道出血。

处理

评估失血量和意识状态。应该评估胎儿状况。确定失血原因。在经超声确定胎盘位置以前避免阴道检查。前置血管、重度胎盘早剥需紧急分娩，而前置胎盘通常在保守治疗后行选择性分娩，通常采用剖宫产。

前置胎盘

从附着于子宫下段的胎盘部位出血。通常无腹痛或者伴有子宫收缩。胎位或胎先露异常常见。

“重度”或“轻度”的分级取决于胎盘边缘是否越过宫颈内口。

危险因素包括既往剖宫产史、多胎妊娠或子宫异常。

通过超声（图 126）、核磁或检查确诊。

胎盘早剥

从位置正常的胎盘处出血。通常有腹痛并伴有宫缩、子宫高张状态、变硬、子宫压痛。阴道流血量不同。超声下不易见到出血。胎心监护图异常、胎死宫内、胎儿窒息常见。分娩后常可见胎盘后凝血块，Kleihauer 试验可能呈阳性（图 128），意味着胎儿红细胞进入母体循环。

前置血管

以异常位置穿行入羊膜的胎儿血管，在自然破膜或人工破膜时发生出血。胎盘帆状附着或副胎盘常可见（图 129）。失血来自胎儿血液循环，围生期死亡率较高。

其他原因

宫颈病变（如宫颈外翻、宫颈癌、继发于感染的宫颈炎）和临产时“见红”。

15 Antepartum haemorrhage

Definition

Bleeding from the genital tract from 24 weeks' gestation and before delivery of the baby.

Management

Assess blood loss and resuscitate. The fetal condition should be assessed. Establish cause. A vaginal examination should be avoided until the placental site is established with ultrasound. Vasa praevia and major abruption demand urgent delivery whereas placenta praevia can more often be managed conservatively with elective delivery later, usually by caesarean section.

Placenta praevia

Bleeding from a placenta encroaching into the lower uterine segment. Often painless or associated with contractions. Abnormal fetal lie/presentation common.

Graded as 'major' or 'minor' depending on whether or not the placental edge actually crosses the internal os.

Risk factors include previous caesarean section, multiple pregnancy and uterine anomaly.

Diagnosis is by ultrasound (Fig 126), MRI or examination in theatre.

Abruption

Bleeding from a normally situated placenta. Usually painful and associated with contractions or hypertonic, hard and tender uterus. The amount of blood passed vaginally can vary. It is unusual to see any bleeding on ultrasound. Cardiotocographic abnormalities and intrauterine fetal death or asphyxia are common. A retroplacental clot is often found at delivery (Fig 127) and a Kleihauer test may be positive (Fig 128), indicating fetomaternal transfusion of fetal red blood cells.

Vasa praevia

Bleeding from abnormally placed fetal vessel coursing through the membranes at the time of spontaneous or artificial membrane rupture. Often found with velamentous insertion or succenturiate lobe (Fig 129). The blood lost is from the fetal circulation and perinatal mortality rates are high.

Other causes

A 'show' at the onset of labor, cervical lesions (e.g. ectropion, cancer, cervicitis secondary to infection).

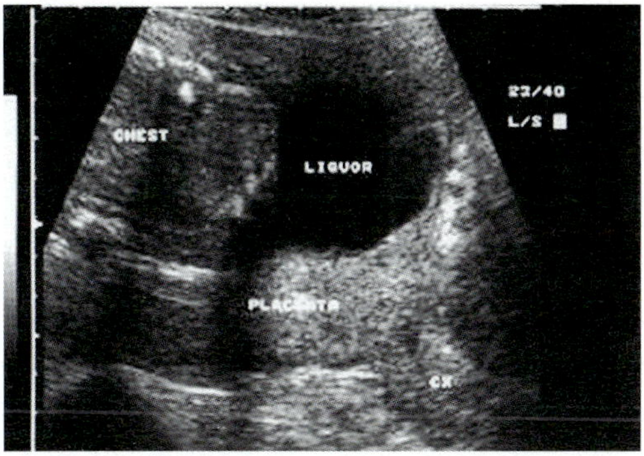

图 126　前置胎盘的超声图像（cx = 宫颈）
Ultrasound image showing placenta praevia (cx = cervix)

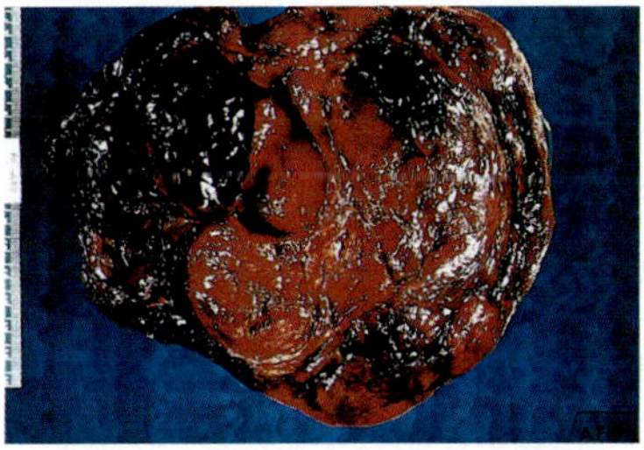

图 127　早剥的胎盘，胎盘后可见凝血块
Abruption with visible retroplacental clot

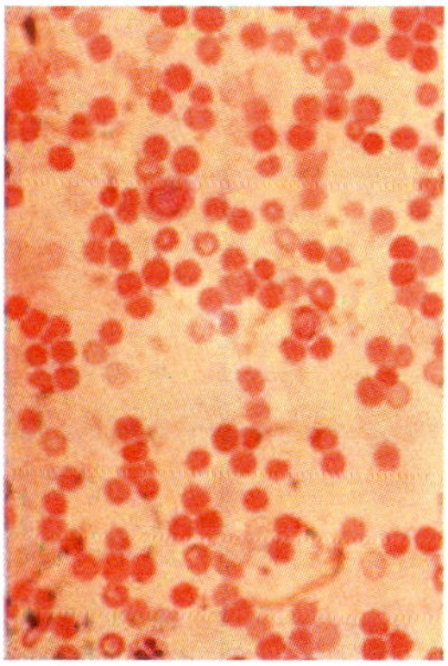

图 128　Kleihauer 试验
Kleihauer test

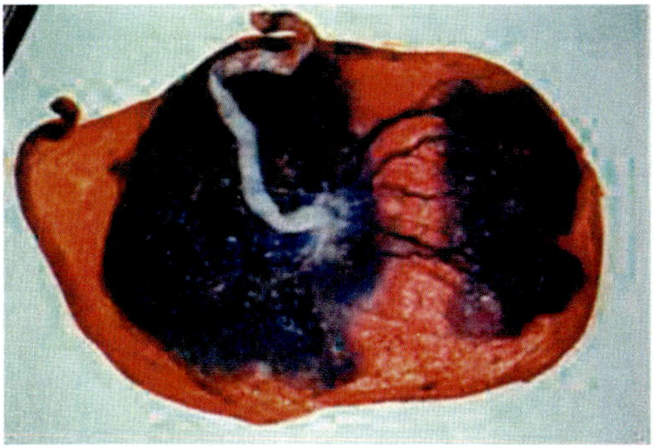

图 129　前置血管
Vasa praevia

分娩

基本原则

处理

参与胎儿分娩的医护人员应当关注产妇及胎儿的安全及健康，努力确保分娩对所有相关者都是一个令人满意的经历。

在许多国家，基本是助产士独自负责或者伴同一个全科医生做咨询。只有出现问题时，产科医生才参与（如胎儿窘迫、产程进展不良、孕妇患病）。然而在其他的国家（如美国），绝大多数分娩由产科医生负责。

监护

临产应该是一个自然过程，包含有监护的处理有助于发现异常。监测包括三个内容，概括在产程图上（为一个图表但是显示了三方面内容）。

- *胎儿情况*（图 130）：每15分钟间断地记录一次胎心，或者用胎心监护仪持续记录。记录经阴道流出液体的颜色，每 4 小时经阴道检查判定胎头位置和 / 或胎头变形的程度。
- *产程进展*（图 131）：记录胎头下降程度（经腹采用五分之一法估测，经阴道则以胎头距坐骨棘的厘米估测），定时做阴道检查记录宫口扩张，记录宫缩强度及频率，以及给予增强 / 诱导分娩的药物。
- *产妇情况*（图 132）：每半小时记录一次产妇一般状态、脉搏、血压。每 4 小时记录一次体温。记录液体入量及尿量。检查尿糖、尿蛋白及尿酮体。给予产妇任何药物都要记录。

General principles

Management

Everyone involved in the birth of a child should be concerned with the safety and health of the mother and baby and should strive to make the birth a satisfying experience for all concerned.

In many countries, overall conduct is the responsibility of a midwife alone or with reference to a general practitioner. An obstetrician is only involved if problems are present (e.g. fetal compromise, poor progress in labour, maternal disease). However, in other countries (e.g. the USA), the great majority of deliveries are conducted by obstetricians.

Monitoring

Labour should be a normal event, and management incorporates a programme of surveillance/monitoring that helps to detect deviation from this. There are three components of this monitoring, summarized on the partogram (one chart but displayed in three sections):

- *Fetal condition* (Fig 130). The fetal heart rate (FHR) is recorded either intermittently, every 15 min, or continuously by cardiotocogram (CTG). The colour of the liquor draining vaginally is recorded, and the degree of caput and/or molding judged from vaginal examinations performed every 4 h.
- *Progress of labour* (Fig 131). Record of the descent of the head (assessed abdominally in fifths, and vaginally in centimetres with respect to the ischial spines), the dilatation of the cervix on regular vaginal examinations, the strength and frequency of contractions, and drugs given to augment/induce labour.
- *Maternal condition* (Fig 132). General well-being, pulse and blood pressure are recorded every half-hour, temperature every 4 h. Fluid intake and urine output are recorded and the urine is also tested for glucose, protein and ketones. Any drugs given to the woman are also noted.

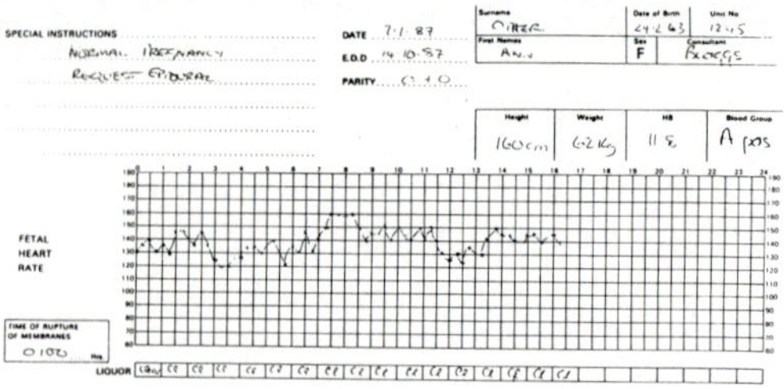

图 130　产程图：胎儿方面
Partogram: fetal section

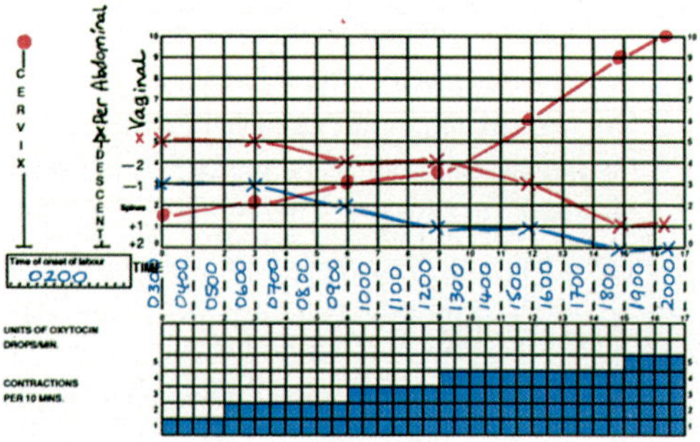

图 131　产程图：产程进展方面
Partogram: progress section

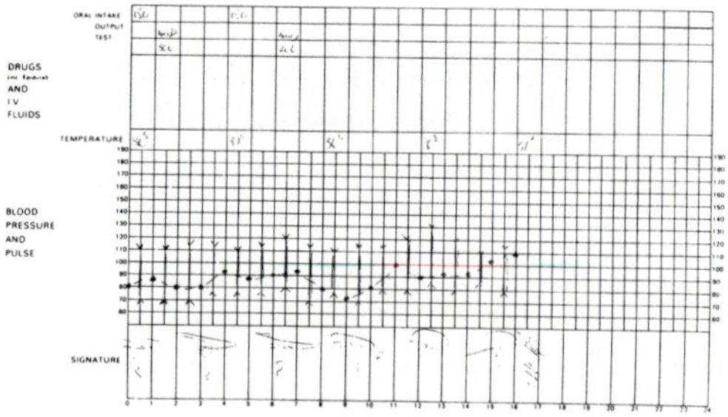

图 132　产程图：产妇方面
Partogram: maternal section

第一产程

定义

从产程发动至宫颈完全扩张。

诊断

分娩发动是回顾性诊断。当一系列阴道检查显示有规律的宫缩的同时出现宫颈进行性改变时（宫颈消失、宫口扩张）判断为分娩发动。通常有见红，即经阴道排出与宫颈粘液相混合的血液。大约仅有10%病例在临产之前发生胎膜破裂。

分期

- *潜伏期*：指分娩发动至宫口扩张3～4cm,宫颈管完全消失。初产妇平均需9小时，经产妇平均需5小时。
- *活跃期*：潜伏期末至宫口开全。初产妇平均需5小时，经产妇平均需2小时。在活跃期宫口每小时至少开大1cm，先露同时下降（图133）。

产程进展不良

第一产程延长有两种形式，可从产程图上看出。原发性宫缩无力（图134）描述的是整个活跃期进展不良。这多见于初产妇，且通常由宫缩不良和胎位异常（如枕后位）引起。继发性停滞（图135）是指产程开始进展良好，而后减慢甚至停止。更常见的原因为先露异常（如额先露）或头盆不称。当胎儿明显大于产妇骨盆时出现头盆不称。

处理

应确定诊断。如原因为宫缩不良，需纠正脱水，如胎膜仍完整行人工破膜。可使用催产素促进宫缩，并使用宫内压力导管监测（图136）。头盆不称或胎位异常可行剖宫产术。

The first stage

Definition

From the onset of labour to full dilatation of the cervix.

Diagnosis

The onset of labour is a retrospective diagnosis made when serial vaginal examinations show progressive cervical change (effacement and dilatation) in the presence of regular contractions. It is often associated with a 'show' —the passage vaginally of a blood-stained mucous plug from the cervix. Membrane rupture precedes labour in only about 10% of cases.

Phases

- *Latent phase*: from the onset of labour to when the cervix is about 3-4 cm dilated and fully effaced. Mean duration is 9 h in primigravidae and 5 h in multigravidae.
- *Active phase*: from the end of the latent phase to full dilatation. The mean duration is 5 h in primigravida and 2 h in multigravida. During this phase the cervix should dilate at least 1cm per hour and the presenting part should descend (Fig 133).

Poor progress

Two patterns of delay in first stage are recognized from the partogram. Primary dysfunctional labour (Fig 134) describes poor progress throughout the active phase. It is more common in primiparous women and is often caused by inefficient uterine activity and fetal malposition (e.g. occipitoposterior). Secondary arrest (Fig 135) occurs when previously good progress slows or comes to a halt. More commonly found with malpresentation (e.g. brow) or cephalopelvic disproportion, which occurs when the fetus is too large for the pelvis.

Management

A diagnosis should be made. If inefficient uterine activity is the cause, dehydration should be corrected and the membranes ruptured if still intact. Augmentation with oxytocin should be considered and can be monitored with an intrauterine pressure catheter (Fig 136). Caesarean section may be indicated for cephalopelvic disproportion or malpresentation.

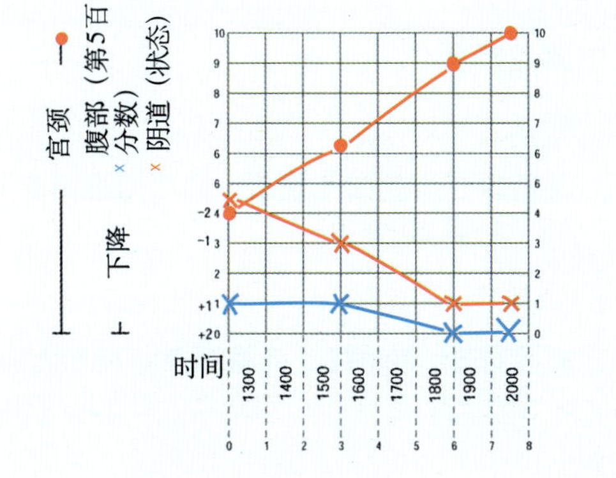

图 133　产程图：正常产程
Partogram: normal progress

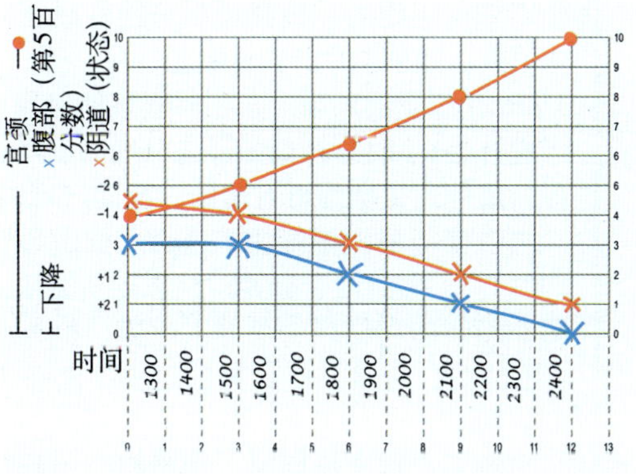

图 134　产程图：产程缓慢
Partogram: slow progress

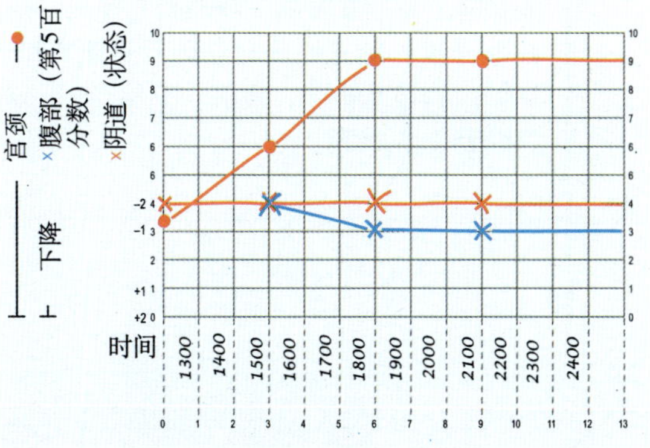

图 135　产程图：继发性停滞
Partogram: secondary arrest

第二产程

定义

从宫口开全到胎儿娩出。初产妇平均需40分钟。经产妇平均需 20 分钟。

分期

- *推进的/被动的*：先露高浮，产妇无向下用力愿望。
- *逼出的/主动的*：先露低，产妇希望向下用力。

处理

当产妇有迫切地想要将胎儿生出来的感觉时，通常鼓励产妇向下用力。该种反射可能在硬膜外麻醉的产妇中消失。如果担忧产妇及胎儿状况，第二产程不应超过3小时并应受到限制，必要时应该使用器械助娩。第二产程开始1小时后产妇如还未分娩，应仔细评估产妇状况。用催产素增强可有帮助，但助产可能为更加适当。

当口变得最大限度的扩张时，据说会发生胎头着冠(图137)。左手防止分娩过快和胎头减压。右手防止会阴非控制的裂伤。一手伸入阴道，检查脐带是否绕颈(图 138)。有脐带绕颈时则钳夹切断脐带或将脐带推到头顶上。

当胎头出现在会阴时，通常将胎头旋转使其与胎肩位于一条轴线上。产妇再次向下用力，助产士双手置于胎儿顶骨隆突，轻轻向下牵引以助胎儿前肩娩出。再托胎颈向上使后肩娩出，继而胎儿娩出。前肩娩出时应肌注催产素。胎儿娩出后立即双重钳夹脐带，剪断（图140)。将婴儿擦干、包裹，交给产妇。采用Apgar评分判断新生儿状态。

Second stage

Definition

From full dilation of the cervix to delivery of the baby. Average duration is 40 min in primiparous women and 20 min in multiparae.

Phases

- *Propulsive/passive*: the presenting part is high and there is no desire to push.
- *Expulsive/active*: the presenting part is low and the mother wishes to push.

Management

The woman is usually encouraged to push when she feels the urge to 'bear down'. This reflex may be blocked in a woman with an epidural. Second stage should last no longer than 3 h and should be limited if there are concerns about maternal or fetal condition, with instrumental delivery if necessary. Women who have not given birth after an hour of active second stage should be carefully assessed. Augmentation with oxytocin may help, but assisted delivery may be more appropriate.

Crowning is said to occur as the introitus becomes maximally stretched (Fig 137). The left hand prevents too rapid a delivery and decompression of the fetal head. The right hand prevents uncontrolled tearing of the perineum. A hand is inserted to check for the presence of the cord around the baby's neck (Fig 138). If found, it is either clamped and cut or pulled over the head.

While the head is on the perineum it usually rotates to realign with the axis of the shoulders. The mother pushes again and, with the hands placed over the baby's parietal eminences, gentle traction is applied posteriorly to encourage the delivery of the anterior shoulder (Fig 139). Anterior traction is then applied, and the posterior shoulder and the body are delivered. An intramuscular injection of an oxytocic agent is given with the delivery of the anterior shoulder. Once the baby is delivered, the cord is double-clamped and cut (Fig 140). The baby is dried and wrapped and handed to the mother. The Apgar score is used to record the condition of the baby at birth.

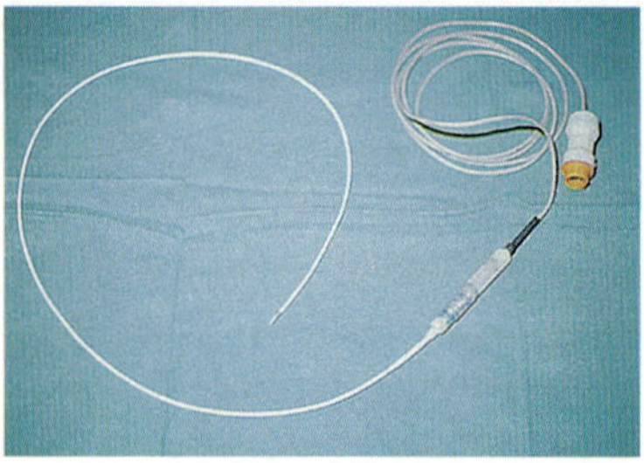

图 136　宫内压力导管
Intrauterine pressure catheter

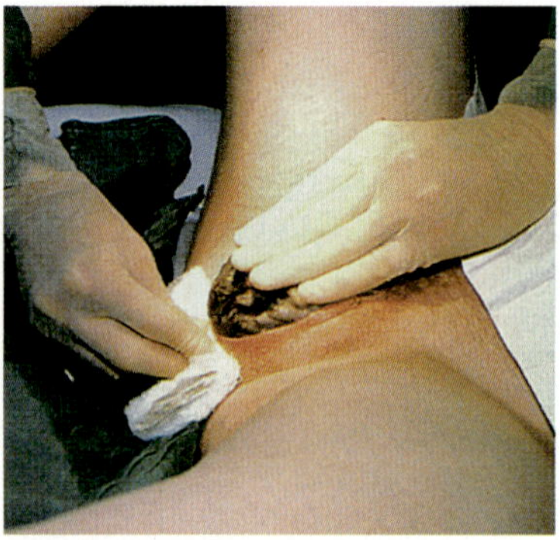

图 137　胎头着冠
Crowning of the fetal head

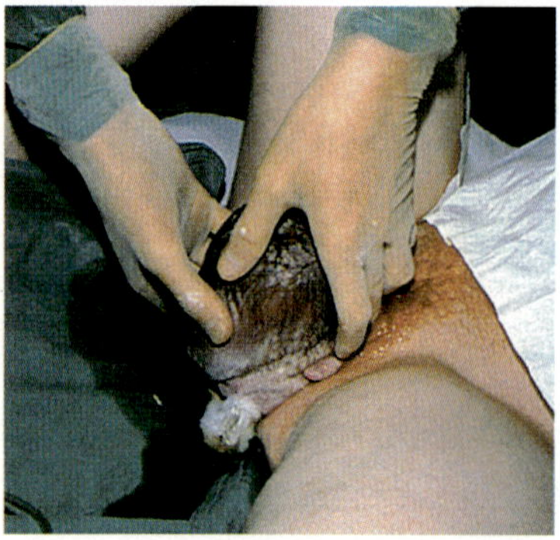

图 138　检查脐带
Checking for umbilical cord

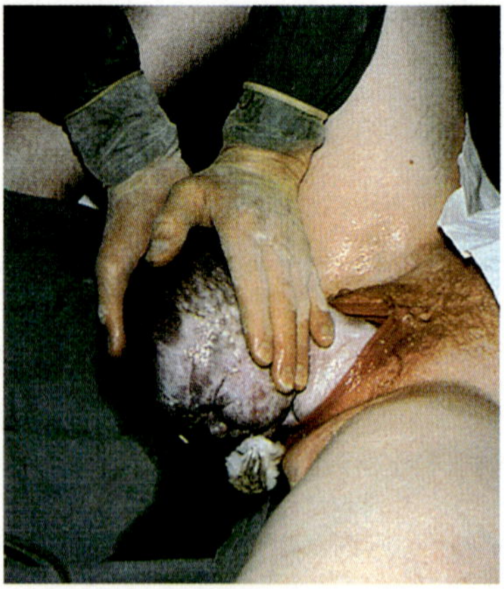

图 139　前肩娩出
Delivery of the anterior shoulder

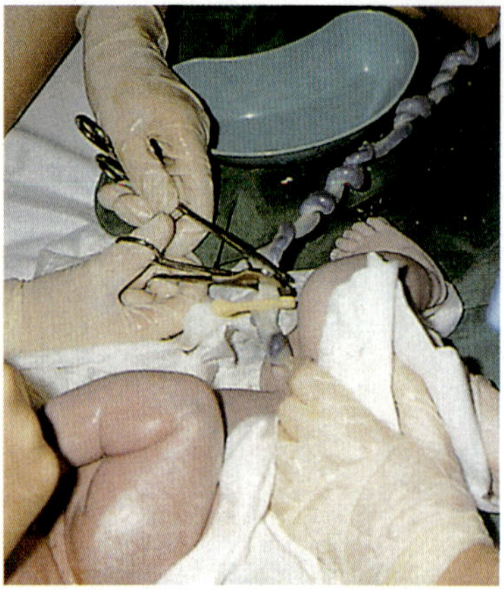

图 140　钳夹、切断脐带
Clamping and cutting umbilical cord

第三产程

定义

从胎儿娩出到胎盘娩出。

处理

积极的处理将减少分娩时出血。前肩娩出、钳夹切断脐带时，使用催产素（如肌注催产素 5U 和麦角新碱 0.5mg，或肌注催产素10U）。有胎盘剥离征象时助胎盘娩出：子宫收缩、血液涌出（图141）、脐带下降/延长。通过控制脐带牵引使胎盘和胎膜娩出（图 142，143）。

生理性的第三产程无需使用催产素或钳夹脐带，胎盘可自然娩出。但原发性产后出血的发生率高。

原发性产后出血

发病率

占分娩总数的 5%。

定义

产后 24 小时内出血量达到或超过 500ml。

病因

子宫收缩乏力（由完全或部分胎盘残留、多胎妊娠、巨大儿、羊水过多、多产导致的子宫松弛）、损伤（如子宫破裂、宫颈或阴道裂伤）、凝血功能障碍。

处理

宫缩乏力者可静脉应用催产素或肌注前列腺素。如病因不明确在麻醉下检查可能是必要的。对于宫缩乏力者特殊子宫缝合（B-Lynch）或子宫内球可以应用。在极少数的情况下髂内动脉结扎或子宫切除可能是必需的。在严重病例需有血液内科医生参与以指导使用血制品。

Third stage

Definition

From the birth of the baby to the delivery of the placenta.

Management

Active management is associated with a reduction in blood loss at delivery. It involves the administration of an oxytocic agent (e.g. intramuscular oxytocin 5 units with ergometrine 0.5 mg, or intramuscular oxytocin 10 units) with the delivery of the anterior shoulder, clamping and cutting the cord, and assisted delivery of the placenta once there are signs of separation: contraction of the uterus, a gush of blood (Fig 141) and descent/lengthening of the cord. The placenta and membranes are delivered by controlled cord traction(Figs 142, 143).

Physiological third stage uses no oxytocic agent or cord clamping and the placenta delivers spontaneously. It carries a higher incidence of primary postpartum haemorrhage.

Primary postpartum haemorrhage

Incidence

Occurs in 5% of births.

Definition

The loss of 500 mL of blood or more within 24 h of delivery.

Causes

Hypotonic uterus (caused by wholly or partially retained placenta, multiple pregnancy, large baby, polyhydramnios, lax uterus associated with high parity), trauma (e.g. uterine rupture, cervical or vaginal lacerations) and clotting disorders.

Management

Uterine atony is treated by intravenous oxytocics or intramuscular prostaglandins. An examination under anaesthesia may be necessary if the cause is uncertain. Special uterine sutures (B-Lynch) or intrauterine balloons may be used for uterine atony. Internal iliac artery ligation or hysterectomy may be necessary on rare occasions. A haematologist should be involved in major cases to advise on the use of blood products.

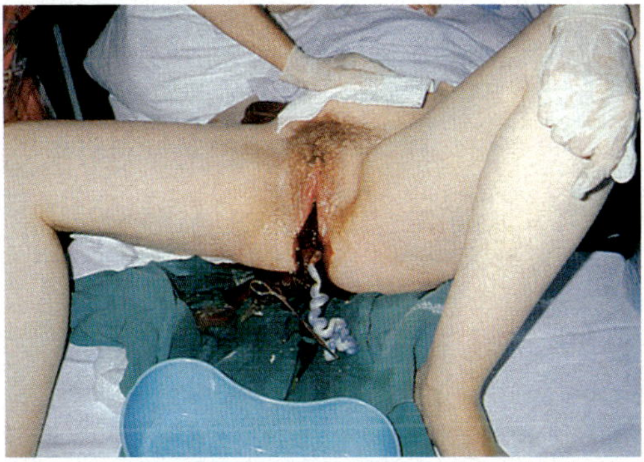

图 141　血液流出，子宫收缩
Blood flow and uterine contraction

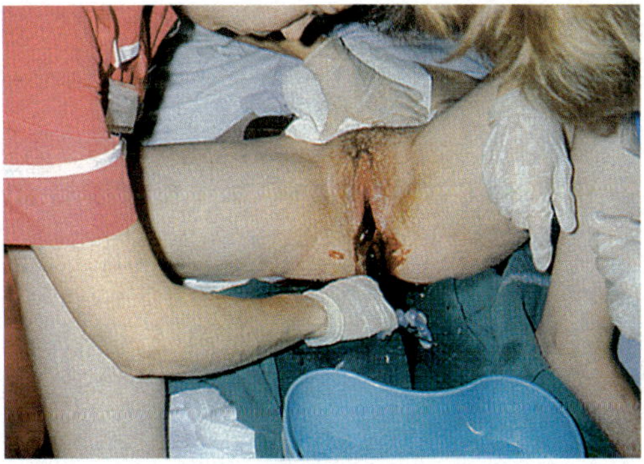

图 142　有控制的脐带牵引
Controlled cord traction

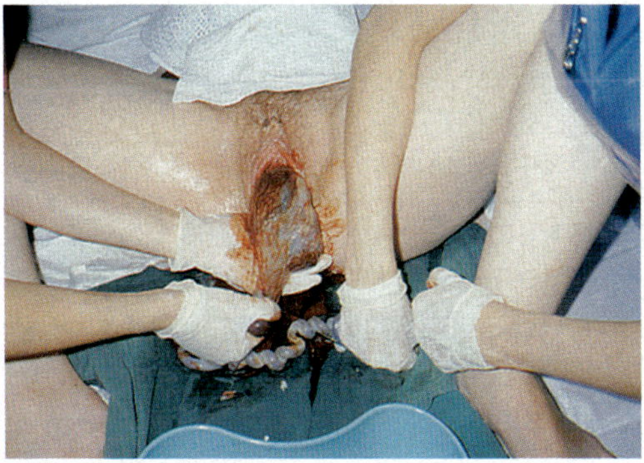

图 143　胎盘娩出
Delivery of the placenta

产时胎儿监护

羊水

通常羊水色清。排出胎粪（图 144）是由缺氧造成的，是持续 FHR 监护的指征。过期妊娠和臀先露可造成胎粪污染羊水。新生儿可发生胎粪吸入，出生时应专门护理以防止胎粪吸入。少量血染可能是“见红”。大量流血可能是由于胎盘早剥、前置胎盘或前置血管引起。

胎心监护

目的

发现产前缺氧与酸中毒。胎儿缺氧引起二氧化碳分压升高，缺氧糖酵解时乳酸堆积可继发代谢性酸中毒。胎儿血pH下降，进而引起胎心异常。许多其他稍轻微的不良原因也可影响胎心，并且判断胎儿窘迫是困难的。采胎儿血测量 pH 经常是必要的。

监护常规

低危妊娠中，胎心在第一产程应每隔 15 分钟记录一次，在第二产程每次宫缩后记录一次。并非所有妊娠都提倡使用持续胎心监护。

持续胎心监护

产时缺氧危险升高（如胎儿生长受限、早产、臀先露、多胎妊娠、硬膜外麻醉、引产或被增强的分娩、糖尿病、高血压、出血、Rh溶血病）、胎心听诊异常或胎粪羊水污染时应采用持续胎心监护。

可使用外置多普勒超声记录仪（图145）或胎儿头皮电极（图 146）。皮肤电极固有的危险（头皮损伤和感染）使外置记录仪更适宜（如果能够获得质量好的记录的话）。

胎心描记图

说明

胎心基线率：正常胎心在 110 ~ 160 次 / 分。如果是过期妊娠，基线降低可能是正常的（105 ~ 110 次 / 分）。胎心率降低，特别是伴随其他不利征象时，可能提示缺氧。胎儿心动过速（基线 > 160 次 / 分）可由缺氧或产妇发热引起。分娩过程中胎心变快（即使胎心在正常范围内）可能也有重要意义。

Intrapartum fetal monitoring

Liquor

Normally the liquor is clear. Passage of meconium (Fig 144) may be due to hypoxia and is an indication for continuous FHR monitoring. Innocent causes are post-dates fetus and breech presentation. Meconium aspiration may occur and expert care is needed at birth to prevent this. Mild blood staining may be just a 'show'. Heavier bleeding may be due to placental abruption, placenta praevia or vasa praevia.

FHR monitoring

Aim

The detection of intrapartum hypoxia and acidosis. Fetal hypoxia causes a rise in pCO_2, and a metabolic acidosis secondary to an accumulation of lactate from anaerobic glycolysis. The fetal blood pH falls. This in turn causes FHR abnormalities. Many other less sinister factors have an impact on the FHR, and recognizing patterns associated with fetal compromise can be difficult. Estimation of fetal pH by fetal blood sampling is often necessary.

Routine

In low-risk pregnancies, the fetal heart is normally recorded intermittently every 15 min in first stage and after every contraction in second stage. The use of continuous FHR monitoring for all pregnancies should be discouraged.

Continuous FHR monitoring

This should be used in pregnancies with an increased risk of intrapartum hypoxia (e.g. fetal growth restriction, prematurity, breech presentation, multiple pregnancy, epidural analgesia, induced or augmented labour, diabetes, hypertension, bleeding, rhesus disease), auscultated FHR abnormalities or meconium staining.

It is performed using external Doppler ultrasound recording (Fig 145) or a fetal scalp electrode (Fig 146). Inherent risks of skin electrodes (scalp trauma and infection) make an external transducer preferable (provided a good-quality recording is obtained).

Cardiotocography

Interpretation

Baseline rate Normal at term is 110-160 beats/min. A low baseline (105-110 beats/min) may be normal if post-dates. Lower rates, especially if accompanied by other adverse features, may indicate hypoxia. Fetal tachycardia (baseline rate >160 beats/min) may be due to hypoxia or maternal pyrexia. A rise over the course of the labour, even if within normal limits, may also be important.

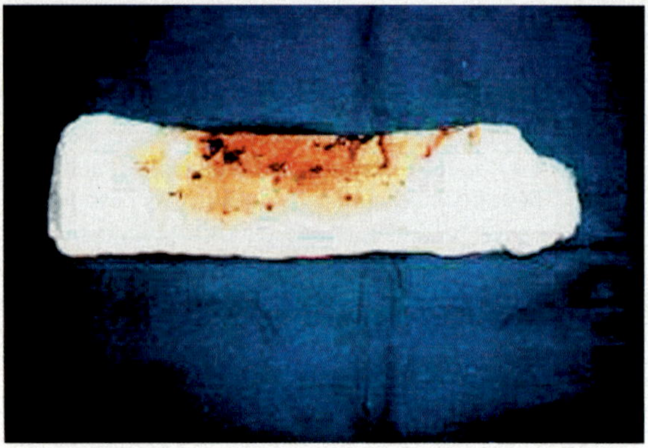

图 144　胎粪
Meconium

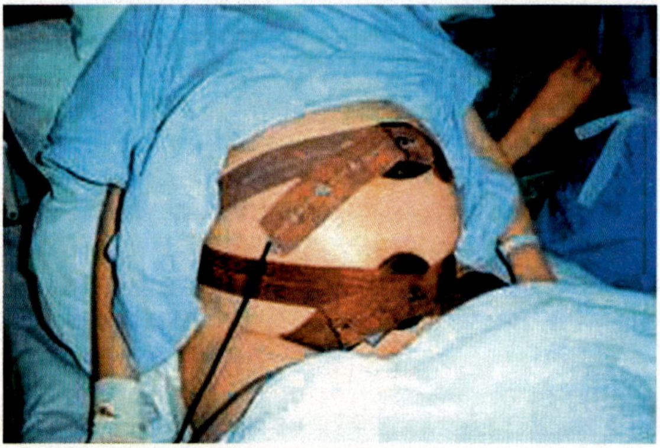

图 145　外置胎心产力描记监护仪
External cardiotocography

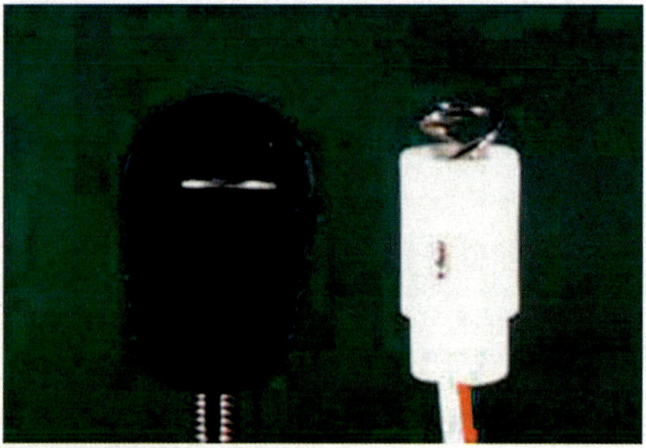

图 146　胎儿头皮电极
Fetal scalp electrodes

基线变异：正常变异 5 ~ 25 次 / 分。基线变异减少可发生在胎儿睡眠、缺氧或产妇使用药物(如哌替啶) 时。

加速：定义为胎心率升高到基线上至少 15 次 / 分，持续至少 15 秒。加速的出现是胎儿状态良好的可靠指征。反应型胎心描记图（图147）在胎动后有2次或更多的加速。

减速：分类如下：

- *早期减速*（图148）：宫缩时开始，宫缩结束后恢复至基线；一般由胎头所受压力的变化引起（衔接、宫口开全）(低 pH 的危险为 5%)。
- *变异减速*（图149）：胎心随着宫缩、深度和持续时间而发生变化。通常由脐带受压引起（低pH的危险为 25%)。
- *晚期减速*（图 150）：胎心减速出现在宫缩高峰之后，通常由胎盘功能不良引起（低pH的危险为50%)。

宫缩：从胎心描记图上可以看出宫缩的频率，而不是强度。

分类

- *正常*：胎心描记图无异常征象。
- *可疑*：有一个异常征象，需持续密切观察。
- *病理*：有一个以上异常征象出现，需采胎儿血样 (fetal blood sampling，FBS) 检测，如不能，需立即分娩。

胎心描记图异常的处理

应该使孕妇左侧卧位，以最大限度增加子宫血流量和胎盘氧供。对有些病例提倡面罩给氧。任何血压降低的情况都应该通过静脉输液以迅速纠正（如硬膜外麻醉后)，如正使用催产素应停用。造成胎心描记图异常的急性的和不可逆的病因（如子宫破裂、脐带脱垂、胎盘早剥）需适当处理。其他情况下，如胎心描记图异常持续存在且器械助娩不可行时，应该检测胎儿血样。

Baseline variability Normal is 5-25 beats/min. Reduced baseline variability may occur with fetal sleep states, hypoxia or maternal drug therapy (e.g. pethidine).

Accelerations Defined as a rise in the FHR above the baseline of at least 15 beats/min, lasting at least 15 s. The presence of accelerations is a reliable sign of fetal well-being. A 'reactive' CTG (Fig 147) has two or more accelerations occurring in response to fetal movement.

Decelerations Various types are recognized:

- *Early* (Fig 148): begins with contraction and returns to baseline by end of contraction; commonly due to change of pressure on fetal head (engagement, full dilation) (5% risk of low pH).
- *Variable* (Fig 149): variable in timing with respect to contraction, depth and duration; often due to cord compression (25% risk of low pH).
- *Late* (Fig 150): deceleration of FHR after the peak of a contraction; commonly due to placental insufficiency (50% risk of low pH).

Contractions The frequency, but not the strength, of contractions can be determined by the CTG.

Classification

- *Normal*: the CTG has no abnormal features.
- *Suspicious*: one feature is abnormal; continued close observation is indicated.
- *Pathological*: more than one abnormal feature is present; the fetal condition needs to be investigated with fetal blood sampling (FBS). If this is not possible, then the baby should be delivered immediately.

Management of pathological CTG

The woman should be turned into a left lateral position to maximize uterine blood flow and placental oxygen transport. Some advocate giving oxygen by face mask. Any hypotension should be corrected swiftly with intravenous fluids (e.g. after an epidural has been sited) and an oxytocin infusion (if present) turned off. Acute and irreversible causes of CTG abnormalities (e.g. uterine rupture, cord prolapse and abruption) should be responded to appropriately. In other situations, if the CTG abnormality persists and an instrumental vaginal delivery is not feasible, then a fetal blood sample should be performed.

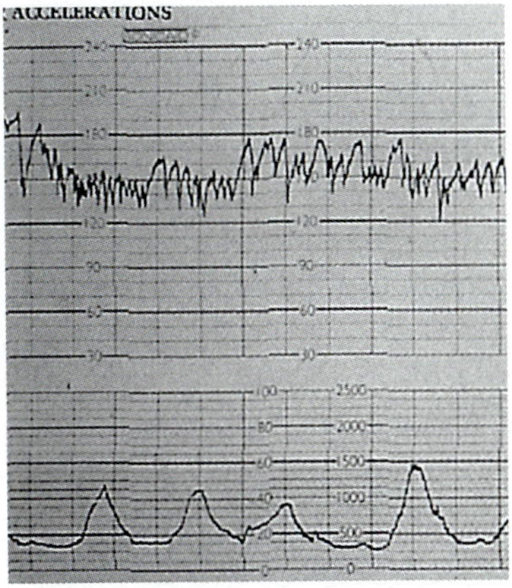

图 147　反应型正常胎心描记图
Reactive normal cardiotocogram

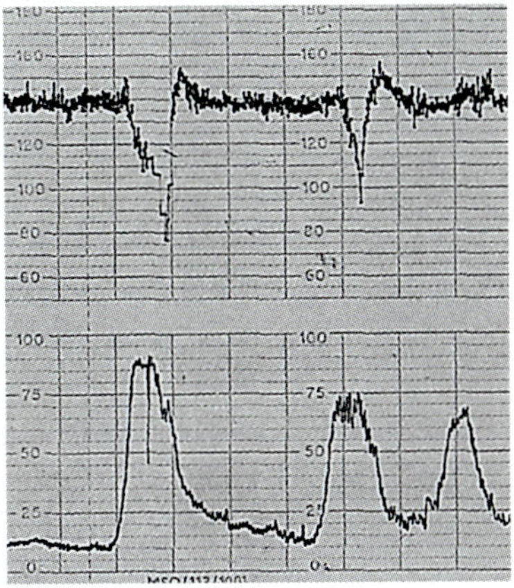

图 148　早期减速
Early decelerations

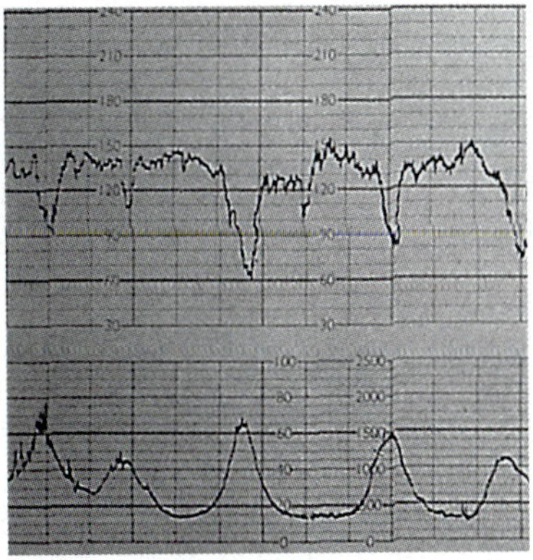

图 149　变异减速
Variable decelerations

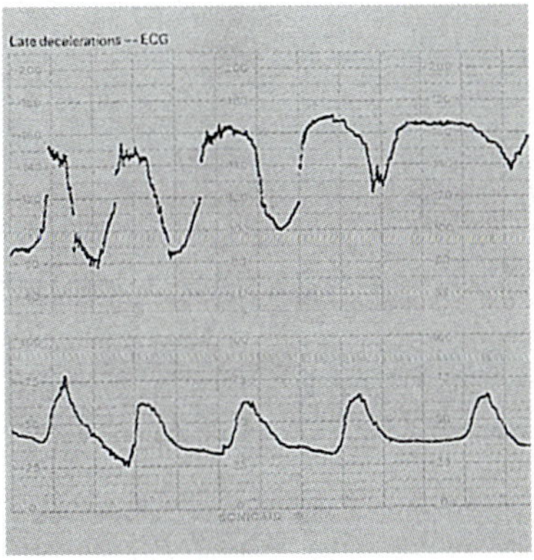

图 150　晚期减速、心动过速、基线变异减少
Late decelerations, tachycardia and reduced baseline variability

胎儿血样采集（fetal blood sampling，FBS）

目的

确定病理性的胎心是否由胎儿缺氧造成。如果确定，应加速分娩，预防严重窒息。

仪器

pH 测量仪、冷光源、氯乙烷喷雾器、杀菌洗剂或杀菌乳剂、硅酮胶、有铁“蚤”的小磁铁以搅拌血样、预先包装好的托盘（羊膜镜、长器械、2mm 长的安全刀片、肝素化的毛细管和拭子）（图 151）。

步骤

使孕妇左侧卧位，清洗外阴及铺单。对着胎儿头皮经宫颈插入适当大小的羊膜镜。接上光源。清洁胎儿头皮，涂抹硅胶。助手在胎儿头皮上喷洒氯乙烷使其充血。使用安全刀片头皮穿刺（图 152）。将没有气泡的连续血柱（10 ~ 30 μl）收集入毛细管（图 153）。压迫胎儿头皮安全止血。

说明

- pH > 7.25，剩余碱 ≤ 10：正常。
- pH 7.20 ~ 7.25：临界；30 分钟内重检一次。
- pH < 7.20 或剩余碱 ≥ 10，或由于技术问题采样失败：分娩应加快。

Fetal blood sampling (FBS)

Aim

To discover whether a pathological FHR is due to fetal hypoxia. If this is confirmed, delivery can be expedited and severe asphyxia prevented.

Equipment

pH meter, a cold light source, ethyl chloride spray, antiseptic lotions and cream, silicone jelly, small magnet with iron 'fleas' to stir the sample and a prepacked tray (amnioscopes, long instruments, 2-mm guarded blade, heparinized capillary tubes and swabs) (Fig 151).

Procedure

Place the mother in the left lateral position. Clean and drape the vulva. Insert an appropriately sized amnioscope through the cervix up against the fetal scalp. Attach the light source. Clean the fetal scalp and smear it with silicone jelly. An assistant sprays the fetal scalp with ethyl chloride to produce hyperaemia. The scalp is stabbed once with the guarded blade (Fig 152). A continuous column of blood (10-30 μL), free of air bubbles, is collected in the capillary tube (Fig 153). Haemostasis is secured by pressure to the fetal scalp.

Interpretation

- pH >7.25, base excess ⩽ 10: normal.
- pH 7.20-7.25: borderline; repeat within 30 min.
- pH <7.20 or base excess ⩾ 10, or if a sample is not achieved due to technical problems: delivery should be expedited.

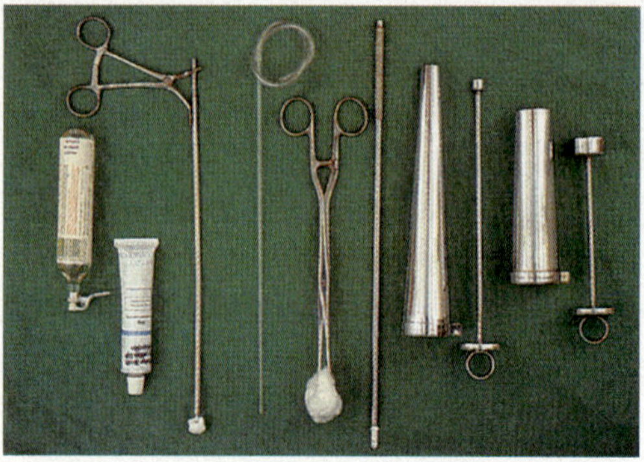

图 151　胎儿头皮 pH 测量采样仪器
Fetal scalp pH instruments

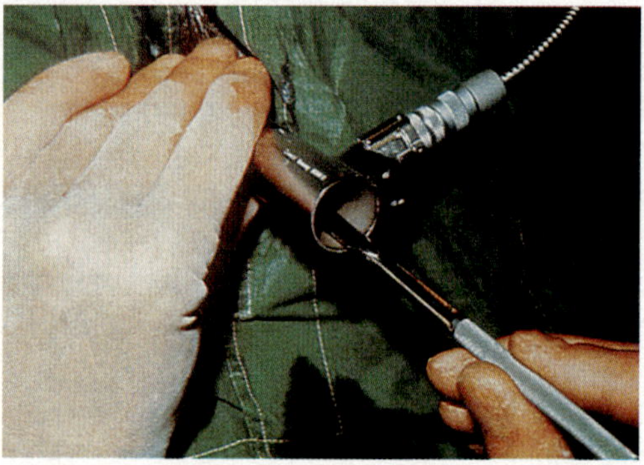

图 152　使用安全刀片穿刺胎儿头皮
Stabbing the fetal scalp with protected blade

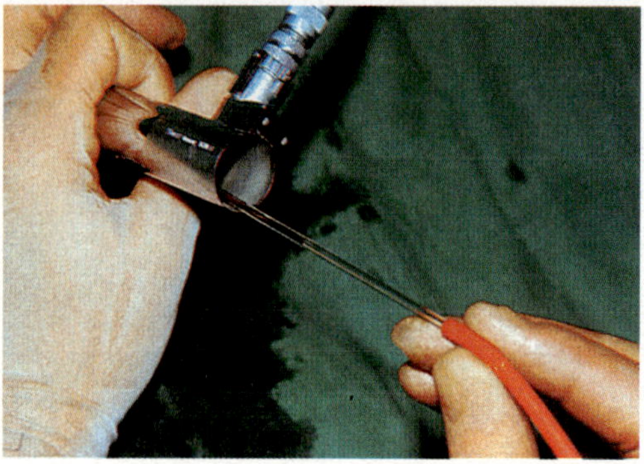

图 153　采胎儿血样
Aspiration of fetal blood

分娩中麻醉

由产妇决定临产时是否需要减轻疼痛，尽管有效性可能不同。鼓励产妇走动和使用分娩球。陪伴分娩经证实有益于分娩。对于低危产妇来说临产、分娩可在温暖的浴盆中进行（图154）。心理/放松的方法可能有助于分娩。产前教育是不可缺少的一部分。

非药物性镇痛

芳香疗法 为由一些助产士开展的新技术（图 155）。

经皮肤神经刺激（transcutaneous nerve stimulation, TENS）（图 156） 只在临产早期有效且有相对较轻的宫缩。该法的理论基础为痛觉的通路控制学说。

药物性镇痛

一氧化二氮—氧混合气 母亲使用一氧化二氮和氧气的1∶1混合物（图157），经常用于第一产程末和第二产程早期。对产妇和宝宝安全、有效，但可能引起恶心、眩晕、失控。

阿片制剂 肌注哌替啶（50～150mg），同时使用或不用止吐药，这种方法广泛应用。阿片制剂的优点是易于给药、起效快、副作用小、可获得拮抗剂。患者控制的阿片制剂静脉给药是可选择的方法。其缺点有 40% 麻醉不充分，呕吐常见。如给药与分娩时间间隔小于2小时，可造成新生儿呼吸窘迫。但可用纳洛酮拮抗。

硬膜外麻醉

硬膜外麻醉是最有效的麻醉方法，但应用时经验非常重要。

适应证

产妇要求、产程延长、臀先露、多胎妊娠、早产、产钳助娩、高血压，产妇痛苦 / 疲惫。

禁忌证

缺乏有经验的工作人员、穿刺部位有感染、脊柱畸形、凝血机制异常、血容量不足、急性胎儿窘迫。

Analgesia in labour

The mother should decide whether she wants pain relief in labour, although the availability may vary. Ambulation and the use of a birthing ball are encouraged. The presence of a supportive birthing partner is of proven benefit. For low-risk women, labour and even delivery can be undertaken in a warm bath (Fig 154). Psychological/relaxation methods may help. Antenatal education is an integral part of the process.

Non-pharmacological

Aromatherapy A newer technique practised by some midwives (Fig 155).

Transcutaneous nerve stimulation 'TENS' (Fig 156) is usually only effective in early labour and with relatively mild contractions. It is based on the 'gate control' theory of pain sensation.

Pharmacological

Entonox® A mixture of nitrous oxide (50%) and oxygen (50%) (Fig 157) is used by the mother, often towards the end of the first stage and during the early part of the second stage. Effective and safe for mother and baby but may cause nausea, giddiness and loss of control.

Opiates Intramuscular pethidine (50-150 mg) with or without an antiemetic is widely used. The advantages of opiates are ease of administration, rapid effect, low incidence of serious side-effects, and antagonists are available. Patient-controlled analgesia with intravenous opiates is an alternative approach. The disadvantages include inadequate analgesia in 40%, and vomiting is common. Neonatal respiratory depression can occur if the administration to delivery interval is less than 2 h. However, the effect is reversible with naloxone.

Epidural anaesthesia

This is the most effective analgesic method, but experience in its use is essential.

Indications

On request, prolonged labour, breech presentation, multiple pregnancy, preterm labour, forceps delivery, hypertension, maternal distress/exhaustion.

Contraindications

Lack of experienced personnel, infection at insertion site, spinal abnormalities, coagulation abnormalities, hypovolaemia, acute fetal compromise.

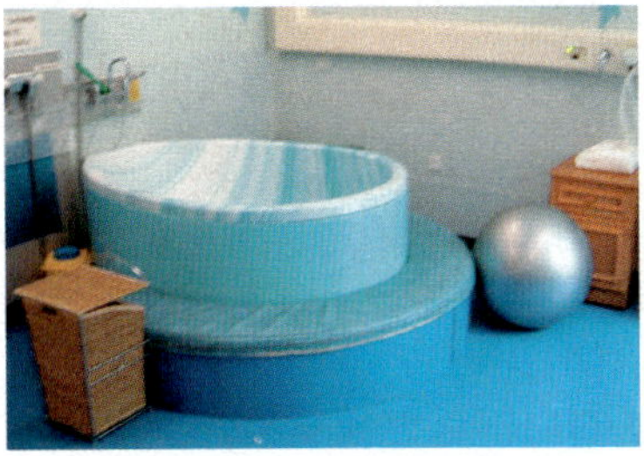

图 154 分娩池
Birthing pool

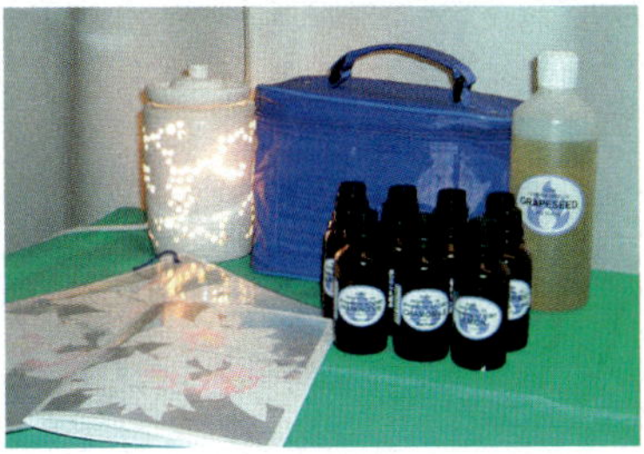

图 155 芳香疗法
Aromatherapy

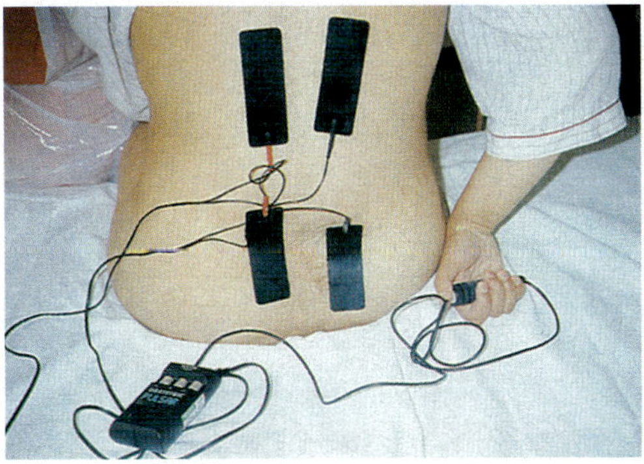

图 156 经皮肤电神经刺激（TENS）
Transcutaneous electrical nerve stimulation (TENS)

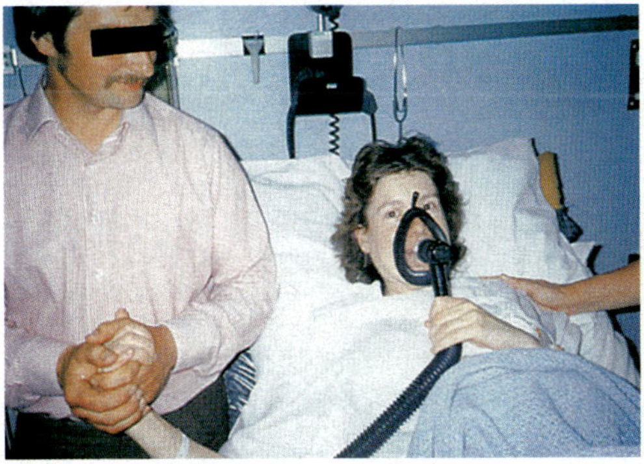

图 157 一氧化二氮—氧混合气
Entonox

技术操作

事先备好使用材料（图 158）。取左侧卧位或直立位穿刺。硬膜外针穿入L3/L4或L4/L5椎间盘间隙直至有落空感（图 159），说明已进入硬膜外。将套管通过穿刺针穿入硬膜外腔（图 160）。

将套管固定在背部和肩部以方便连接细菌过滤器（图161）。单独使用布比卡因（重复注射或灌注以持续麻醉）或合用阿片制剂（如芬太尼）是经常使用的药物。剂量取决于患者身高与对药物的反应。

血压、呼吸、胎心率（持续的）被密切监测。麻醉目的是阻滞（麻醉）T10 ~ L1 神经根。硬膜外或单纯蛛网膜下腔/鞘内（“脊柱”）注射麻醉药可提供局部麻醉以便实施徒手剥离胎盘或剖宫产。

并发症

- 脑脊膜刺破（头痛）。
- 全脊柱麻醉（感觉运动功能丧失、无意识、低血压、呼吸暂停）。
- 低血压（由于腔静脉受压、静脉回流减少、心输出量减少、内脏血流淤积）。
- 运动神经麻痹。
- 尿潴留。
- 毒性反应。
- 少见无菌性脊膜炎。

Technique

The materials used are prepacked (Fig 158). Insertion is in the left lateral or upright positions. The epidural needle is inserted through the L3/L4 or L4/L5 intervertebral disc space until there is a loss of resistance (Fig 159), indicating that the epidural (extradural) space has been reached. The cannula is then threaded through the needle into this space (Fig 160).

Externally, the cannula is strapped up over the back and shoulder for ease of access (Fig 161) with a bacterial filter attached. Bupivacaine alone (repeated injections or as an infusion for continuous analgesia) or with opiates (e.g. fentanyl) are the drugs commonly used. The dose is tailored to the patient's size and response.

Blood pressure, respiration and FHR (continuous) are carefully monitored. The aim is to 'block' (anaesthetize) T10-L1. An epidural or a single subarachnoid/intrathecal ('spinal') injection can provide regional analgesia for procedures such as manual removal of placenta or caesarean section.

Complications

- Dural puncture (headache).
- Total spinal block (loss of sensory and motor function, unconsciousness, hypotension, apnoea).
- Hypotension (due to caval compression, reduced venous return and cardiac output, and pooled blood in splanchnic bed).
- Motor paralysis.
- Urinary retention.
- Toxic reactions.
- Rarely, an aseptic meningitis.

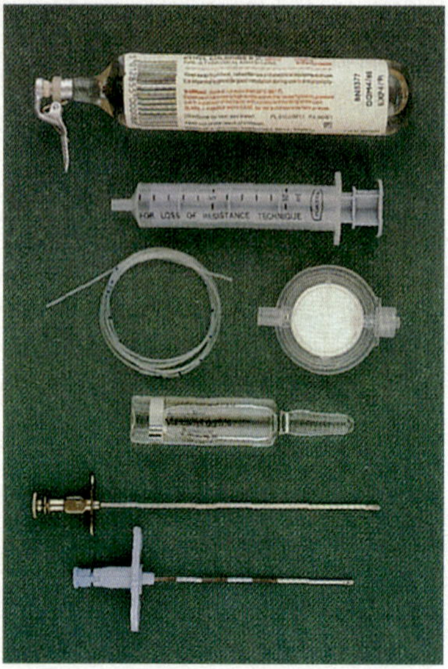

图 158　硬膜外麻醉需要的器械
Equipment needed for an epidural

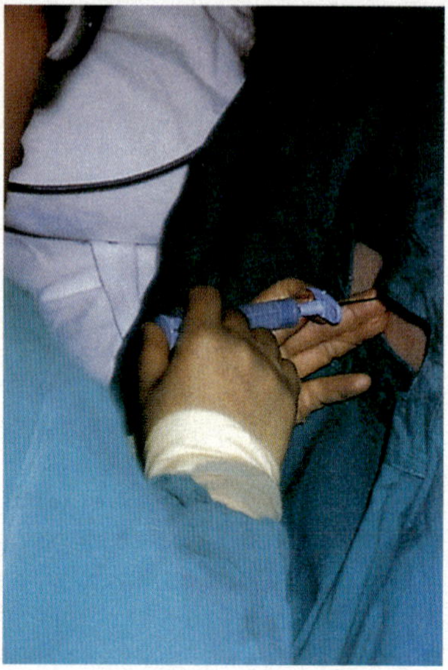

图 159　硬膜外麻醉：穿刺
Epidural anaesthesia: insertion of needle

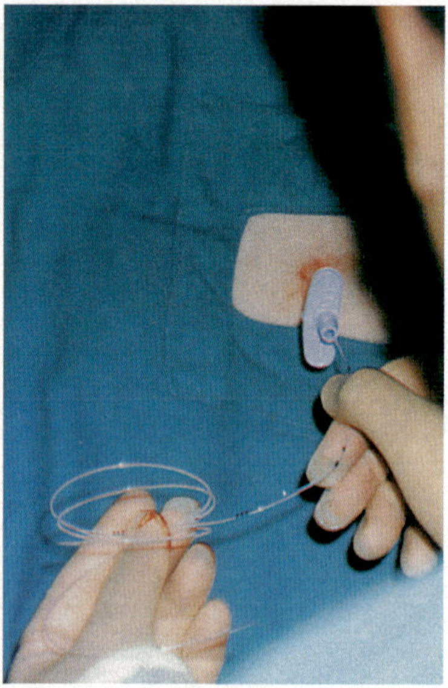

图 160　硬膜外麻醉：将套管通过穿刺针穿入
Epidural anaesthesia: threading the cannula through the needle

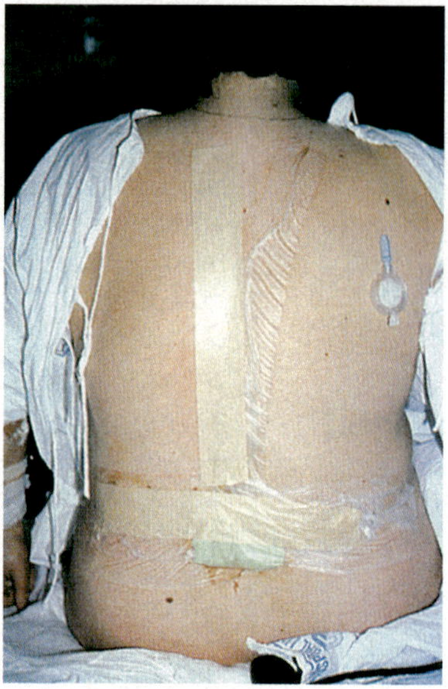

图 161　硬膜外麻醉：位置
Epidural anaesthesia:in situ

决定行会阴切开术需要有丰富的经验和判断力。不是所有的母亲都会发生严重的会阴裂伤，而且可以很确定的是大多数的经产妇分娩都会保持会阴完整。以往工作中对所有的初产妇行会阴切开术是没有充分根据的，是不应该鼓励的。

适应证

避免严重的外阴裂伤；有胎儿窘迫证据时在第二产程后期加速分娩过程；大多数的产钳助产(为避免严重的外阴裂伤)和臀位分娩。

操作技巧

行会阴切开术（后外侧）时应该用锋利的剪子在正确的时间进行(太早会导致不必要的失血，而太晚会导致会阴裂伤)，并给予充分的局部麻醉和区域性麻醉（如硬膜外麻醉或脊髓阻滞)，分娩后应尽快修复。

如行会阴切开术是必要的，在会阴膨隆时应给予10ml的1%利多卡因（利诺卡因）浸润麻醉（图162)。

行会阴切开术时，选择中间外侧方向切开（从阴唇系带的后侧面）会减少裂伤达肛门括约肌的风险（图163)。应在宫缩并在会阴膨隆达最大程度时进行侧切。

会阴切开术的修复

操作技巧

病人处于膀胱截石位，会阴体和外阴部予以清洁及铺巾，照明及视野的暴露应充分。运用局部或区域性麻醉使充分止痛。

阴道粘膜　应清晰地确认阴道切口的尖端（图164)。阴道粘膜可用聚乙醇酸缝合线连续缝合，并且在切口尖的上缘开始缝合（图165)。必须很小心地确保阴道粘膜缘整齐的对合。缝线在处女膜痕的水平打结。

Episiotomy

The decision to perform an episiotomy requires considerable experience and judgement. Not all mothers will experience a severe perineal tear, and certainly most multiparae will be able to have a delivery with an intact perineum. The previous practice of episiotomy for all primigravidae was not evidence-based and should be discouraged.

Indications

Avoidance of inevitable severe perineal tear, to expedite delivery late in second stage when there is evidence of fetal compromise, most forceps deliveries (to avoid severe tears) and breech delivery.

Technique

The episiotomy (posterolateral) should be performed with sharp scissors at the correct time (too early results in unnecessary blood loss, while too late may end with a perineal tear anyway), with adequate local or regional (epidural or spinal block) analgesia and repaired properly as quickly as possible after delivery.

If episiotomy is necessary, then the perineum initially is infiltrated with 10 mL of 1% lidocaine (lignocaine) as it becomes distended (Fig 162).

A mediolateral direction for the episiotomy (extending posterolaterally from the fourchette) is chosen as this limits the risk of extension into the anal sphincter (Fig 163). The episiotomy should be performed during a contraction when the perineum is maximally distended.

Episiotomy repair

Technique

The patient is placed in the lithotomy position and the vulva and perineum cleaned and gowned. Lighting and the field of view should be adequate. There should be adequate analgesia using local anaesthetic or regional analgesia.

Vaginal skin The apex of the vaginal incision must be clearly identified (Fig 164). The vaginal skin is repaired with a continuous suture of polyglycolic acid, starting just above the apex of the incision (Fig 165). Care must be taken to ensure an even apposition of the vaginal skin edges. The suture is tied at the level of the hymenal remnants.

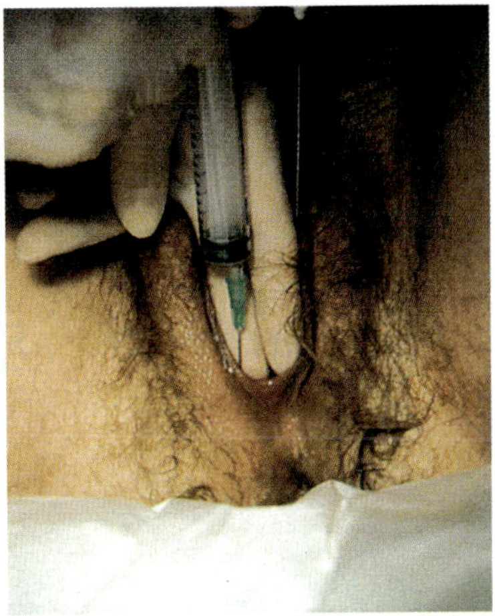

图 162　会阴浸润性局部麻醉
Infiltration of perineum with local anaesthetic

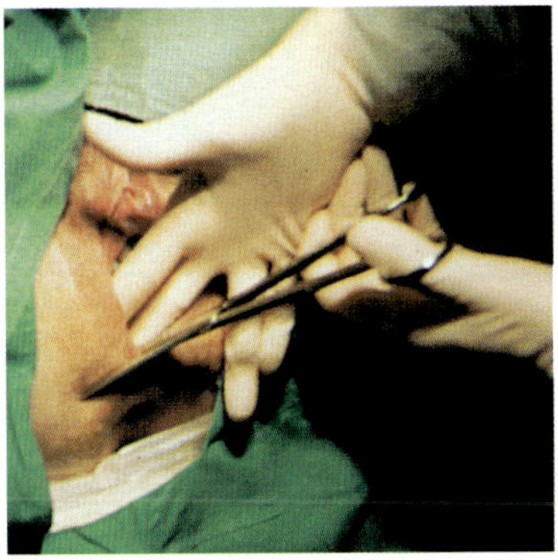

图 163　会阴右侧中间切口
Cutting a right mediolateral episiotomy

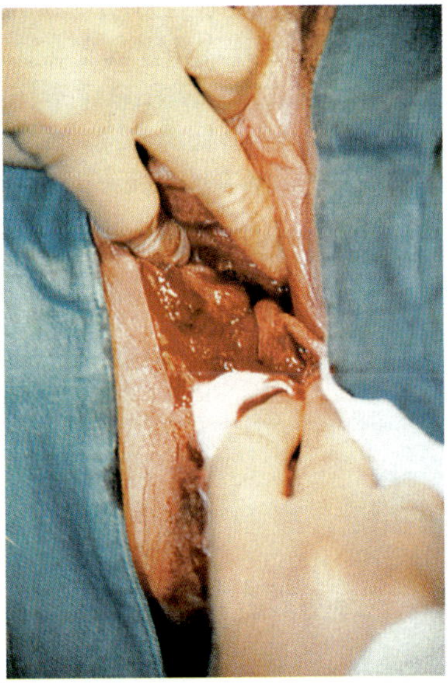

图 164　查看阴道切口的顶端
Inspection of apex of vaginal incision

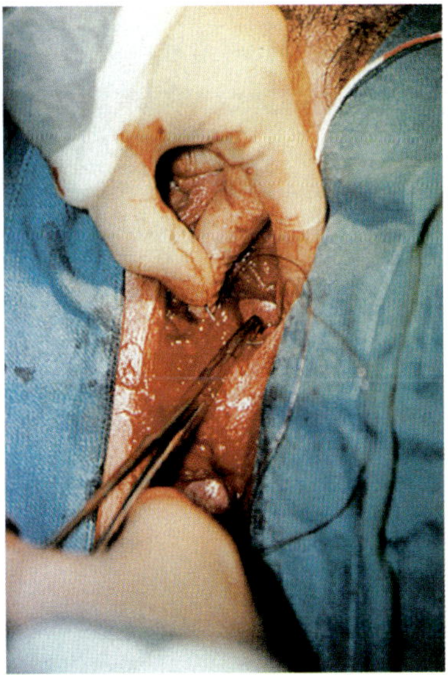

图 165　阴道缝合
Vaginal suture

会阴组织　在完成阴道壁的缝合后，会阴部的切口应该大约呈椭圆形。会阴部深部组织应用聚乙醇酸缝线间断缝合。缝合会阴体时（图 166）要小心避免缝入直肠，而且要与切口的长轴呈直角。

会阴皮肤　应该用快速溶解的聚乙醇酸缝线缝合，间断缝合（图167）或可以采用表皮下缝合技术。修复完毕后，应进行一次阴道检查（图168）以确定没有将药拭子留在阴道内以及没有残留的缺口或血肿。最后应行直肠检查以确定无缝合线穿透直肠粘膜（图 169）。

术后护理

应给予产妇充分止痛，可以是全身用药(经口或经直肠给镇痛药)，也可以是局部用药(冰块冷敷，北美金缕梅 /hemalis水)。并发症包括出血、裂开、感染和瘘管形成。

会阴裂伤

处理

Ⅰ度(仅皮肤裂伤)和Ⅱ度(皮肤和会阴体裂伤)会阴裂伤时采取与会阴切开（见上）相同的处理和修复方法。

更加严重的裂伤包括肛门括约肌的裂伤(Ⅲ度裂伤)和 / 或直肠裂伤（Ⅳ度裂伤）。通常需要由有经验的产科医生在全身和区域性麻醉下在手术室进行修复。应用聚乙醇酸缝线间断缝合直肠和肛门(把线结打在肠腔内)，然后将括约肌的边缘用不吸收的缝线交叠缝合，其余的Ⅱ度裂伤可依常法缝合。产妇术后需进高纤维素饮食，事后给予缓泻剂 / 轻泻剂和抗生素治疗。

Perineal tissues On completion of the vaginal suturing the defect in the perineum should be approximately elliptical. The deep tissues of the perineum are repaired with interrupted sutures of polyglycolic acid. The perineal body sutures (Fig 166) are inserted with care to avoid penetration of the rectum and at right-angles to the axis of the defect.

Perineal skin The perineal skin should be repaired with a rapidly dissolving polyglycolic acid suture. Interrupted sutures (Fig 167) or a subcuticular technique may be used. After the repair has been completed, a vaginal examination is performed (Fig 168) to check that no swabs have been left in the vagina and that there is no remaining defect or haematoma. Finally, a rectal examination is performed to confirm that no sutures have penetrated the rectal mucosa (Fig 169).

Aftercare

Adequate analgesia should be offered to the mother, both systemic (oral or per rectum analgesics) and topical (ice-packs, witch hazel/hemalis water). Complications include haemorrhage, dehiscence, infection and fistula formation.

Perineal tears

Management

First-degree (skin only) and second-degree (skin and perineal body) perineal tears are managed and repaired in the same way as an episiotomy (above).

More serious tears include the anal sphincter (third-degree) and/or rectum (fourth-degree). They are repaired usually in the operating room under general or regional anesthesia by an experienced obstetrician. The rectum and anus are first repaired with fine interrupted polyglycolic acid sutures (leaving the knots in the rectal lumen), and then the edges of the sphincter are overlapped with non-dissolvable sutures. The residual second-degree tear is then repaired in the usual manner. The mother is given a high-fibre diet, laxative/aperient and antibiotics afterwards.

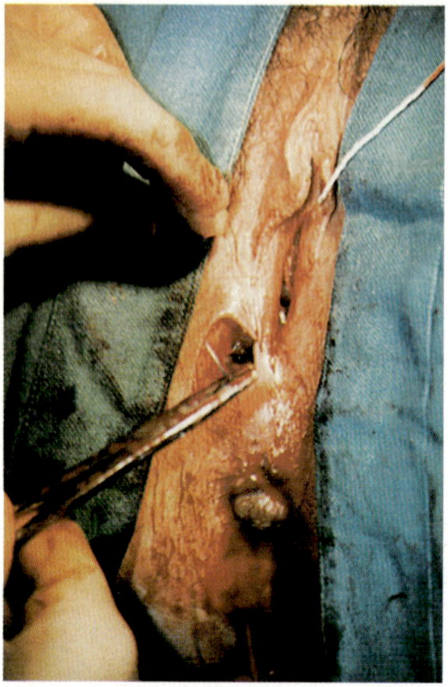

图 166 会阴体的缝合
Suturing the perineal body

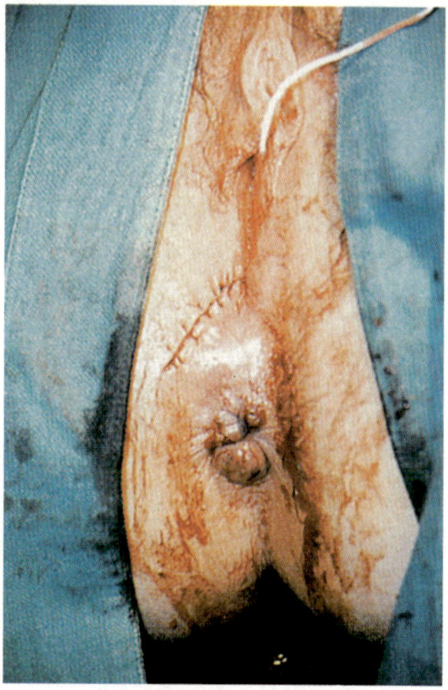

图 167 会阴皮肤的缝合
Sutured perineal skin

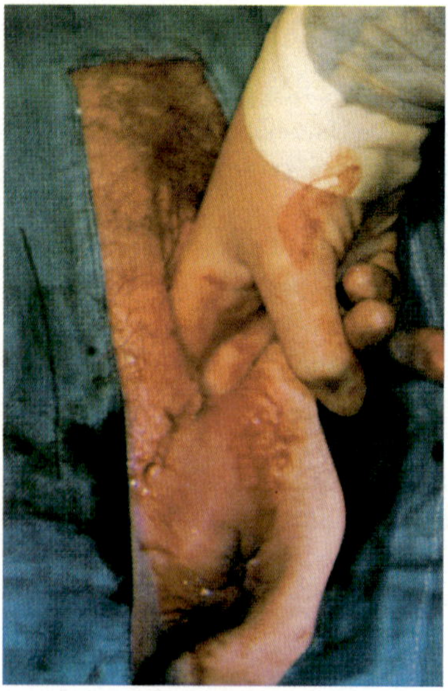

图 168 阴道的检查
Vaginal examination

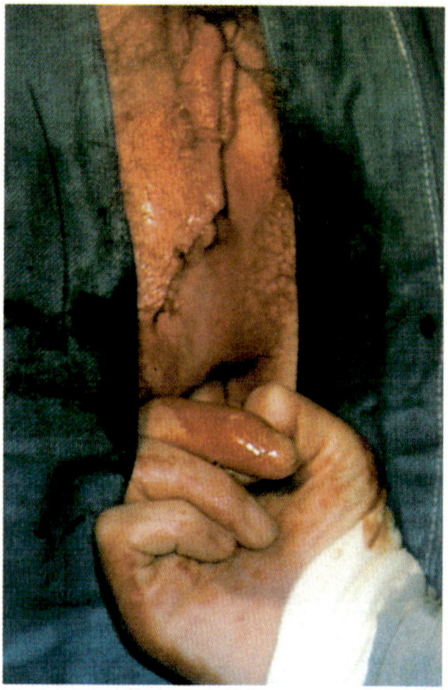

图 169 直肠检查
Rectal examination

适应证

当考虑到分娩后新生儿更为安全，或者继续妊娠对母亲的危害超过了分娩对胎儿的危害，就应该决定终止妊娠。

如果无法承受分娩的风险则需行剖宫产术。在其他的病例中也可行引产术。母亲的适应证可包括高血压、糖尿病和心脏疾病；胎儿的适应证包括生长受限、多胎妊娠和足月妊娠时的胎膜早破。

禁忌证

- *绝对禁忌证* 包括不是纵产式的胎产式、胎儿情况较危险、如阴式分娩有不可避免的梗阻（比如下段的纤维瘤）/既往上段剖宫产（经典剖宫产）或有子宫破裂史。
- *相对禁忌证*：多产、以往子宫下段的瘢痕、臀先露、早产＜34周。

方法

如果宫颈成熟度良好，可用羊膜钩破膜（羊膜穿刺术）（图170）。在破膜后给予催产素静点通常是必要的。

绝大多数的引产由不同类型的前列腺素E_2启动；多数引产应用阴道的片剂或栓剂或凝胶（图171）。可能有必要多次给药，使宫颈成熟以允许破膜和运用催产素。经阴道分娩死婴或有致死性畸形的婴儿可用其他的方法（如前列腺素E_2经羊膜外宫颈管内导管给药，或联合应用抗孕激素和前列腺素E_2，可经口服和经阴道给药）。

并发症

早产、过度刺激（图172）、感染、引产失败。大剂量合成的催产素可导致新生儿黄疸及母亲和婴儿的水中毒。

Induction of labour

Indications

The decision to end a pregnancy is taken when it is considered that the infant will be safer if delivered, or the risk to the maternal health of continuing with the pregnancy outweighs the risk of delivery to the baby.

If the risk of labour is unacceptable, then delivery should be by caesarean section. In other cases, labour can be induced. Maternal indications may include hypertension, diabetes and cardiac disease. Fetal indications may include growth retardation, multiple pregnancy and premature rupture of the membranes at term.

Contraindications

- *Absolute*: include a fetal lie that is not longitudinal, poor fetal condition, an unavoidable obstruction to vaginal delivery (e.g. lower segment fibroid), a previous upper segment caesarean section ('classical') or history of uterine rupture.
- *Relative*: grand multiparity, previous lower segment uterine scar, breech presentation, prematurity (less than 34weeks).

Methods

If the cervix is very favourable for induction, membrane rupture (amniotomy) with an amnihook (Fig 170) may be all that is required. An intravenous infusion of an oxytocic agent is often necessary after an amniotomy.

Most inductions are initiated with prostaglandin E_2 in various formulations; the majority of inductions use vaginal tablets or pessaries, or gel (Fig 171). Repeated doses may be necessary to bring the cervix to a point that will allow amniotomy and commencement of oxytocin. Vaginal delivery of a dead fetus or one with a lethal malformation can be undertaken using other methods (e.g.extra-amniotic prostaglandin E_2 administered via an endocervical catheter, or a combination of antiprogesterone and prostaglandin E_2 given orally and vaginally).

Complications

Iatrogenic prematurity, hyperstimulation (Fig 172), infection, or failed induction. Large doses of synthetic oxytocin can produce neonatal jaundice and water intoxication of mother and baby.

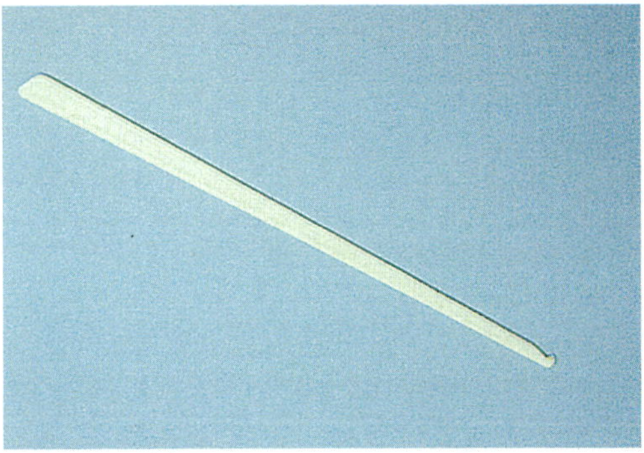

图 170　羊膜钩
Amnihook

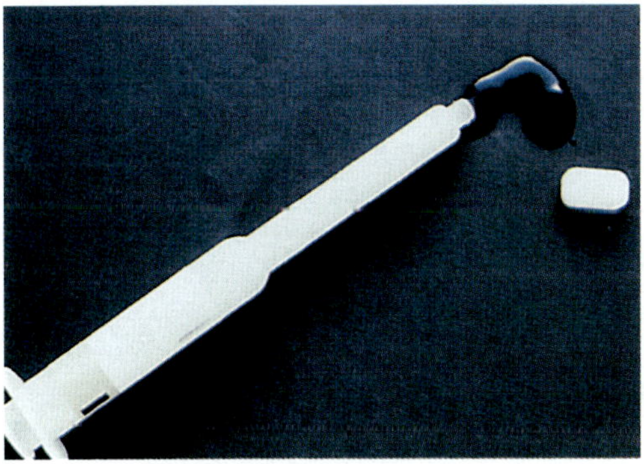

图 171　凝胶和片剂前列腺素
Gel and tablet prostaglandin formulations

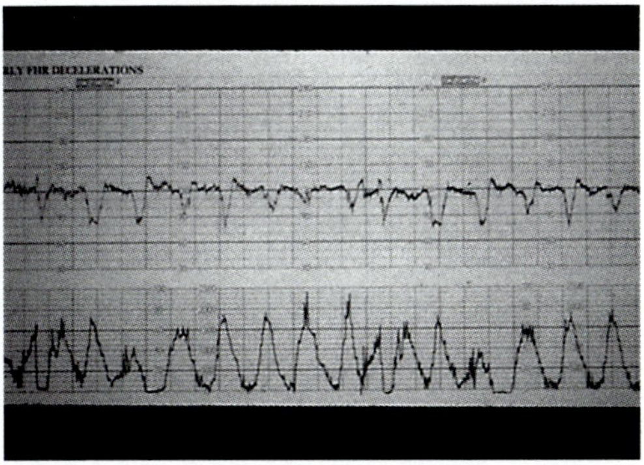

图 172　子宫过度刺激（每 10 分钟超过 5 次宫缩）
Uterine hyperstimulation (more than five contractions every 10 min)

产钳术

前提条件

- 必须有合格的适应证（见下）。
- 合适的先露。
- 无头盆不称或儿头的过度变形。
- 经腹部触摸不到胎头。
- 了解胎头的方位。
- 宫口开全。
- 麻醉充分。
- 排空膀胱。
- 充分的宫缩。

适应证

- 母亲身体状况无法耐受长时间的逼出的努力(心脏病、高血压和硬脊膜穿刺)。
- 在第二产程中可能或确定存在胎儿窘迫。
- 第二产程中出现脐带脱垂。
- 由于产妇体力衰竭或枕后位而造成第二产程进展缓慢。
- 臀位分娩时胎头的娩出。

尚无证据表明选择性产钳术能给低体重儿带来任何益处。

产钳的种类（图 173）

- *非旋转型产钳*：适用于枕前位的胎头，它们具有一个头曲和一个骨盆曲(比如Neville Barnes型、Wriglry型、Simpson 型)。
- *旋转型产钳*：适于将枕横位和枕后位胎头旋转为枕前位，该产钳仅具有头曲(比如 Kielland 型)。

操作过程(非旋转型产钳)

验证检查的发现，并将产妇置于膀胱截石位。清洁外阴，铺无菌巾并留置尿管。麻醉必须充分：可用区域性麻醉（如硬膜外麻醉），也可用 1% 利多卡因（利诺卡因）行局部麻醉（阴部和会阴部阻滞）。润滑产钳叶，置于胎头一侧以牵引(先置入左叶)(图 174)。应在宫缩和产妇用力屏气时行牵引（图175）。需行会阴切开术，在胎头娩出时应像正常分娩那样保护会阴（图 176），同时使胎头缓缓娩出，然后取出产钳。

Prerequisites

- A valid indication must exist (see below).
- Suitable presentation.
- Absence of cephalopelvic disproportion or excessive moulding.
- No fetal head palpable per abdomen.
- Known position of the fetal head.
- Full dilatation of the cervix.
- Adequate analgesia.
- Empty bladder.
- Adequate uterine contractions.

Indications

- Maternal conditions in which prolonged expulsive efforts may be contraindicated (e.g. cardiac disease, hypertension,dural puncture).
- Presumed/confirmed fetal compromise in the second stage.
- Cord prolapse in the second stage.
- Poor progress in the second stage due to maternal exhaustion or occipitoposterior position.
- For delivery of the head in a breech delivery.

There is no evidence that elective forceps delivery of low-birthweight infants confers any benefits to the baby.

Types of forceps (Fig173)

- *Non-rotational*: suitable for occipitoanterior fetal head positions. They have a cephalic curve and a pelvic curve (e.g. Neville Barnes, Wrigley's, Simpson's).
- *Rotational*: suitable for rotating transverse or occipitoposterior positions to occipitoanterior. They only have a cephalic curve (e.g. Kielland's).

Procedure (non-rotational)

Check examination findings and place the mother into the lithotomy position. Clean, gown and catheterize. Analgesia must be adequate: regional analgesia (e.g. epidural) or local anaesthetic with 1% lidocaine (lignocaine) (pudendal and perineal blocks). The forceps blades are lubricated and guided alongside the fetal head (left blade first) (Fig 174). Traction is applied with a contraction and maternal effort (Fig 175). An episiotomy is normally performed and the head delivered gently with protection of the perineum as for a normal delivery (Fig 176). The forceps blades are removed.

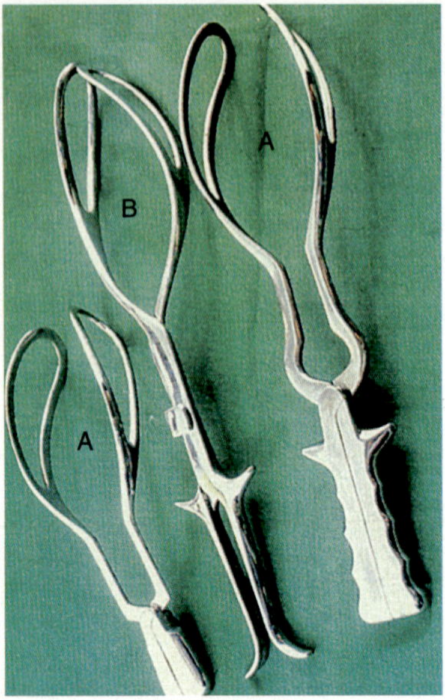

图 173　不同类型的产钳
Different kinds of forceps

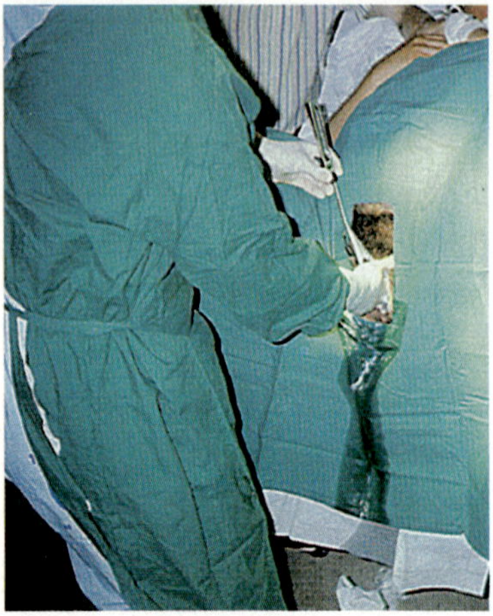

图 174　放置左手产钳叶
Applying the left hand forceps blade

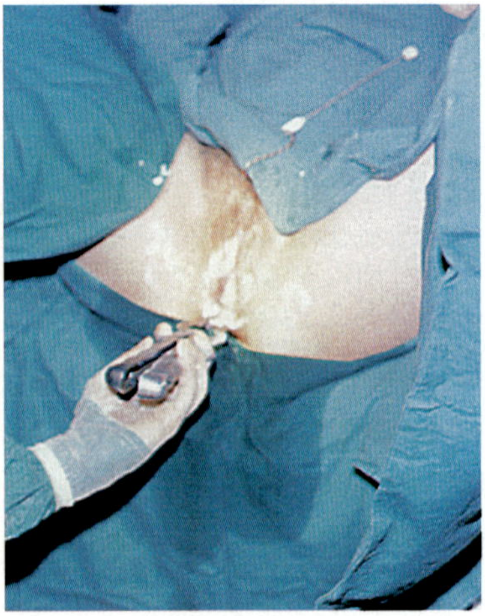

图 175　用产钳牵引
Applying traction with forceps

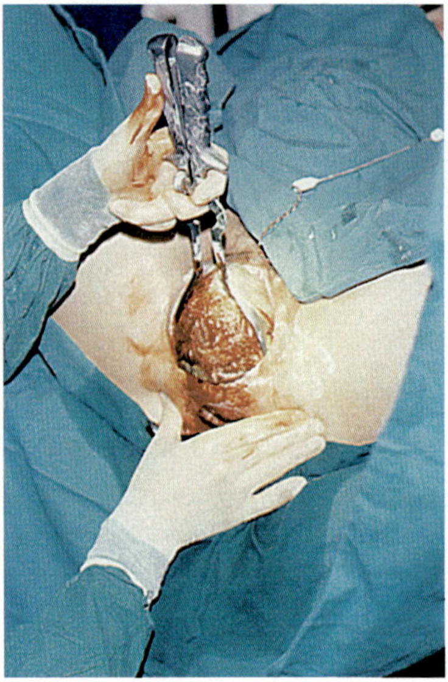

图 176　胎头着冠
Head crowning

适应证

同产钳术，但在臀位分娩时不可应用。美国和许多其他地区的产科专家不赞成在宫口未开全时使用胎头吸引器。

器械

不锈钢或塑料的罩杯，配有吸引管，有时还有链子。有不同的杯罩直径(40mm、50mm或者60mm)。虽然新式的吸罐是手提式的而且有内置的吸引泵，但通常都配有抽吸机。而特别设计的可旋转的胎头吸引器罩杯通常在一侧配有吸引臂。当胎头位置并非枕前位时，这些也适合（图 177）。

操作技术

用大小适宜的杯罩以尽可能贴近俯屈点（恰好在后囟的前方），并可用手动或电动的泵来产生真空（图 178）。起初的压力可增加到$0.2kg/cm^2$，然后当检查确定吸引器的边缘无阴道或宫颈组织时，压力可逐步增加到 $0.8kg/cm^2$。此操作过程超过 2 分钟则没有好处。然后在宫缩和产妇用力的同时进行牵引，当胎头通过阴道口时可停止吸引。

并发症

胎儿头皮擦伤和头皮出血很常见。视网膜出血、颅内出血和头皮坏死很少见。当胎儿有任何出血障碍性疾病的风险时应避免使用胎头吸引器。

优点

与产钳相比，吸引器需要麻醉少，而且产妇创伤的风险也低，仅在时间上比产钳助产稍微长一点。

弊端

一些人认为当胎头旋转异常时，使用相对无效。失败率要比产钳术高。并且不能用于面先露和臀位阴式分娩后出胎头的助产。

Vacuum/ventouse

Indications

Same as for forceps, but cannot be used during a breech delivery. Use at less than full dilatation is not accepted in the USA or by many obstetricians elsewhere.

Instruments

Stainless steel or plastic cup with suction tube and sometimes a chain. Variable cup diameter (40 mm, 50 mm, or 60 mm). A suction machine is usually required, although newer ventouse cups are hand-held with a built-in suction pump. Specially designed rotational ventouse cups are available with side-fitting suction arms. These are suitable when the position is any other than occipitoanterior (Fig 177).

Technique

A suitably sized cup is applied as near to the flexion point as possible (just anterior to the posterior fontanelle) and a vacuum is created by means of a hand or electric pump (Fig 178). The pressure is initially increased to 0.2 kg/cm^2, then, after having checked there is no vagina or cervix included under the rim, the pressure is increased gradually to 0.8 kg/cm^2. There is no advantage in making this process take longer than 2 min. Traction is then applied (Fig 179), coinciding with uterine contractions and maternal pushing; the suction is released when the head passes through the introitus.

Complications

Fetal scalp abrasions and cephalohaematomas are common. Retinal haemorrhages, intracranial haemorrhage and scalp necrosis occur rarely. The ventouse should not be used if there is any risk of a fetal bleeding disorder.

Advantages

The vacuum requires less analgesia and carries less risk of maternal trauma than the forceps. It takes only marginally longer to perform than a forceps delivery.

Disadvantages

Some argue that it is relatively inefficient in cases of malrotation. Failure rates with the ventouse are higher than with forceps. It cannot be used in face presentation or in a vaginal breech delivery for delivering the aftercoming head.

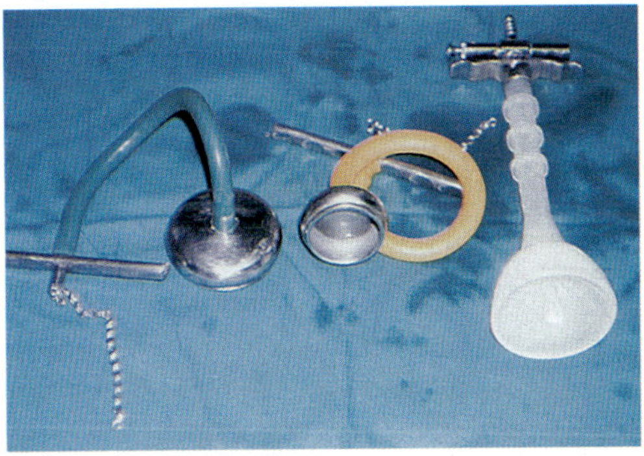

图 177　不同种类的胎头吸引器罩杯
Different kinds of ventouse cups

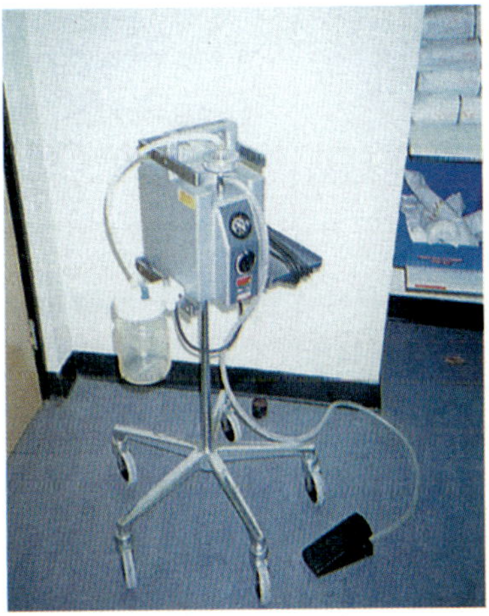

图 178　抽吸机
Suction machine

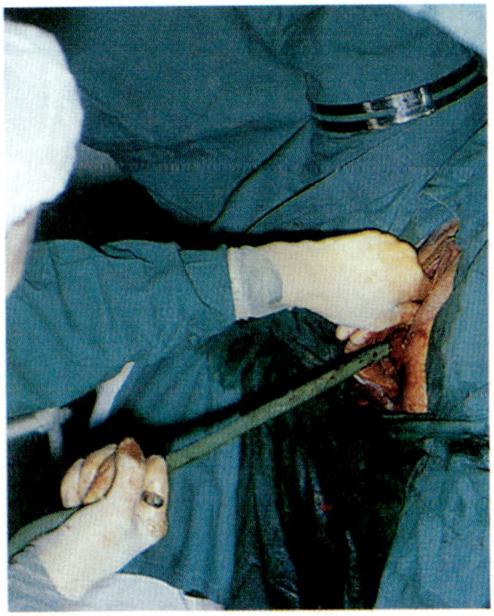

图 179　用胎头吸引器施行牵引
Applying traction with a ventouse

剖宫产术

发生率

由于政策的不同和所处于不同的民族而异：现在，在英国的发生率为 20%，在北美的发生率为 25%。可以是选择性剖宫产（事先计划的）和急诊剖宫产。在急诊手术时产妇和围生儿发病率和死亡率均较高。

适应证

常规 / 选择性剖宫产（caesarean section, CS）

- 既往剖宫产的病因持续存在(如真性头盆不称)。
- 两次或两次以上的剖宫产史。
- 臀先露。
- 前置胎盘。
- 不稳定的胎产式。
- 母体的疾病(如：严重的心脏病、未治疗的颅内小动脉瘤、近期的视网膜剥离)。
- 产妇选择（高度争议）。
- 双胎当其中第一个胎儿不是头先露，以及更多的多胎妊娠。

急诊剖宫产

- 推测或已确定的胎儿窘迫：比如不正常的胎心监测，胎儿血样出现酸中毒，脐带脱垂或在第一产程前或第一产程中出现胎盘早剥。
- 产程受阻(如盆腔囊肿和平滑肌瘤)。
- 由于子宫收缩机能异常、胎位不正或真性头盆不称而引起的产程延长。
- 前置胎盘出血。
- 存在分娩对母亲的风险（如不可控制的高血压、子痫）在不能迅速经阴道结束分娩时（通常早产）。
- 由任何以上原因拟定日期择期剖宫产的患者有宫缩/进入产程。

操作技术

在全身或区域（脊椎的）麻醉下行手术，病人给予插导尿管，以抗菌剂清洁腹部皮肤（图180）并铺以无菌巾。切开腹部皮肤时可用下腹低位横切口（图 181），也可行脐下正中切口。

Incidence

Varies with policies and populations at different centres: currently, 20% in the UK and 20-25% in North America. May be elective (planned in advance) or an emergency. Maternal and perinatal mortality and morbidity are higher when the operation is an emergency.

Indications

Routine/elective caesarean section (CS)

- Previous CS with recurrent cause (e.g. true cephalopelvic disproportion).
- Two or more previous CS.
- Breech presentation.
- Placenta praevia.
- Unstable lie.
- Maternal disease (e.g. severe cardiac disease, untreated berry aneurysm, recent retinal detachment).
- Maternal choice (highly controversial).
- Twins when the first twin is anything other than a vertex presentation, and higher-order multiple gestations.

Emergency CS

- Presumed/confirmed fetal compromise ('fetal distress'): i.e. abnormal cardiotocography, acidosis on fetal blood sampling, cord prolapse or abruption before or during the first stage of labour.
- Obstructed labour (e.g. pelvic cyst/fibroid).
- Prolonged labour due to dysfunctional uterine activity, malposition or true cephalopelvic disproportion.
- Bleeding from placenta praevia.
- Delivery for maternal risk (e.g. uncontrollable hypertension, eclampsia) where prompt vaginal delivery is not feasible (usually preterm).
- Contractions/labour in a pregnancy with a date for elective CS for any of the reasons listed above.

Technique

Following induction of general or regional (spinal) anaesthesia, the patient is catheterized, the abdomen is cleaned with antiseptic (Fig 180) and draped with sterile towels. The abdomen is opened with either a lower transverse incision (Fig 181) or a midline subumbilical incision.

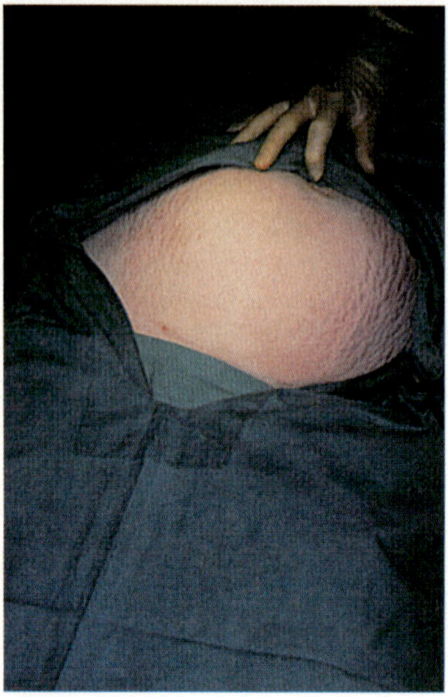

图 180 准备
Preparation

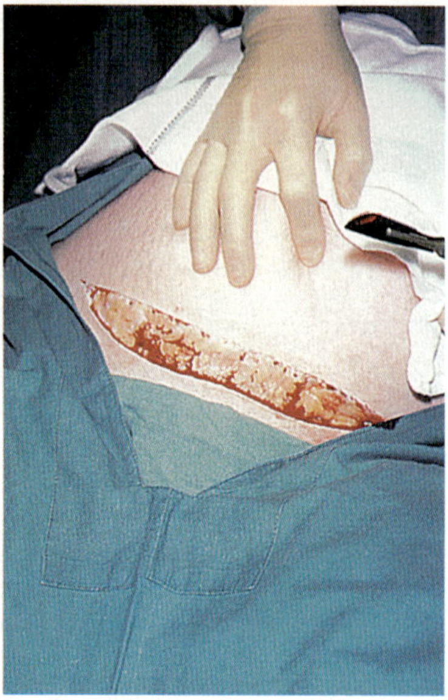

图 181 切口
Incision

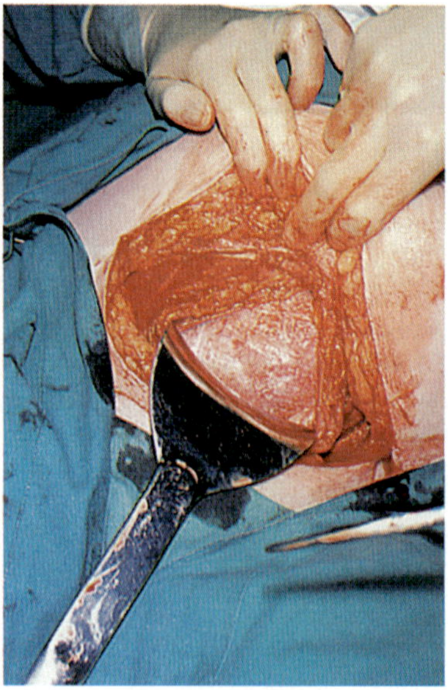

图 182 子宫下段的暴露
Exposure of the lower uterine segment

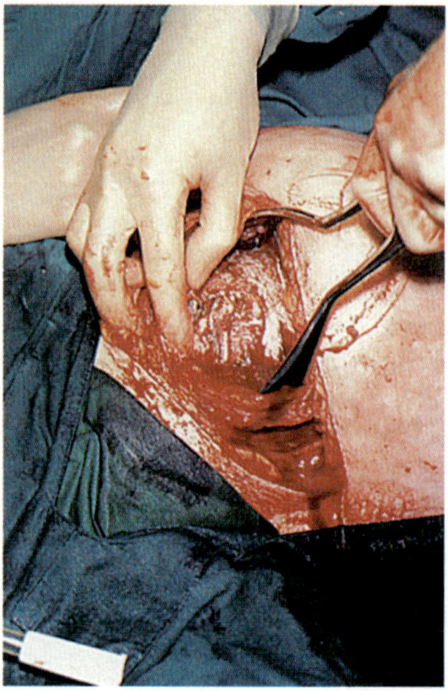

图 183 用产钳娩出胎头
Delivery of the head with forceps

手术的种类

下段剖宫产：这是最常见的方法，可在高达99%的病例中应用。膀胱子宫腹膜是反折的，而且子宫下段被横行打开。在以后的分娩中发生子宫破裂的危险较低（大约0.3%）。

上段剖宫产：这一方法已运用了几个世纪，因此也被称为经典剖宫产。在子宫上段施行纵切口。通常有更多的失血，以后的分娩中较高的子宫破裂风险（4%～9%）以及高的肠粘连发病率和术后肠梗阻。

经典剖宫产的适应证：

- 无法转变为纵产式的横产式（如有手臂脱垂）。
- 某些子宫异常（如有肌瘤存在于子宫下段）。
- 一些前置胎盘的病例。
- 为助娩一些低体重儿（尤其是伴有羊水过少）；对子宫下段形成不佳的病人施行横切口可能会造成分娩困难和裂伤。
- 粘连严重使子宫下段难以暴露者。

操作过程

可用手或产钳娩出胎头（图183、184）。予以产妇静脉点滴催产素，牵拉脐带娩出胎盘（图185）。子宫修复可用可吸收线分两层缝合（图186）。腹腔也应逐层缝合（图187）。关闭子宫和腹腔的方法各异。手术后应注意止痛、理疗、活动和帮助哺喂婴儿。

并发症

包括流血、感染（如切口、尿道）、血栓栓塞性疾病、内脏损伤、麻痹性肠梗阻、不孕以及再次妊娠剖宫产率增高、前置胎盘的发生率增加。

Types of operation

Lower segment This is the most common approach, used in 99% of cases. The uterovesical peritoneum is reflected (Fig 182) and the lower segment opened with a transverse incision. The risk of rupture in subsequent labour is low (about 0.3%).

Upper segment This approach was used for several centuries, hence its description as 'classical'. A vertical incision is made in the upper segment of the uterus. It is associated with a greater blood loss, higher risk of rupture in a subsequent labour (4-9%) and greater risk of bowel adhesions and postoperative ileus.

Indications for classical CS are:

- Transverse lie which cannot readily be converted to longitudinal (e.g. prolapsed arm).
- Certain uterine abnormalities (e.g. fibroids in the lower segment).
- Some cases of placenta praevia.
- For delivery of some low-birthweight babies (particularly with oligohydramnios). A poorly formed lower segment may make delivery difficult and traumatic through a transverse incision.
- Dense adhesions obscuring the lower segment.

Procedure

The head is delivered either manually or with forceps (Figs 183, 184). An oxytocic agent is administered intravenously to the mother and the placenta is delivered by cord traction (Fig 185). The uterus is repaired in two layers of continuous absorbable sutures (Fig 186). The abdomen is closed in layers (Fig 187). There are variations in the technique of closure of both uterus and abdomen. Postoperative attention is paid to analgesia, physiotherapy, mobilization and assistance with feeding.

Complications

These include haemorrhage, infection (e.g. wound, urinary), thromboembolic disease, visceral damage, paralytic ileus, infertility and increased risk of CS and placenta praevia in a future pregnancy.

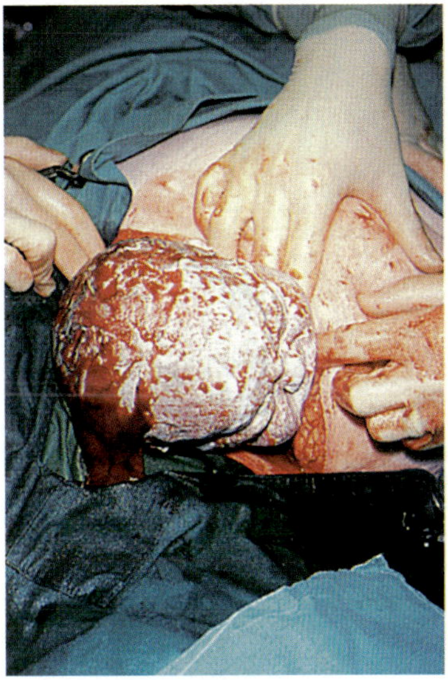

图 184　胎头娩出
Head delivered

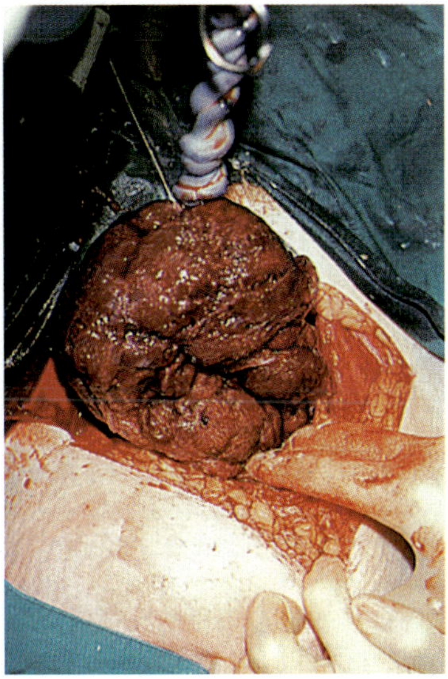

图 185　胎盘娩出
Delivery of the placenta

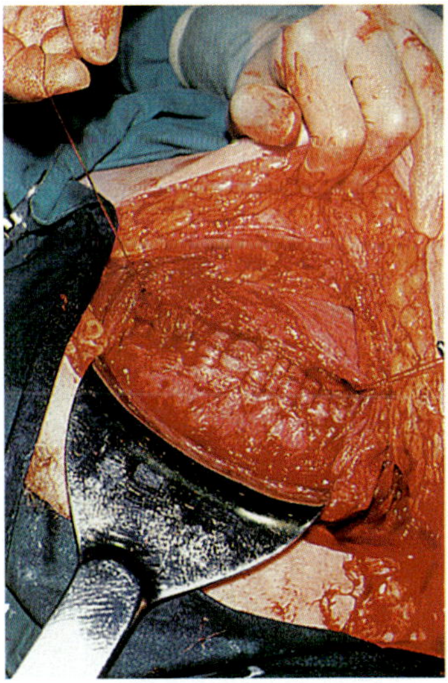

图 186　子宫修复
Uterine repair

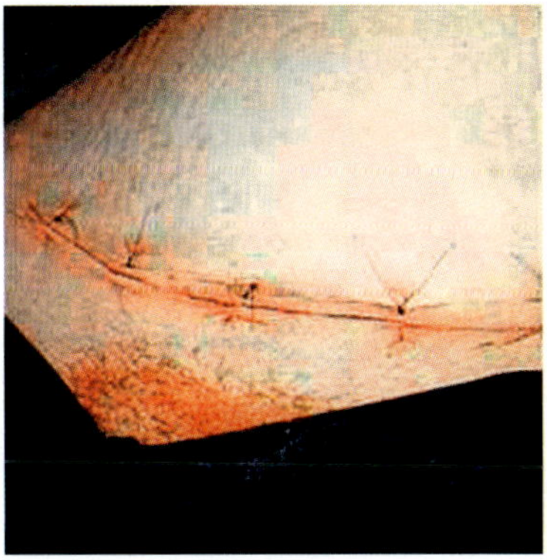

图 187　皮肤缝合
Skin sutures

22 双胎

发生率

自发（自然发生）双胎的发生大约为每80例妊娠中发生1例。自然发生的更多胎的妊娠较少见：每8000例妊娠中有1例三胎妊娠，每80 000例妊娠中有一例四胎妊娠。辅助生殖技术（如克罗米酚的应用和体外受精）使多胎妊娠数大大超过了以上的估计。

种类

单绒毛膜双胎（monochorionic, MC, 相同的双胎）
是由于单个的卵细胞受精并分裂成两个胚胎而形成的，共用同一羊膜囊较罕见（单羊膜囊双胎，1%），更罕见的是连体儿（图188）。没有种族和家族诱因，妊娠头三个月末超声图像的特点是薄的分割性的羊膜连接宫壁，如嵌入的T型（图189）。

双绒毛膜双胎（dichorionic， DC， 不同/异卵双胎）
是由多个卵细胞受精而来。有较强的家族和种族（如尼日利亚人）诱因。母亲的年龄越大、产次越多、身材越高、越胖，则越可能发生多胎。单卵双胎/双卵双胎的比例1∶4。妊娠头三个月末超声图像的特点是厚的分割性的羊膜连接宫壁，如V型或λ型。

诊断

通常在预约的或常规的超声检查中发现。也可表现为腹型大于相应停经月份、妊娠剧吐、血清甲胎蛋白升高或早期高血压/先兆子痫。临床可根据触及多个胎体或发现两个胎心而获此诊断。

常见并发症

除了过度成熟以外，妊娠期的其他并发症都明显增多，包括早产、先兆子痫、胎儿宫内生长受限，造成了大约10%的围生儿死亡。单卵双胎具有更高的围生儿死亡率，因为他们有双胎输血综合征的危险。

Incidence

The incidence of spontaneous (naturally occurring) twins is about 1 in 80 pregnancies. Spontaneous higher-order multiples are much less common: triplets 1 in 8000, quadruplets 1 in 80 000. Assisted reproductive techniques (e. g. use of clomifene and in vitro fertilization) have increased the numbers of multiple gestations above these estimates.

Types

Monochorionic (MC, identical) Result from fertilization of single ovum that divides into two embryos. Rarely share the same sac (monoamniotic, 1%) and very rarely are conjoined (Fig 188). No racial or familial predisposition. Characterized on ultrasound at the end of the first trimester by a thin dividing membrane which joins the uterine wall as a 'T'-shaped insertion (Fig 189).

Dichorionic (DC, non-identical/fraternal) Result from multiple ovulation and fertilization. Strong familial and racial (e.g. Nigerian) predisposition. More frequent with greater maternal age, parity, height and obesity. The MC/DC ratio is 1:4. Characterized on ultrasound at the end of the first trimester by a thick dividing membrane that joins the uterine wall as a 'V' or 'lambda' sign (Fig 190).

Diagnosis

Usually detected now at the dating or routine detailed ultrasound. May also present as 'large-for-dates', hyperemesis, a raised serum α-fetoprotein, or early hypertension/pre-eclampsia. Clinical diagnosis is made by palpating more than two poles or detecting two fetal hearts.

General complications

With the exception of postmaturity, every complication of pregnancy is increased, including preterm labour, pre-eclampsia and fetal growth restriction, accounting for about 10% of perinatal deaths. Monochorionic twins have a much higher perinatal mortality as they run the risk of twin-twin transfusion syndrome.

Specific complications

Twin-twin transfusion syndrome Complicates only monochorionic twin pregnancies. A mismatch in

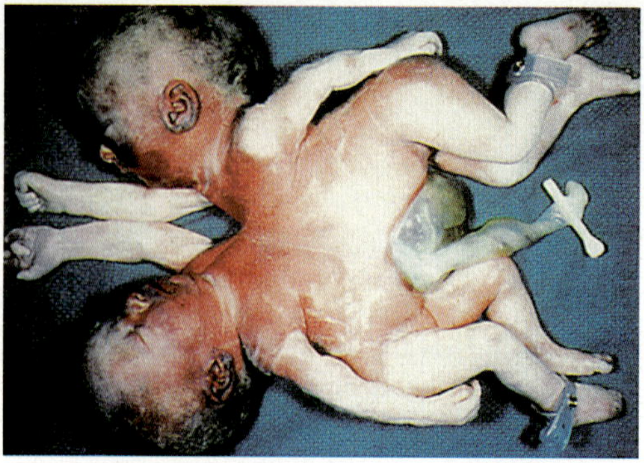

图 188　连体双胎
Conjoined twins

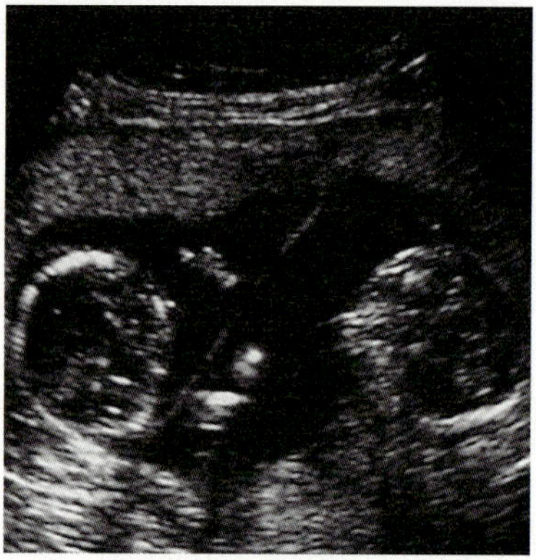

图 189　单绒毛膜双胎的 T 征象
The ‘T’ sign of monochorionic twins

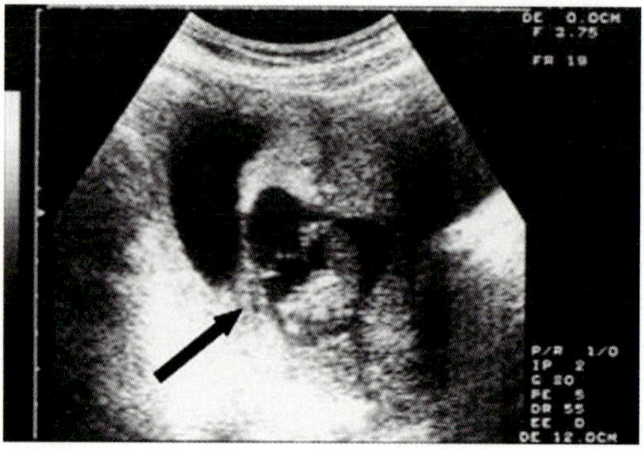

图 190　双绒毛膜双胎的 λ 征象
The lambda sign of dichorionic twins

特殊并发症

双胎输血综合征　仅存于单绒毛膜双胎的妊娠。在共同的胎盘内动静脉连接的不匹配导致血液的不平等分配。“供血儿”会出现贫血和生长受限，并伴羊水过少。“受血儿”则出现血量增多／红细胞增多和大于相应月份，并伴羊水过多。在分娩时这种效果会非常明显（图191）。如不经治疗，早产和围产期死亡率显著升高。此病可用对胎盘的激光治疗给予纠正。

单羊膜囊双胎　占病例的1%。能够引起脐带缠绕（图192）和分娩时的胎儿绞锁。

产前护理

除了常规的产前护理，还包括：

- 饮食上补充铁剂和叶酸。
- 进行更频繁的产前检查。
- 在妊20周时应行详尽的筛查（有更高的胎儿畸形率）。
- 此后应每月行一次详细检查（如出现生长不协调应增加监测次数）。
- 警惕早产的发生（大约10%的双胎在妊28周前会分娩，约30%的双胎在妊37周前分娩）。

  很多人主张加强单绒毛膜双胎的监护（从妊18周开始）。如果已达妊娠38～40周仍未动产应引产。

分娩方式

大多数产科专家对双胎均为顶先露者建议行阴式分娩。如果第一个胎儿不是头位而是其他胎方位，或者任何一个胎儿受到危害时应建议行剖宫产术。

生产和分娩

持续监测两个胎儿。硬膜外封闭可作为首选的麻醉方式。第一个胎儿的分娩同单胎分娩。第二个胎儿的分娩时间延长会增加其发生窒息的危险度。应准备好催产素输注（在第一个胎儿娩出后往往会出现宫缩减退）。可通过腹部触诊来判断第二个胎儿的胎产式和胎先露。可通过外倒转和经阴道牵引胎足行内倒转将横产式转为纵产式。随着下一个宫缩，产妇又开始屏气用力，并且破膜。第二个胎儿的分娩可以是自然分娩或经助产。在分娩时应需要两位儿科医生和双套的复苏设备。原发性产后出血的风险增高。

arteriovenous connections across the shared placenta causes an unequal distribution of blood. The 'donor' twin is anaemic and growth-restricted, with oligohydramnios. The 'recipient' twin becomes plethoric/polycythaemic and large-for-dates, with polyhydramnios. The effect is obvious at delivery (Fig 191). Untreated, the preterm delivery and perinatal mortality rates are extremely high. The problem can be corrected by laser treatment to the placenta.

Monoamniotic twins Comprise 1% of cases. Can result in cord entanglement (Fig 192) and twin entrapment at delivery.

Antenatal care

In addition to routine antenatal care:

- Dietary supplementation of iron and folate.
- More frequent antenatal checks.
- Detailed scan at 20 weeks (higher rate of fetal anomalies) (Fig 193).
- Monthly growth scans thereafter (more often if discordant).
- Vigilance for preterm labour (approximately 10% deliver at less than 28 weeks; 30% deliver at less than 37 weeks).

Many advocate increased surveillance of monochorionic twins (from 18 weeks). Induction of labour at 38-40 weeks is often advised if spontaneous delivery has not occurred.

Mode of delivery

Most obstetricians would advise a vaginal delivery with a vertex/vertex presentation. A caesarean section is recommended if the first twin is any other presentation than cephalic or if either twin is compromised.

Labour and delivery

Continuously monitor both fetuses. Epidural block is the preferred mode of analgesia. Delivery of the first twin is as for a singleton. Delay in delivery of the second twin carries an increased risk of asphyxia. An oxytocin infusion should be ready (contractions tend to subside after delivery of the first baby). The abdomen is palpated to determine the lie and presentation of the second twin. A transverse lie is converted to longitudinal either by external version or by grasping a foot vaginally. With the next contraction, the mother recommences pushing and the membranes are ruptured. Delivery of the second twin may be spontaneous or assisted. Two paediatricians and double resuscitation facilities should be available at delivery. There is an increased risk of primary postpartum haemorrhage.

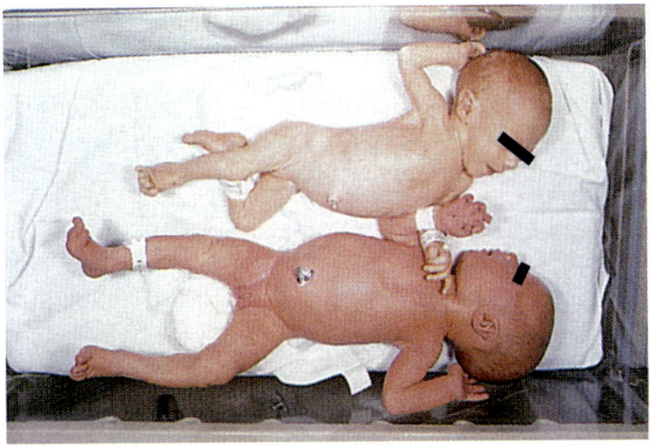

图 191　双胎输血综合征
Twin-twin transfusion syndrome

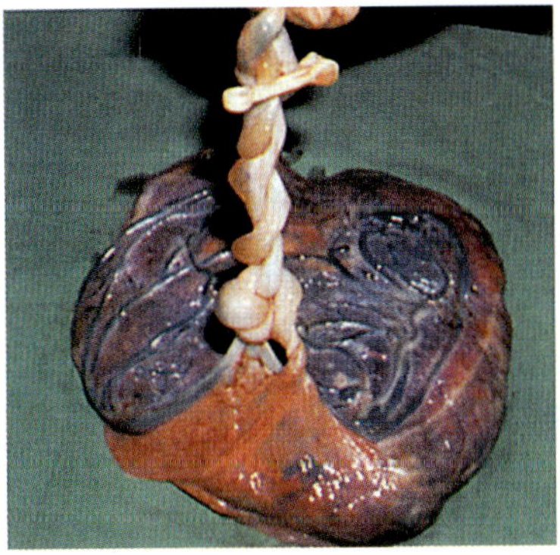

图 192　单绒毛膜双胎的脐带缠绕
Cord entanglement of monoamniotic twins

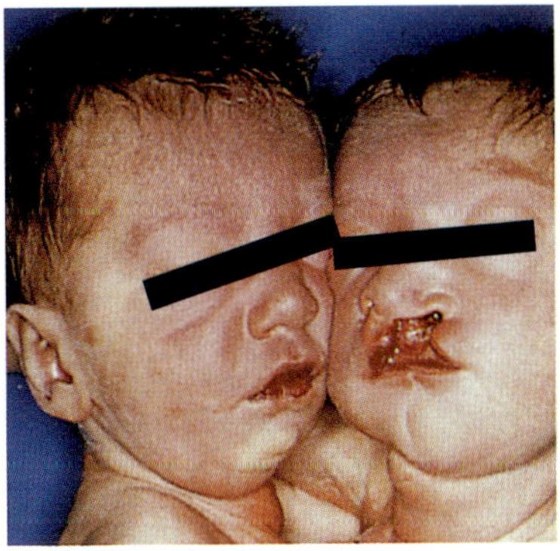

图 193　先天异常的危险
Risk of congenital anomaly

臀先露

发病率

随着妊娠周数的增加而降低：在妊娠 30 周时为 25%，在妊娠 40 周时为 3%。

病因学

- 子宫异常（如子宫肌瘤、双角子宫）。
- 胎儿异常（如脑积水、无脑畸形）。
- 多胎妊娠。
- 前置胎盘。

在很多病例中，无确切的病因。

治疗

在妊36周可通过超声确诊并除外明显的病因（见上），可选择方案包括：

- *外倒转术*：在无其他并发症的妊娠此方法应该鼓励使用。可通过腹前壁和子宫壁来转动胎儿成头位，并辅以宫缩抑制剂，成功率为 40% ~ 60%。
- *选择性剖宫产*：如外倒转术失败可行此术，有证据表明剖宫产术对胎儿的危险性最小。
- *臀位阴式分娩*：有更高的围产期发病率和死亡（尤其是巨大儿、初产妇或为足先露者）。如产程进展缓慢或胎儿窘迫应尽早行急诊剖宫产术。

臀位阴式分娩

建议在产程中持续监测胎心率。如进展缓慢和出现异常胎心图通常行剖宫产术，即使在第二产程也应如此。对从胎臀取血样测定pH和应用催产素问题颇有争议。行硬膜外麻醉可有效抑制过早地向下屏气用力并允许在阴道的操作。当看见胎臀或胎足时鼓励屏气用力（图 194），而且臀位分娩通常需行会阴切开术。脐的娩出以后可由母亲独立完成。如果腿是伸展的，可通过膝部的外展和屈曲来协助娩出（图 195）。上臂通常交叉于胸前，母亲的产力足以使胎肩娩出。助产者手指置于胎儿的肘窝处可使伸展的上肢放下（图 196）。术者可上提胎体或将胎体放低置于助手的胳膊上直至可看到胎儿的发际线。娩出可用 Mauriceau-Smellie-Veit 手法或在助手手提胎足后应用产钳使其娩出（图 197）。

并发症

将在第 24 章探讨。

Incidence

Falls with advancing gestation: 25% at 30 weeks, 3% at 40 weeks.

Aetiology

- Uterine anomalies (e.g. fibroids, bicornate uterus).
- Fetal anomalies (e.g. hydrocephalus, anencephaly).
- Multiple pregnancy.
- Placenta praevia.

In most cases, no cause is identified.

Management

Confirm with ultrasound from 36 weeks and exclude obvious causes (see above). Options include:

- *External cephalic version*: this approach should be encouraged in otherwise uncomplicated pregnancies. The fetus is manipulated through the anterior abdominal and uterine walls into a cephalic presentation, aided by tocolysis. 40-60% success rates.
- *Elective caesarean section (CS)*: should be advised if external cephalic version fails, as the evidence suggests this carries least fetal risk.
- *Vaginal breech delivery*: has higher perinatal morbidity/mortality rates (especially if macrosomia, primiparity or a footling presentation). Early recourse to emergency CS if poor progress or fetal compromise.

Vaginal breech delivery

Continuous fetal heart rate monitoring should be instigated. Slow progress and abnormal cardiotocogram are commonly managed by CS, even in the second stage. Fetal buttock sampling for pH and use of oxytocin are controversial. An epidural prevents premature pushing and allows manipulation. Pushing is encouraged once the buttocks/feet (Fig 194) are visible, and a generous episiotomy is made with their delivery. Delivery to the umbilicus is by maternal effort alone. If the legs are extended, their delivery is assisted by abduction and flexion at the knees (Fig 195). The arms usually lie across the chest, and maternal effort is sufficient to deliver the shoulders. A finger in the antecubital fossa can be used to bring down extended arms (Fig 196). The fetus is either allowed to hang or delivered along the attendant's arm until the hairline is visible. Delivery of the head is controlled by the Mauriceau-Smellie-Veit manoeuvre or by applying forceps after an assistant has lifted the feet (Fig 197).

Complications

These are discussed in Chapter 24.

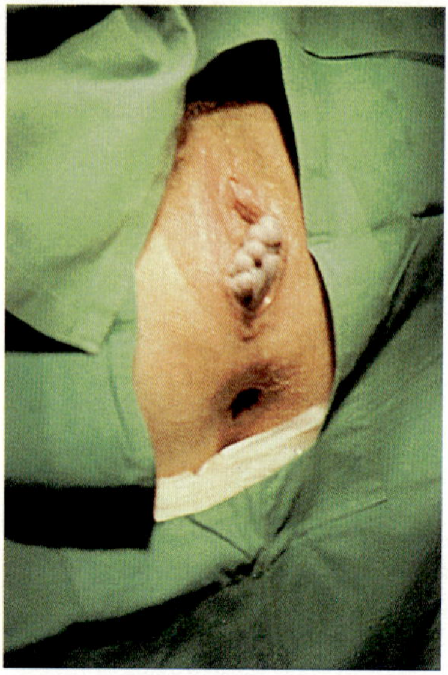

图 194　阴道口的脚
Feet at the introitus

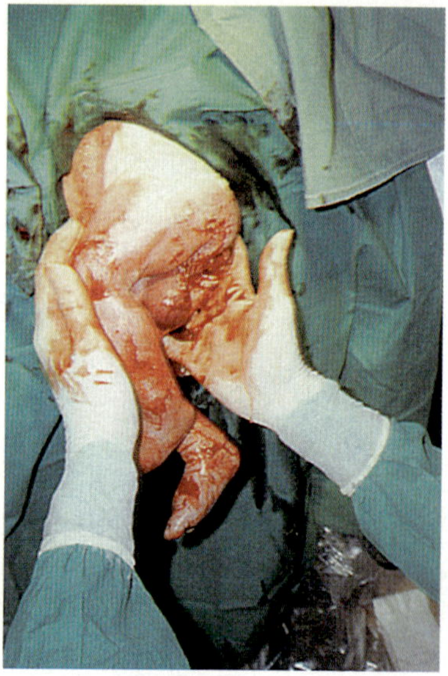

图 195　腿的娩出
Delivery of the legs

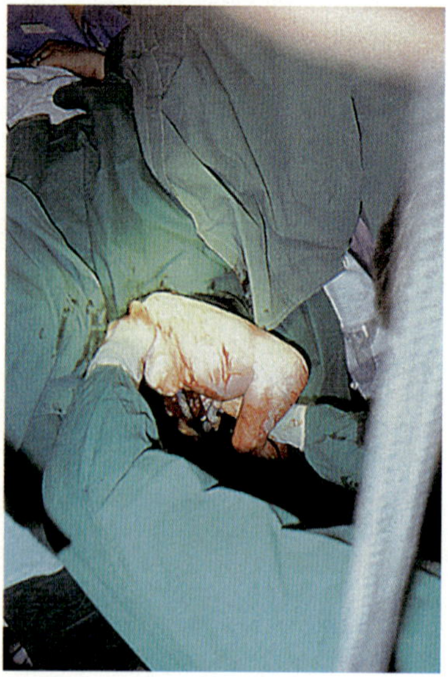

图 196　胳膊的娩出
Delivery of the arms

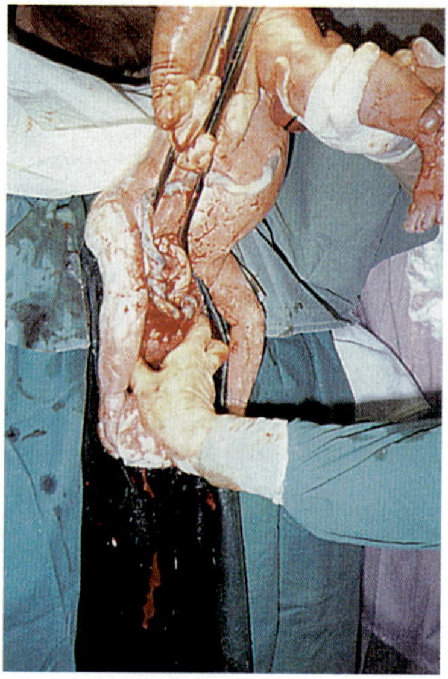

图 197　产钳的帮助下头的娩出
Delivery of the head with the aid of forceps

头部出血

定义

为位于颅骨（通常是顶骨）骨膜下与其较疏松相连的并具有波动性的肿物，且不越过骨缝（图 198）。可导致贫血和黄疸，通常几周后可消退。

发病率

阴道分娩中约为 0.5% ～ 2.5% 的发病率。

病因学

可发生于自然分娩后，但更多见于产钳术和胎头吸引术（3%）。

面神经麻痹

在哭闹时面部出现不对称（图 199），多数病例可在数天内消退。

发病率

约占出生婴儿的 0.25%。

病因学

在产程／分娩时由于压迫了面神经远端至茎乳突孔部分。更常见于经产钳助娩的新生儿，但在自然分娩时，由于母体骨的隆凸或胎儿肩膀的压迫，也可发生。

治疗

注意保护无法闭合的眼睛（由于下位运动神经元受损）。

器械助产所致的损伤

胎头吸引器

头皮瘀斑和人工产瘤（假髻）通常发生于胎吸助产。头皮擦伤易发生于有金属杯罩的吸引器（8%）和牵引时间延长者（最长的时间为 15 分钟）（图 200）。他们需要更长的时间方可愈合，而且容易发生坏死。也有报道可通过开放的囟门抽吸出脑组织。

产钳

面部的压痕很常见（图 201），擦伤少见。骨折是一种较罕见却比较严重的并发症。

Fetal birth trauma

Cephalohaematoma

Definition

Fluctuant mass loosely attached under the periosteum of cranial bones (commonly parietal) and not crossing the suture lines (Fig 198). May contribute to anaemia and jaundice but usually resolves over several weeks.

Incidence

0.5-2.5% of vaginal deliveries.

Aetiology

May follow spontaneous delivery but more commonly follows forceps or ventouse (3%).

Facial nerve palsy

Presents as asymmetry of the face on crying (Fig 199). Most cases resolve within days.

Incidence

Approximately 0.25% of births

Aetiology

Compression of the facial nerve distal to the stylomastoid foramen during labour or delivery. More common with forceps, but can follow normal delivery due to pressure on a maternal bony prominence or the fetal shoulder.

Management

Protect the eye which cannot be closed (lower motor neuron lesion).

Injuries confined to instrumental delivery

Ventouse

Scalp ecchymoses and artificial caput (the chignon) always occur with ventouse delivery. Scalp abrasions (8%) are more likely with metal cups and if the application time is prolonged (maximum duration should be 15 min) (Fig 200); they take longer to heal and necrosis can occur. Aspiration of cerebral tissue through open fontanelles has also been reported.

Forceps

Facial pressure marks are common (Fig 201), abrasions less so. Skull fracture is a rare but very serious complication.

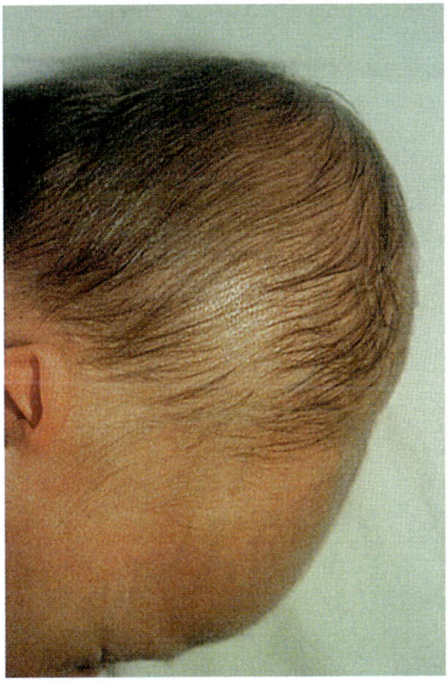

图 198　头颅血肿
Cephalohaematoma

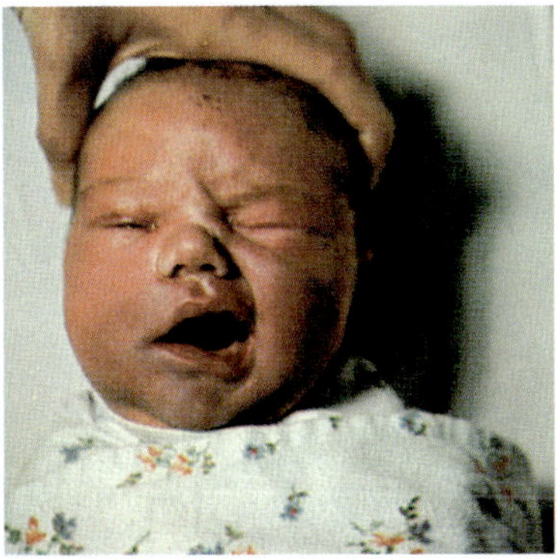

图 199　面神经麻痹
Facial nerve palsy

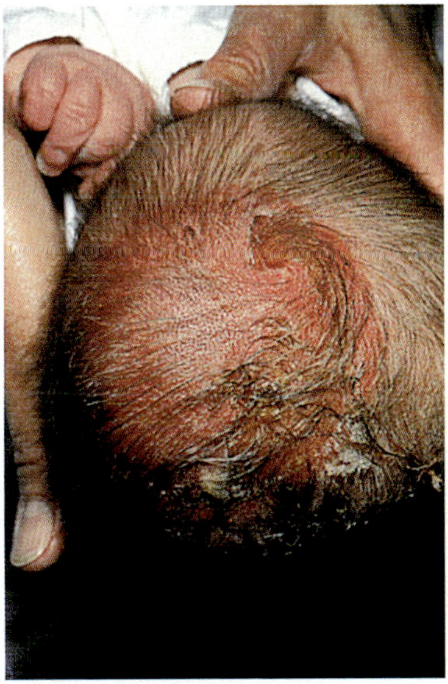

图 200　胎头吸引器擦伤
Ventouse abrasion

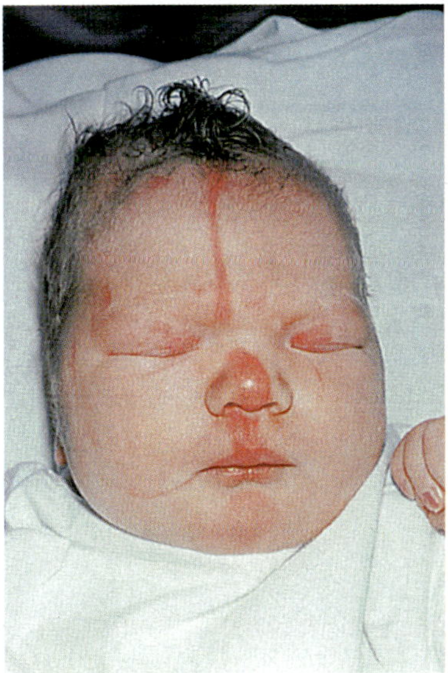

图 200　产钳印迹
Forceps mark

臀位阴式分娩的相关损伤

臀位阴式分娩可导致某些类型的损伤，包括外生殖器的擦伤、脊髓的损害和外周神经瘫痪、骨折和颅内出血。肝（图202）和脾的损伤可通过减少对臀部操作而得以避免。

臂丛损伤

种类

Erb 瘫痪　发病率为 97%。由于 C5 或 C6 神经根的伸展、擦伤和撕脱而导致手臂内旋转，伴有手的伸展和内收（图 90）。偶尔也会发生膈神经瘫痪。

Klumple 瘫痪　发病率 3%，出现 C8 和 T1 的损害。手无力。伴有 Horner 综合征罕见。

病因学

由于分娩时牵拉臂丛引起。在肩难产和臀位助产后更常见。

预后

80% 的病例可在 3 ～ 6 个月完全恢复正常。偶尔可发生严重的永久缺陷，导致无功能的短肢。

小脑幕撕裂

病因学

缺氧使脑组织水肿及其支持膜较坚硬且易于破裂（图203）。过度的胎头变形、早产、臀位和器械助产是此病更进一步的素因性因素。

临床特点

新生儿表现为肌张力松弛、苍白，出生时很难复苏。幸存者常有较高的神经系统后遗症发病率。

其他损害

结膜下出血、在胎儿头皮电极放置部位出现撕脱或感染（图204）以及剖宫产时发生的割破（图205），这些大多数可避免。

Injuries associated with vaginal breech delivery

Vaginal breech delivery predisposes to certain types of injury, including bruising to genitalia, spinal cord lesions, peripheral nerve palsies, fractured bones and intracranial bleeding. Injuries to the liver (Fig 202) or spleen can be avoided by minimizing handling of the breech.

Brachial plexus injuries

Types

Erb's palsy Incidence 97%. Stretching, bruising or avulsion of C5 and C6 nerve roots causes internal rotation of the arm with extension and adduction of the hand (Fig 90). Rarely, a phrenic nerve palsy also occurs.

Klumpke's palsy Incidence 3%. Lesion of C8 and T1. Weakness of hand. Rarely with Horner syndrome.

Aetiology

Traction on brachial plexus during delivery. More common after shoulder dystocia and vaginal breech delivery.

Prognosis

80% recover completely in 3-6 months. Occasionally there is severe permanent deficit, resulting in a functionless short limb.

Tentorial tear

Aetiology

Hypoxia renders the brain oedematous and its supporting membranes rigid and prone to damage (Fig 203). Excessive moulding, prematurity, breech and instrumental delivery are further predisposing factors.

Clinical features

The infant is usually flaccid, pale and difficult to resuscitate at birth. Survivors have a high incidence of neurological sequelae.

Other injuries

Subconjunctival haemorrhages, avulsion or infection at the site of fetal scalp electrodes (Fig 204) and lacerations at the time of caesarean section (Fig 205) many of which are avoidable.

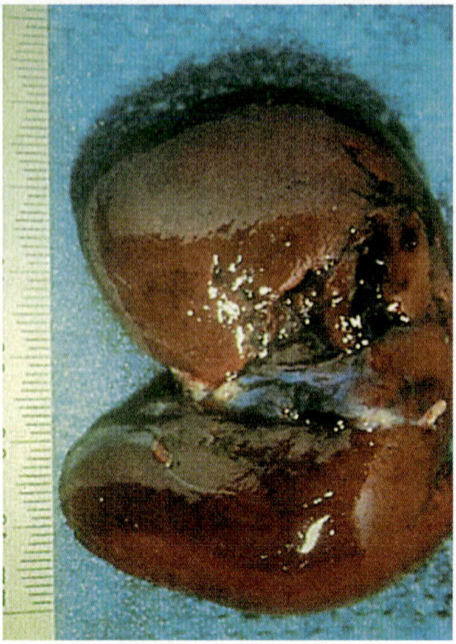

图 202　肝撕裂
Ruptured liver

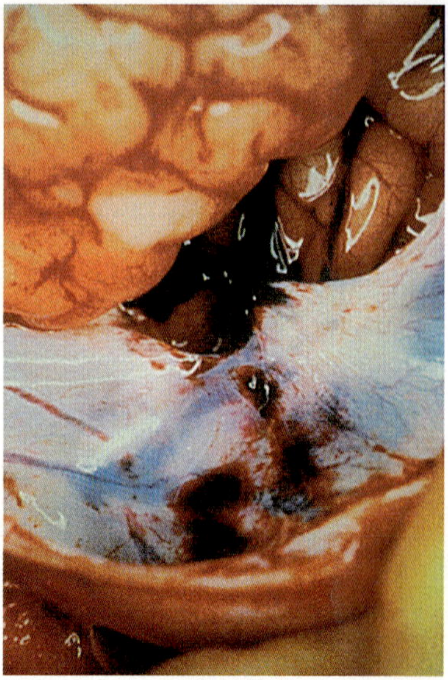

图 203　小脑幕撕裂
Tentorial tear

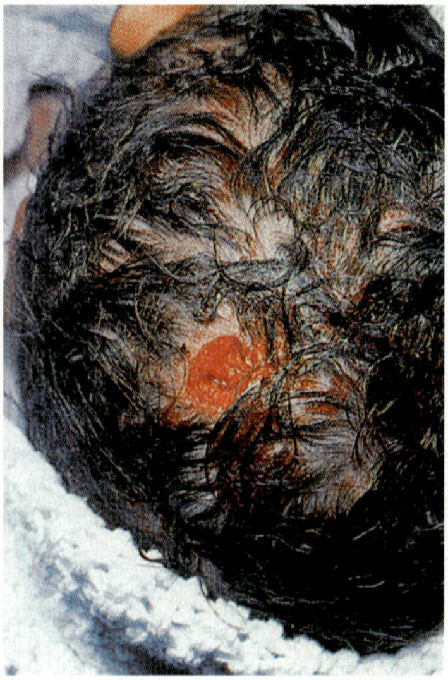

图 204　胎儿头皮电极使头皮撕脱
Avulsion of scalp skin by fetal scalp electrode

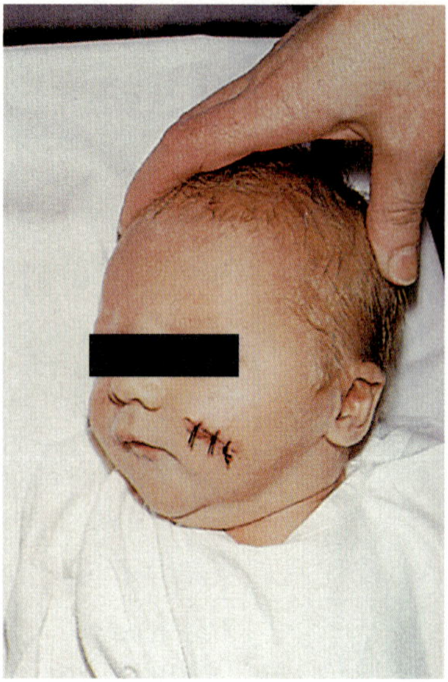

图 205　剖宫产时面部割伤
Facial laceration at caesarean section

定义

是指产后恢复到正常未孕状态的这一时期。在不同国家其定义有差异。许多国家定为6周，虽然大多数解剖学改变在2周内完成。在英国，法律要求产妇需由助产士每日探视达10～14天，常规测血压、体温，检查切口、恶露、乳房和子宫的复旧情况（图206）。助产士也同时检查新生儿并对喂养上的困难进行指导。

并发症

产后脓毒症 表现为产后14天内体温达到或超过38℃。常见的病因包括以下：

- 乳腺感染。
- 尿道感染。
- 创口感染（剖宫产后）。
- 血栓性静脉炎（腿部或静点部位）。
- 血栓栓子疾病。
- 盆腔感染（伴或不伴胎盘残留）。

会阴部的并发症 自觉会阴部疼痛是阴式分娩最常见的症状，是由擦伤（图207）、水肿（图208）和感染导致的。止痛、增加冲洗次数和拆去过紧的缝线都可使症状减轻。

阴道的并发症 阴道血肿（图209）不常见。表现为越来越严重的阴道痛／直肠痛，通常在产后6小时内出现。鸦片镇痛通常对这种疼痛效果不佳。血肿可通过阴道或直肠检查触到。可通过手术去除凝血块，止血并再次缝合阴道和外阴。血肿的出血量可能足可以致使病人出现贫血。小的血肿可保守治疗。

Definition

The interval taken to return to the normal non-pregnant state following delivery. Definitions vary in different countries. For many it is taken as 6 weeks, although most anatomical changes are complete within 2 weeks. In the UK, it is a statutory requirement for mothers to be seen daily for 10-14 days by a midwife who routinely checks blood pressure, temperature, scars, lochia, breasts and involution of the uterus (Fig 206). The midwife also checks that the infant is well and advises on feeding difficulties.

Complications

Puerperal sepsis Defined as a temperature of 38℃ or more within 14 days of delivery. The usual causes include:

- Breast infection.
- Urinary infection.
- Wound infection (following caesarean section).
- Thrombophlebitis (legs or drip sites).
- Thromboembolic disease.
- Pelvic infection (with or without retained placental tissue).

Perineal complications Perineal pain is extremely common following vaginal delivery and results from bruising (Fig 207), oedema (Fig 208) and infection. Analgesia, frequent bathing and removal of any tight sutures provide symptomatic relief.

Vaginal complications Vaginal haematomas (Fig 209) are less common. Presentation is with increasingly severe vaginal/rectal pain, usually within 6 h of delivery. The pain is often refractory to opiate analgesia, and the haematoma is palpable on vaginal or rectal examination. Management is by surgical evacuation of the clot, haemostasis and resuturing of the vagina and perineum. The amount of blood contained may be sufficient to make the patient anaemic. Small haematomas can be treated conservatively.

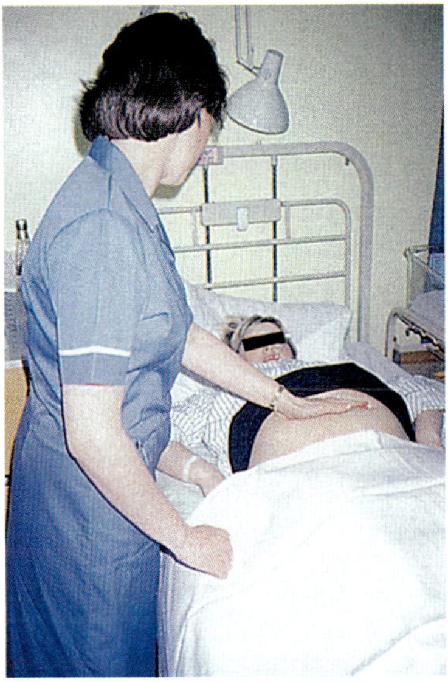

图 206　产后检查
A postnatal check

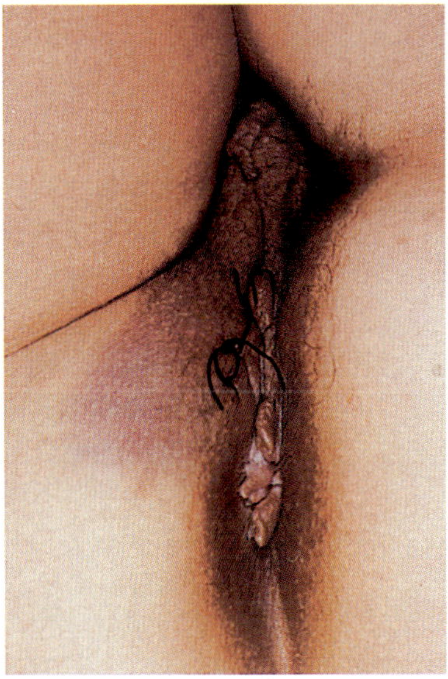

图 207　会阴擦伤
Perineal bruising

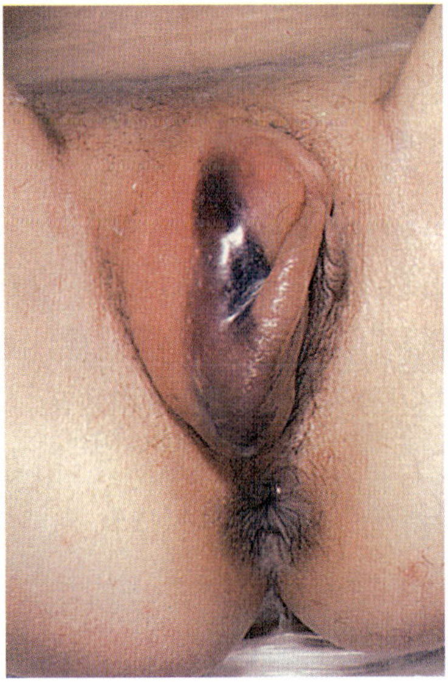

图 208　会阴水肿
Perineal oedema

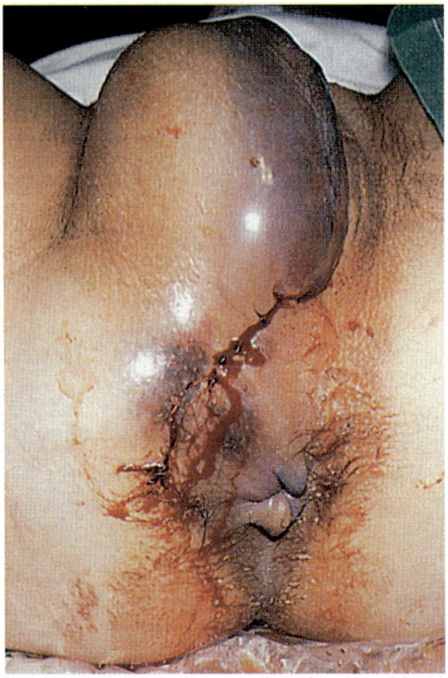

图 209　外阴 / 阴道血肿
Vulval/vaginal haematoma

其他并发症

- 痔核易于发生栓塞而且于分娩时脱出，引起疼痛和刺激（图 210）。
- 母亲在第二产程用力屏气可导致结膜下出血（图 211），可无任何症状，能自行消退。
- 切口感染或血肿（图212）占剖宫产手术的10%。它它使愈合延迟，而且为纵切口时常会引起切口裂开（横切口罕见）。胸部感染、血栓栓塞、肠梗阻、泌尿系感染和贫血也比阴式分娩常见。
- 子宫的感染（子宫内膜炎）通常发生在胎盘附着的部位，表现为发热、腹部不适和阴道流血。可用抗生素和止痛治疗。
- 深部静脉血栓形成和肺栓子更易发生于剖宫产术后。肺栓子是导致产妇死亡的首要病因。

母乳喂养的并发症

乳房肿胀通常发生在产后 2 ~ 4 天，乳腺炎（图 213）相对较常见，最初表现为乳房发红，有触痛。进而表现为水肿的硬结并伴发热及不适。

病因学

葡萄球菌或链球菌感染，通常由婴儿吸吮母乳时引起，尤其在乳头皲裂并合并有乳腺小叶或乳腺导管堵塞的乳汁淤积者更易发生。

治疗

抗生素治疗（氟氯青霉素）、止痛和规律地排空乳房（感染不是给健康的婴儿哺乳的禁忌证）。被忽略的乳腺炎可进一步发展成为脓肿形成，需手术引流或行抽吸术。

Other complications

- Haemorrhoids are prone to thrombosis and prolapse at delivery, resulting in pain and irritation (Fig 210).
- Subconjunctival haemorrhages (Fig 211) may result from maternal expulsive efforts during the second stage. They are asymptomatic and resolve spontaneously.
- Wound infection or haematoma (Fig 212) follow 10% of caesarean sections. They delay healing and, when associated with a vertical incision, occasionally give rise to wound dehiscence (rare with a transverse incision). Chest infection, thromboembolism, ileus, urinary tract infection and anaemia are also more common than following vaginal delivery.
- Uterine infection (endometritis) is usually at the placental site and presents with pyrexia, abdominal discomfort and vaginal bleeding. Treatment is with antibiotics and analgesia.
- Deep venous thrombosis and pulmonary embolus are more common following caesarean section. Pulmonary embolus is a leading cause of maternal mortality.

Complications of breastfeeding

Engorgement of the breasts normally occurs on days 2-4. Mastitis (Fig 213) is relatively common and starts with reddening and tenderness, progressing to an oedematous induration with fever and malaise.

Aetiology

Staphylococci or streptococci, often from the baby during suckling, particularly with a cracked nipple and associated stasis of milk in breast lobule or blocked duct.

Management

Antibiotics (flucloxacillin), analgesia and regular breast-emptying (infection is not a contraindication to continuing breastfeeding in a healthy baby). Neglected mastitis can progress to abscess formation requiring surgical drainage or aspiration.

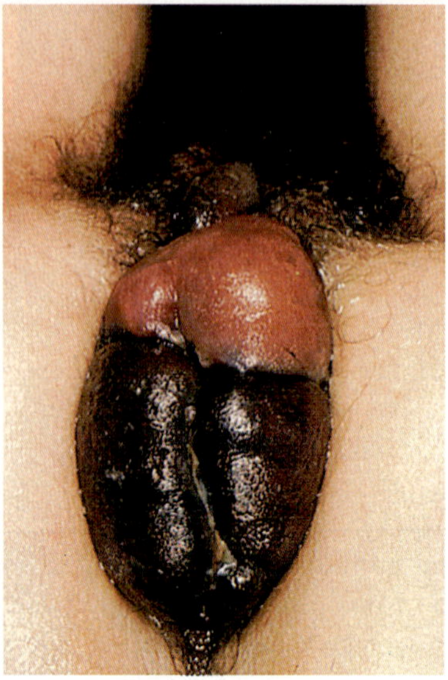

图 210 痔疮
Haemorrhoids

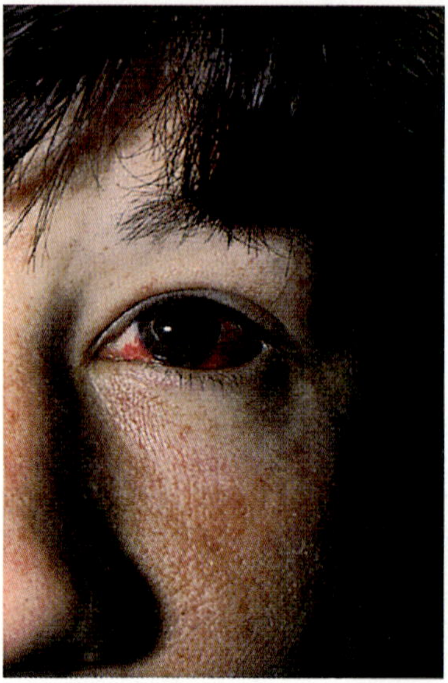

图 211 结膜下出血
Subconjunctival haemorrhages

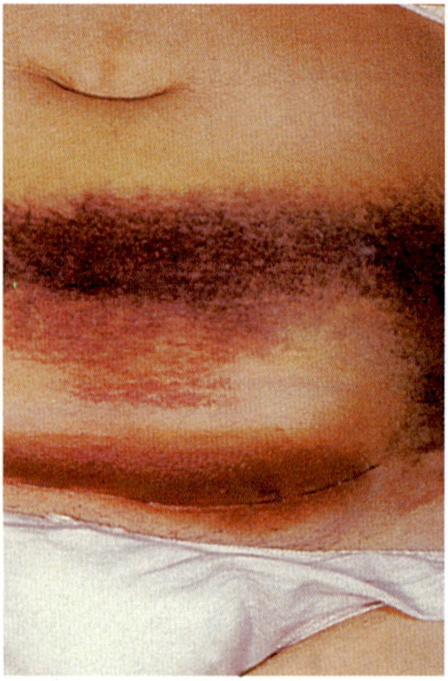

图 212 创口血肿和擦伤
Wound haematoma and bruising

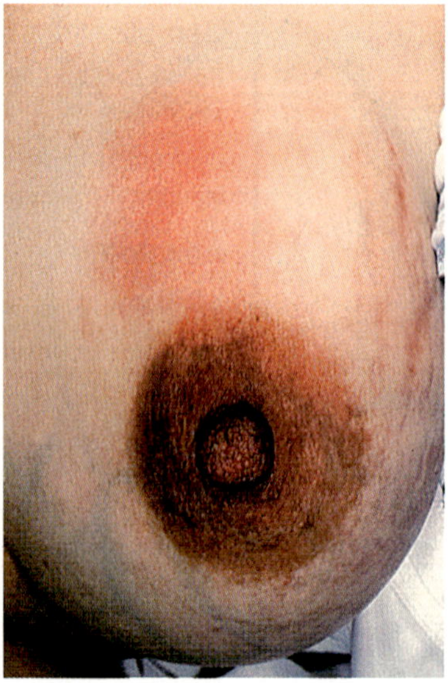

图 213 乳腺炎
Mastitis

随着妊娠过后，一旦觉得性生活舒适，性生活就可以重新开始。如果产妇已行会阴修补，则需要数周的时间。绝大多数由于妊娠而发生的解剖学变化可在2～4周内恢复正常。内分泌的变化则需更长的时间。恢复到能受孕的时间因人而异，如哺乳则可推迟数月。不哺乳的妇女可在产后4周内排卵，月经周期的恢复平均为58天。对全母乳喂养的妇女来说出现排卵和月经是很罕见的。然而单纯的母乳喂养并不是一种推荐的避孕方法。

激素法

在图 214 中可见一些典型的例子。复合的口服避孕药（combined oral contraceptive pill, COCP）应避免在哺乳期间使用，因为药物中的雌激素成分会抑制泌乳。由于在产褥期自然增加血栓形成的风险，不哺乳的妇女开始口服避孕药的时间不应早于产后3周。在通常情况下使用口服避孕药的禁忌证也需考虑到（如既往有血栓栓塞的疾病、脑血管意外和肝疾病）。

以孕激素为主的制剂（如仅含孕激素的药剂、孕激素的埋植剂）不影响泌乳，可即刻给予。但起初可导致不规律的阴道流血，而这在产褥期后是令人困惑及令人烦恼的事。

宫内避孕器

可在产褥期的任何时候置入节育器（图215、216）。一般来讲，放置节育器越早，脱落率越高，因此通常推迟至6周。含孕激素节育器（Mirena）具有较低的失败率（与口服避孕药相比），但可导致放置节育器后不规则流血3～6个月。更多传统的含铜线圈可导致月经过多和痛经，而且易于发生盆腔感染。带节育器失败增加了宫外孕或者早期流产/早产的机会。

26 Contraception after pregnancy

Following pregnancy, sexual activity may be resumed as soon as it is comfortable to do so. This may take several weeks if a woman has had a perineal repair. Most anatomical changes of pregnancy have regressed by 2-4 weeks. Endocrine changes take longer; return to fertility is variable and may be delayed for months by lactation. Non-lactating women may ovulate within 4 weeks of delivery, and return of menstruation occurs, on average, at 58 days. It is extremely rare for fully breastfeeding women to ovulate or menstruate. However, breastfeeding alone is not a recommended contraceptive method.

Hormonal methods

Some typical examples are shown in Fig 214. The combined oral contraceptive pill (COCP) should be avoided in breastfeeding women as the oestrogen content may suppress lactation. Non-lactating women may commence the COCP no sooner than 3 weeks postpartum due to the natural increase in thrombotic risk during the puerperium. The usual contraindications to the use of the COCP must also be considered (e.g. history of prior thromboembolism, cerebrovascular accident, liver disease).

Progestogen-based preparations (e.g. progestogen-only pill, progestogenic implants) do not interfere with lactation and can be started immediately. They may, however, cause erratic bleeding initially and this can be confusing and an annoyance in the postpartum period.

Intrauterine contraceptive devices

Insertion can be undertaken at any time in the puerperium (Figs 215, 216). In general, however, expulsion rates are higher when insertion is earlier and thus this is usually deferred until 6 weeks. The progestogen-based intrauterine system (Mirena) has a very low failure rate (comparable with the COCP), but can cause irregular bleeding for 3-6 months postinsertion. More traditional copper-based coils can cause menorrhagia and dysmenorrhoea and are associated with a higher risk of pelvic infection. Failure of the device increases the chances of an ectopic pregnancy or preterm miscarriage/labour.

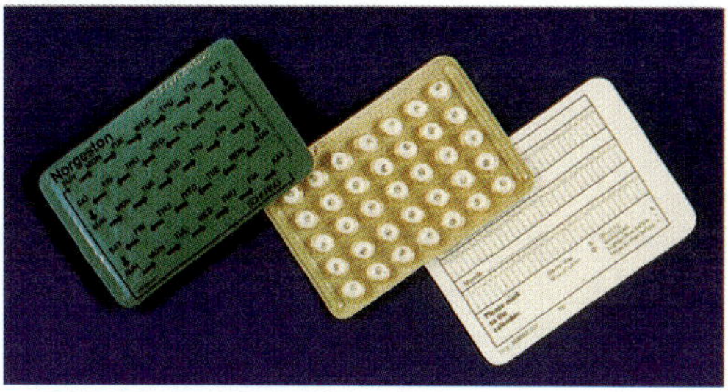

图 214　不同的避孕药
Various contraceptive pills

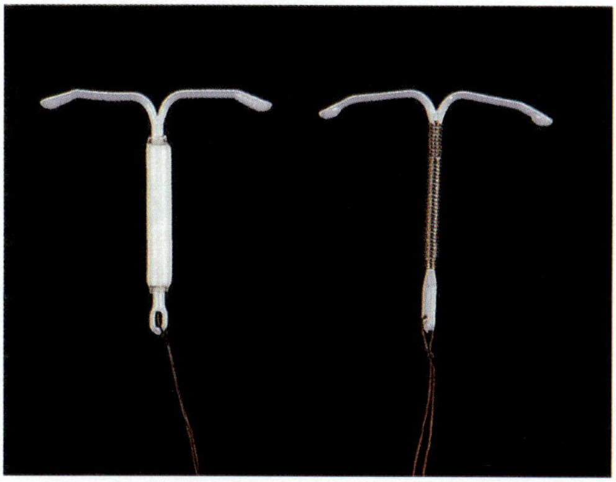

图 215　宫内避孕器
Intrautcrine contraceptive devices

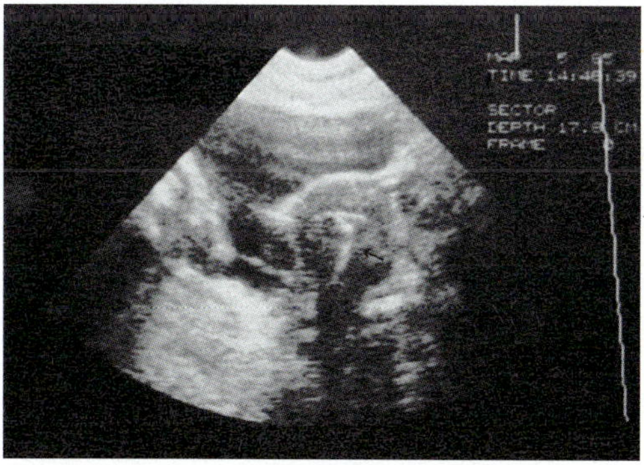

图 216　超声图像显示宫内避孕器
Ultrasound image showing an intrauterine contraceptive device

屏障法

避孕套（图217）是通常在产后使用的一种短期的避孕工具（比如直到哺乳期结束并且可给予复合避孕药，或直到产后6周可放置宫内节育器，或直到能行间期绝育手术）。在怀孕前使用隔膜（图 218）避孕的妇女在分娩后会需要不同的尺寸，可在产后 6 周重新评估。

绝育术

女性

对那些需要永久节育的妇女，在行剖宫产时可行输卵管闭塞术，虽然与距妊娠时间较长的绝育术（1∶300）相比其失败率明显增高（1∶200）。这可能是因为输卵管过厚和血管过于丰富。

女性的绝育术现通常在腹腔镜下完成。失败率约为1∶300。夹和环用于闭塞输卵管（图 219）。对那些在绝育术后怀孕的妇女，患宫外孕的风险相当地增加了。

绝育术应被视为不可逆的一个过程。仅有40%～60%的绝育术后再通可获得宫内孕。在腹腔镜下行绝育术时发生内脏损伤（如肠管）的比例是1∶1000，而这是威胁生命的并发症。

男性

男性绝育术与女性绝育术相比具有更多的优点，失败率低于10倍，也不需要全身麻醉，而且手术的并发症也较轻。当然这种情况不会控制女性的生育。

Barrier methods

The sheath (Fig 217) is commonly used as a short-term contraceptive in the puerperium (e.g. until breastfeeding ceases and the combined pill can be prescribed, or until an intrauterine contraceptive device can be inserted at 6 weeks, or until an interval sterilization is performed). Women who have used a diaphragm (Fig 218) before pregnancy may need a different size after childbirth; this can be reassessed after 6 weeks.

Sterilization

Female

Tubal occlusion for those women wanting permanent contraception can be performed at caesarean section, although a higher failure rate is quoted (1 in 200) than for sterilizations performed at a time distant to pregnancy (1 in 300). This is probably because of the greater thickness and vascularity of the tubes.

Female sterilization is more usually performed laparoscopically. The failure rate is quoted as 1 in 300. Clips or rings are used to occlude the fallopian tubes (Fig 219). For those women conceiving after sterilization, the risk of ectopic pregnancy is substantially increased.

Sterilization should be considered an irreversible procedure. Only 40-60% of sterilization reversals are followed by an intrauterine pregnancy. Visceral (e.g. bowel) damage during laparoscopic sterilization occurs in 1 in 1000 cases and is a life-threatening complication.

Male

Male sterilization has many advantages over female procedures. The failure rate is 10 times lower, no general anaesthetic is required and the surgical complications are less serious. It does not, of course, provide the woman with control over her fertility.

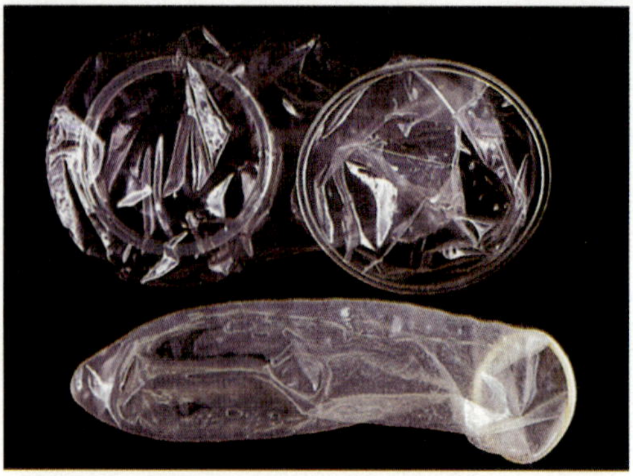

图 217　男用或女用避孕套
Male and female condoms

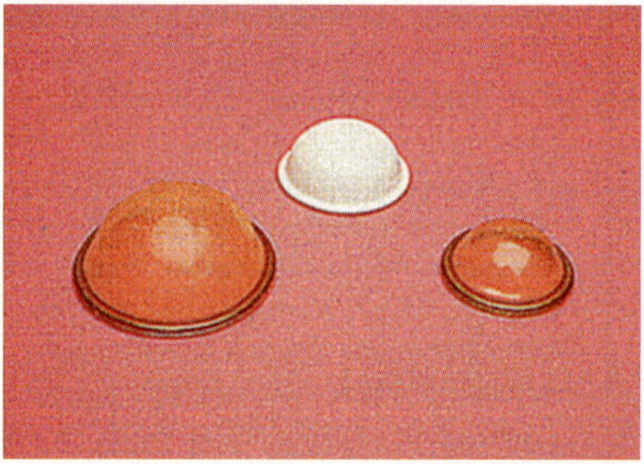

图 218　避孕隔膜和帽
Contraceptive diaphragms and caps

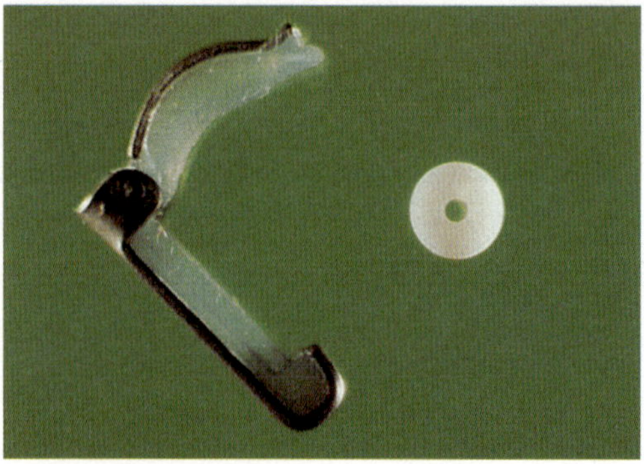

图 219　绝育夹和环
Sterilization clips and rings

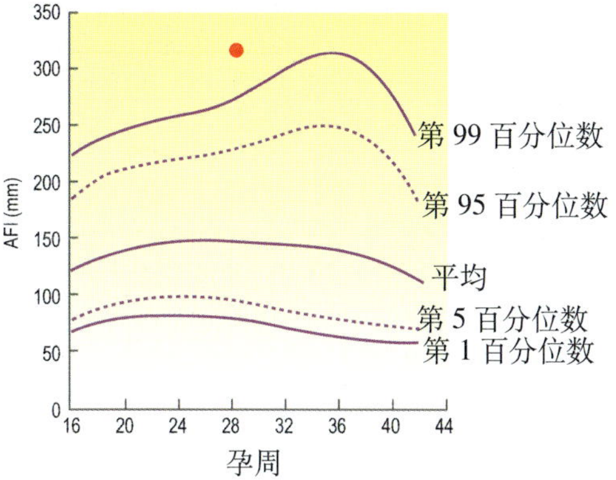

1. 该羊水指数（AFI）图中显示的是妊娠 28 周时的羊水量
a. 诊断是什么?
b. 写出四项诊断依据。
c. 写出相应的 2 个症状及体征。

This amniotic fluid index (AFI) chart shows the liquor volume of a pregnancy at 28 weeks' gestation.
a. What is the diagnosis?
b. Name four causes of this.
c. Name two symptoms and two signs associated with this diagnosis.

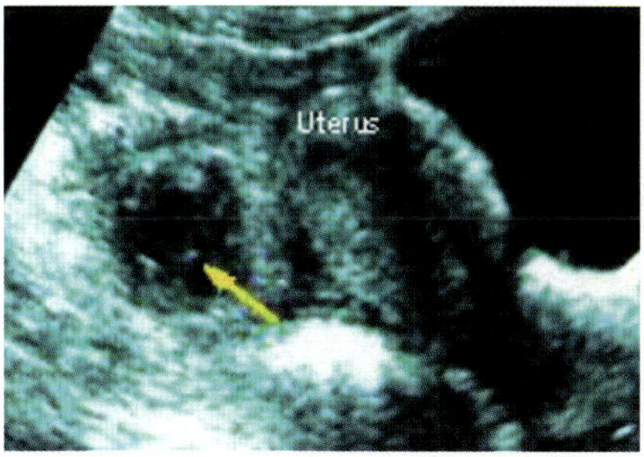

2. 该图为妊娠 7 周妇女的超声图像。该妇女停经 7 周，少量阴道流血，血清 hCG 值为 3500IU/L。
a. 诊断是什么?
b. 写出该疾病的四个高危因素。
c. 列举 3 种治疗选择。

This is an ultrasound scan of a woman with 7 weeks of amenorrhoea, minor vaginal bleeding and a serum hCG of 3500 IU/L.
a. What is the diagnosis?
b. Name four risk factors for this condition.
c. Give three treatment options.

3．该图显示的是从停经 8 周妇女宫腔内刮出的宫内容物。该妇女有阴道流血，血清 hCG 值为 80 000 IU/L。

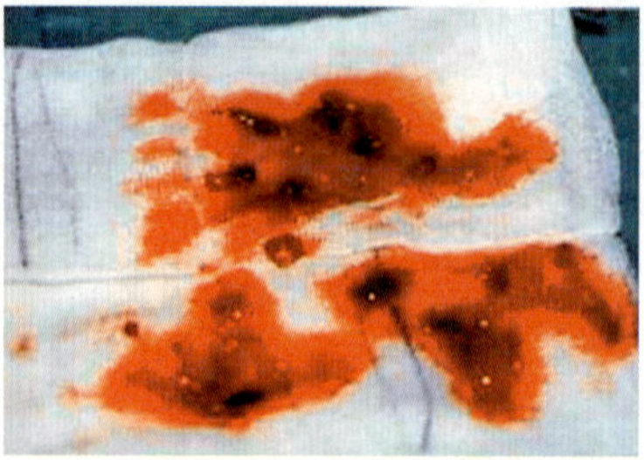

a．诊断是什么？

b．该妇女行超声检查可能会发现什么异常？

c．该患者应如何处置？

These are curettings removed from the uterus of a woman presenting at 8 weeks'amenorrhoea with vaginal bleeding and a serum hCG of 80 000 IU/L.

a．What is the diagnosis?

b．What might have been found on the ultrasound scan?

c．How would she be managed from this point onwards?

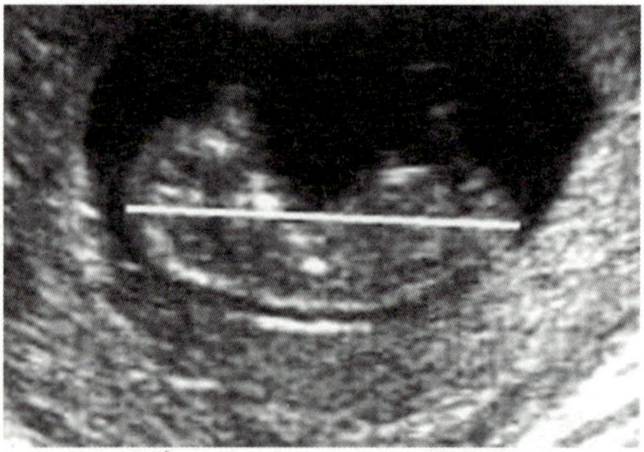

4．此图为妊娠 11 周时的超声图像。

a．图中所示的胎儿生物测量称为什么？

b．使用该径线判断妊娠周数的误差（± 2 个偏差）在于什么？

c．可用于描述妊娠 16 周时的 2 个测量径线是什么？

This is an ultrasound scan of an 11-week fetus.

a．What is this fetal biometric measurement called?

b．What is the error (i.e. ± 2 standard deviations) of the prediction of gestational age made using this measurement?

c．What two measurements can be used at 16 weeks' gestation to date a pregnancy?

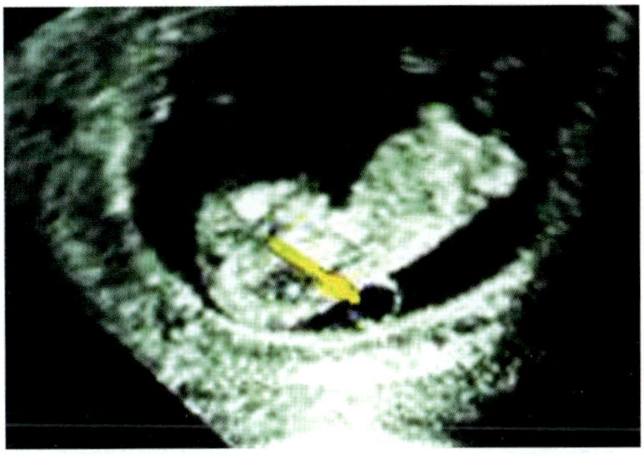

5．该图显示的是妊娠 10 周时的超声图像。
a．黄色箭头所指的是何种结构？
b．该结构何时初现？何时消失？
c．该结构的功能为何？

This ultrasound picture shows a fetus at 10 weeks' gestation.
a．What normal structure is the yellow arrow pointing to?
b．When does this first become visible and when does it disappear?
c．What is the function of this structure?

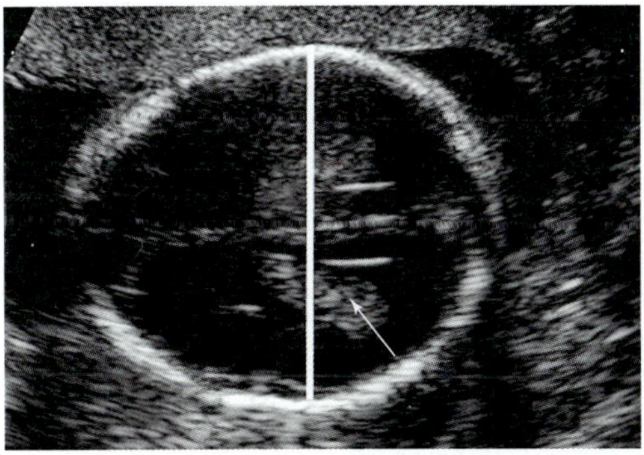

6．该超声图显示的是妊娠 20 周时通过胎头的横断面。
a．图中白线所测量的是何结构？
b．箭头所指的为何种颅内结构？
c．该结构有何功能？

This ultrasound picture shows a cross-section through the fetal head at 20 weeks' gestation.
a．What measurement is shown by the white line?
b．What intracranial structure is indicated by the arrow?
c．What function does this structure have?

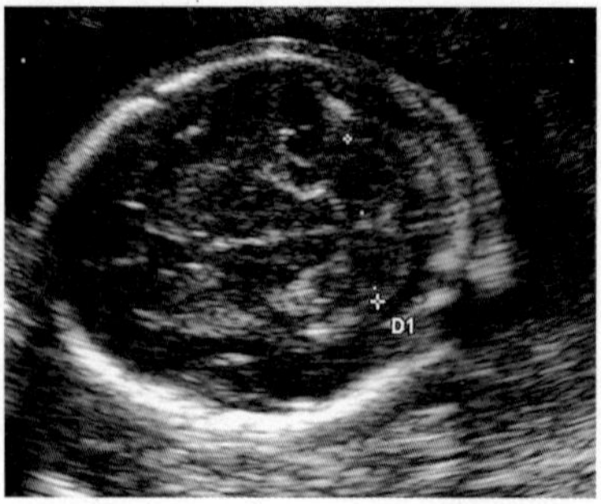

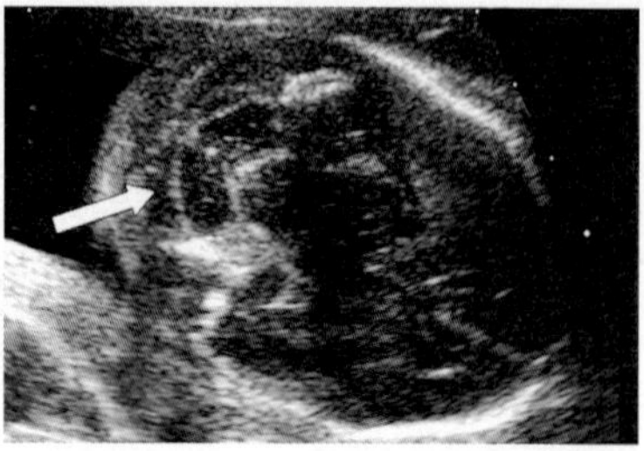

7．图 A 中的测径器和图 B 中的箭头所示的为胎儿脑内的同一结构。
a．该结构是什么？
b．两幅图中哪一个是正常的？
c．异常图中的胎儿可能出现哪些情况？

The calipers in image A and the arrow in image B are identifying the same structure within the fetal brain.

a．What structure is this?

b．Which of the two images is normal?

c．What condition might the fetus with the abnormal image have?

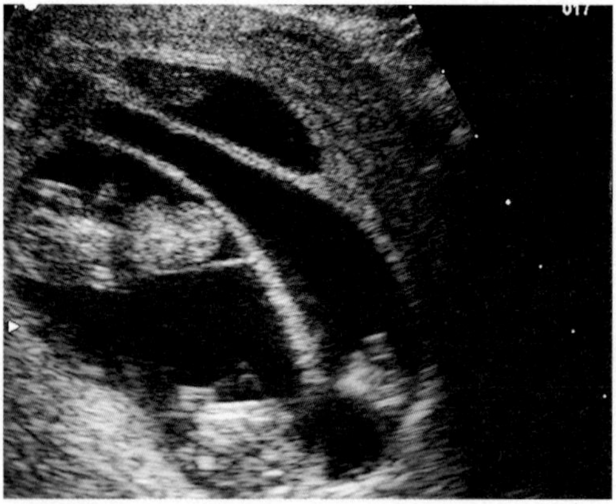

8．该超声图为大约妊娠 9 周时所摄。
a．该超声图显示的是什么？
b．出现该情况可能的原因是什么？
c．写出该种妊娠最有可能发生的 6 种并发症。

This ultrasound picture was taken at approximately 9 weeks' gestation.

a．What does this ultrasound picture show?

b．How might this condition have been caused?

c．Name six complications more likely in this pregnancy?

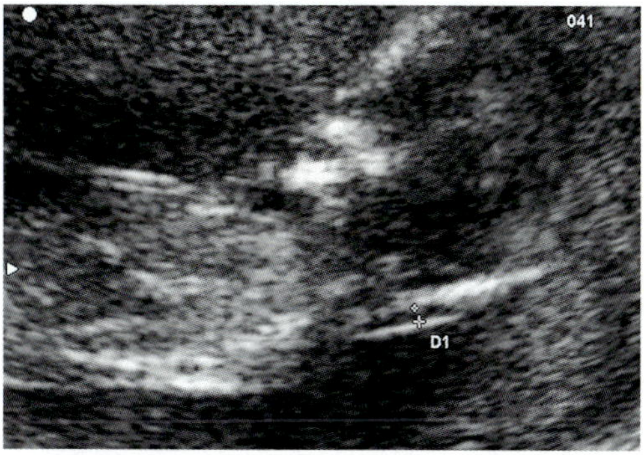

9．该超声图摄于妊娠 12 周时。

a．被测量部位的是何名字？

b．测量该处的目的是什么？

c．还可进行什么其他检查方法？何时进行？

This ultrasound image was taken at 12 weeks' gestation.

a. What is the name of the area being measured?

b. What is the main indication for taking this measurement?

c. What alternative tests might be offered and when?

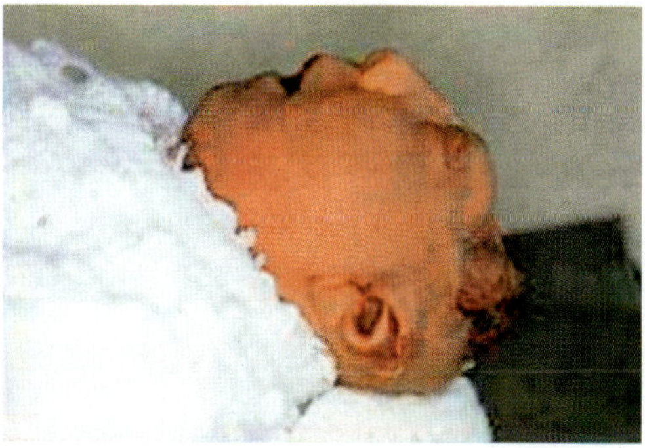

10．该婴儿的母亲拒绝所有形式的产前筛查，妊娠 33 周时耻上宫高达 39cm。

a．此为何种畸形？

b．产前应该进行什么检查有可能发现？

c．为何该产妇子宫大小超过相应妊娠周数？

This baby was born to a woman who declined all forms of antenatal screening and presented at 33 weeks with a symphysiofundal height of 39 cm.

a. What abnormality is shown here?

b. How might it have been detected antenatally?

c. What caused her to have a large-for-dates uterus?

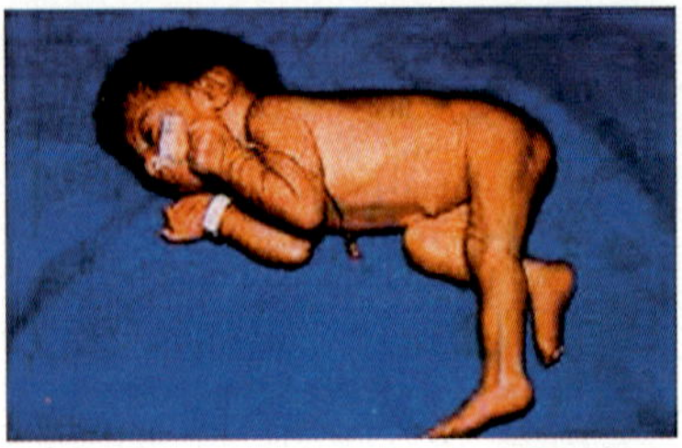

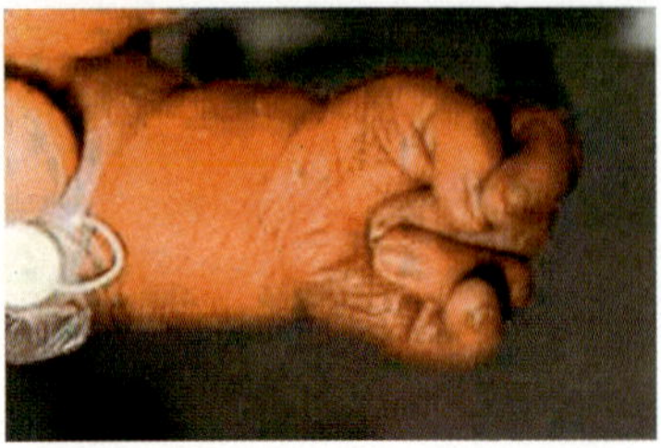

11．该患儿有生长受限，关节挛缩，手呈指交叉握拳状，妊娠 20 周时行超声检查提示双侧脉络膜囊肿。

a．诊断是什么?

b．该患儿染色体核型为什么?

c．列举另外三种与该病有关的畸形。

This baby was born with growth restriction, joint contractures and overlapping fingers with clenched fists. Antenatal scans had shown bilateral choroids plexus cysts at 20 weeks' gestation.

a．What is the diagnosis?

b．What would the karyotype be?

c．Name three other abnormalities associated with this condition.

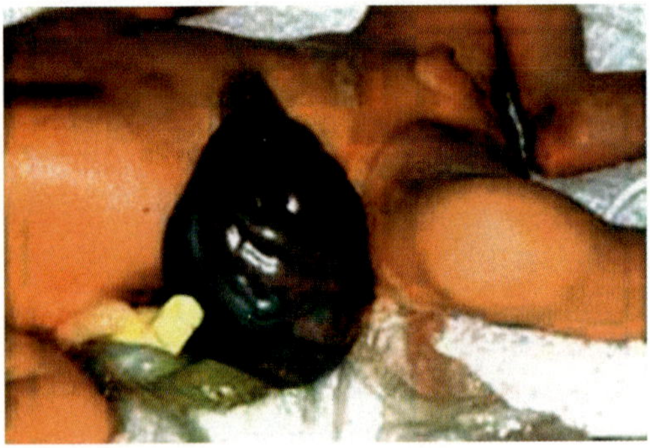

12．该足月儿的父母在妊娠 20 周时拒绝做详细的超声检查。

a．诊断为什么?

b．如果该情况在产前通过超声检查出来，应进行何种检查以确诊?

c．此种畸形常见什么症候群和情况?

This baby was born at term to a couple who had declined detailed ultrasound scanning at 20 weeks' gestation.

a．What is the diagnosis?

b．If this had been detected antenatally by ultrasound what diagnostic test might have been offered?

c．What syndromes and conditions are associated with this anomaly?

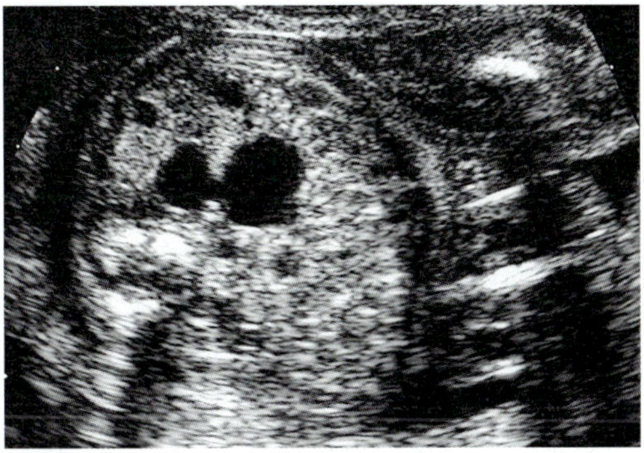

13．该超声图像摄于妊娠 21 周，显示的是通过胎儿腹部的横断面。
a．图中所见的特征性图像称为什么?
b．何种结构畸形可引起该情况?
c．该异常常见于何种疾病?

This ultrasound image, taken at 21 weeks' gestation, shows a cross-section through the fetal abdomen.
a．What is the name of the abnormal ultrasound feature shown here?
b．What structural abnormality causes this to occur?
c．With which syndrome is it commonly associated?

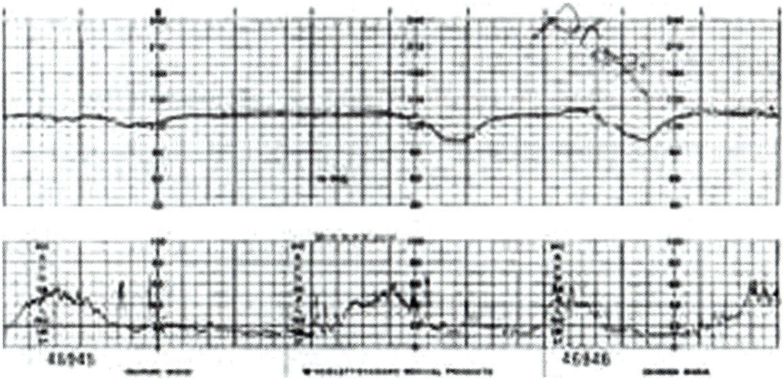

14．该胎心产力图是妊娠 38 周妇女临产,宫口开大 2cm 时。胎心基线为 140 次 / 分。
a．列出图中所示的三个异常征象。
b．你如何描述该胎心图?
c．人工破膜后你认为能发现什么状况?

This cardiotocogram (CTG) is taken from a woman in labour at 38 weeks' gestation, at 2 cm dilatation. The baseline rate is 140 beats/min.
a．Name the three abnormal features shown here.
b．How would you describe this CTG?
c．What might you expect to find if you artificially ruptured the membranes?

15．该女孩身材矮小。

a．诊断为什么？

b．列出其他四种特征。

c．产前超声检查最可能发现什么情况？

This young girl is of short stature.

a．What is the diagnosis?

b．Name four other characteristic features.

c．What would be the most common antenatal ultrasound finding?

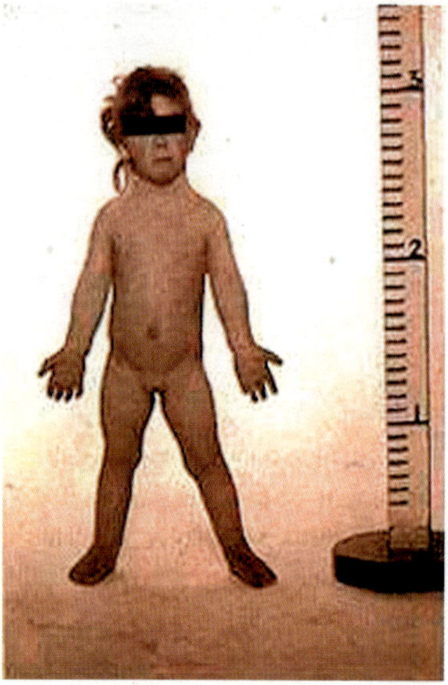

16．图示的婴儿刚出生数小时。

a．图中所示的是何问题？

b．最可能的分娩方式是什么？

c．大多数情况下此症状是永久性的吗？

This baby is only a few hours old.

a．What problem is illustrated here?

b．What was the most likely method of delivery?

c．In most cases, is this permanent?

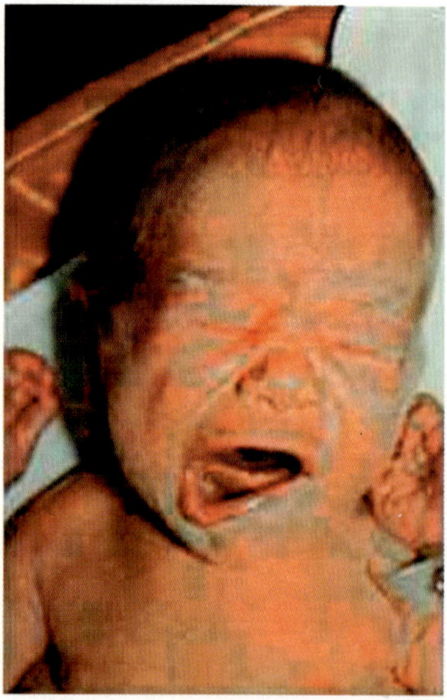

17．该足月儿出生时有缺氧、酸中毒，随后在新生儿期有癫痫发作。

a．该临床症状称为什么？

b．正在进行的是何种检查？

c．如果该婴儿进一步发作，其预后如何？

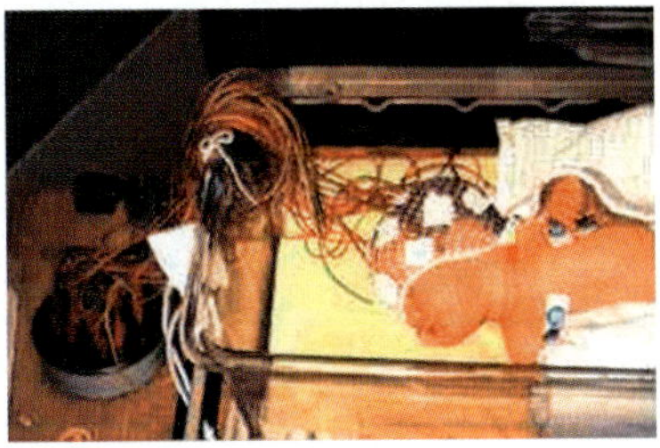

This term baby was born hypoxic and acidotic and subsequently developed seizures in the neonatal period.

a．What is the clinical syndrome called?

b．What investigation is being performed?

c．What is the prognosis if the baby suffers seizures?

18．该婴儿早产后数天出现腹部膨隆，其早产原因为其母亲先兆子痫恶化。

a．诊断为什么？

b．何种产前治疗可以减少该情况的发病率？

c．如何进行保守治疗？

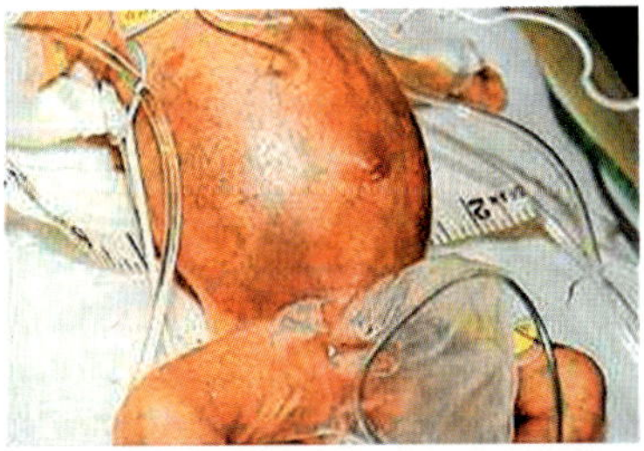

This infant developed a distended abdomen a few days after it was delivered prematurely for worsening maternal pre-eclampsia.

a．What is the diagnosis?

b．Which antenatal treatment can reduce the incidence of this condition?

c．How would you manage this conservatively?

19．该新生儿为刚刚选择性剖宫产出生。

a．该图显示的是何种先天畸形？

b．该情况属何种缺陷？

c．哪两种影像学技术可用于妊娠期间以发现此种结构？

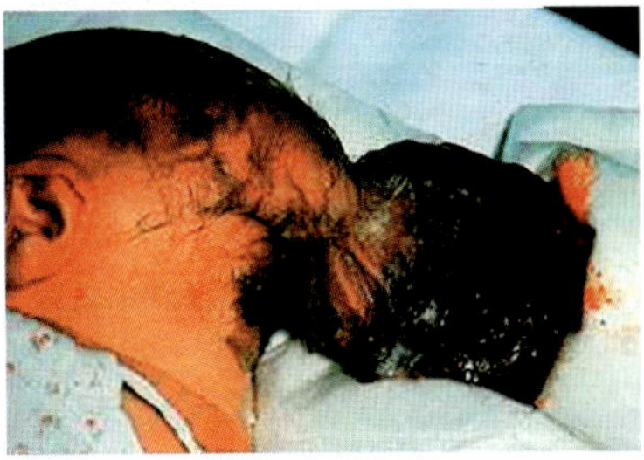

This newborn infant has recently been delivered by elective caesarean section.

a．What congenital abnormality is present?

b．To which group of defects does this belong?

c．Which two imaging techniques would be useful in assessing this structure during pregnancy?

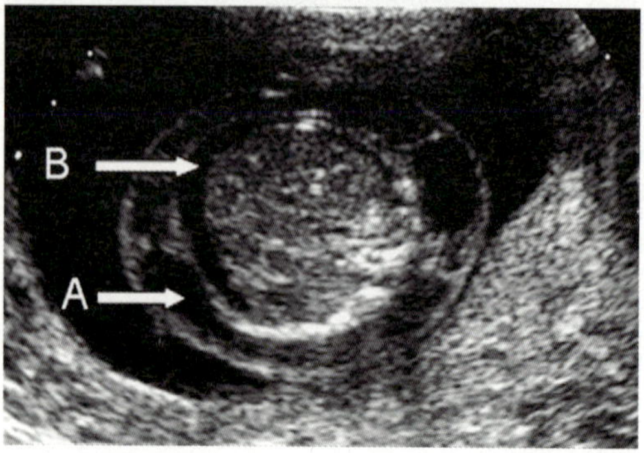

20．该超声图摄于妊娠22周，显示的是胎儿腹部的横断面。

a．诊断为什么？

b．箭头A和箭头B所示的各为何异常？

c．列举5种病因。

This ultrasound image was taken at 22 weeks' gestation and shows a cross-section through the fetal abdomen.

a. What is the diagnosis?

b. What abnormalities are indicated by the arrows A and B?

c. Name five causes.

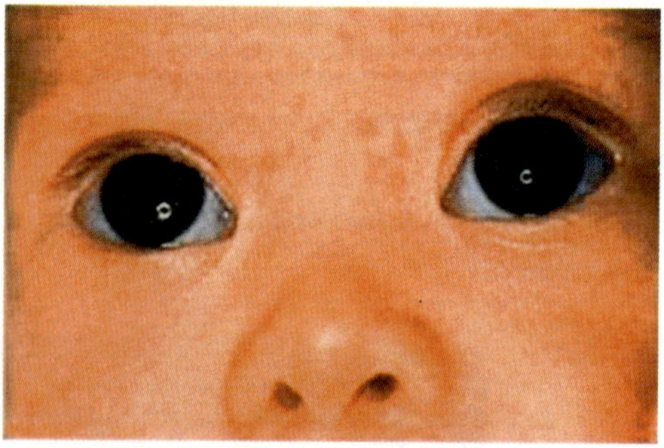

21．该婴儿于新生儿期被发现张力降低。仔细的检查显示轻微的异常征象。

a．列举图中所示的三种面部异常征象。

b．最可能的诊断为什么？

c．再次妊娠时该情况的再发风险是什么？

This baby was found to be hypotonic in the newborn period. Close examination revealed subtle dysmorphic features.

a. Name three abnormal facial features shown here.

b. What is the likely diagnosis?

c. What is the recurrence risk for this condition in a future pregnancy?

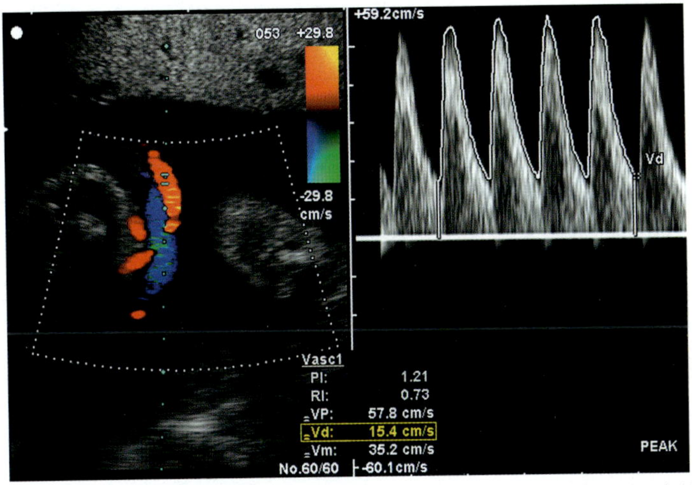

22．图为妊娠 31 周的妇女，由于先兆子痫入院以观察及行胎儿监护。

a．正进行的是何种产前检查？

b．图中所示的波形显示的是什么？

c．为什么在先兆子痫这可能是异常的？

A woman at 31 weeks' gestation is admitted with pre-eclampsia for observation and fetal surveillance.

a．Which antenatal investigation is being performed here?

b．What does the waveform pattern show?

c．Why might this be abnormal in pre-eclampsia?

23．该婴儿难产，体重 4.5kg。

a．图中所示的是何种产伤？

b．此种产伤产生的机理为什么？

c．除外胎儿大小，与该情况相关的其他高危因素是什么？

This baby was born weighing 4.5 kg following a difficult delivery.

a．What birth injury is shown in this image?

b．What is the underlying nature and mechanism of the injury?

c．Apart from fetal size, what other risk factor is associated with this condition?

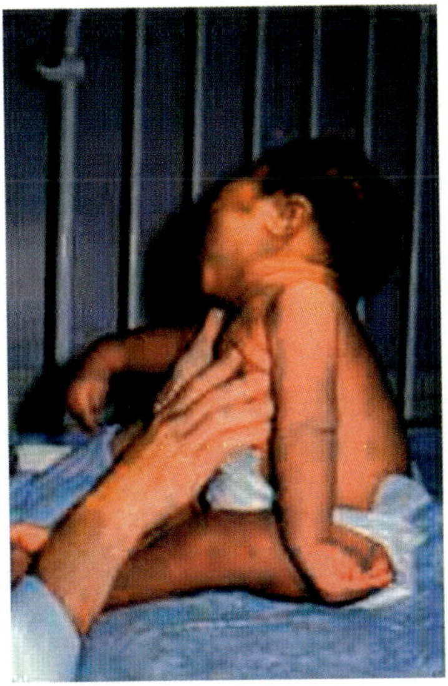

24．该孕妇妊娠 14 周，伴广泛分布的泡状皮疹。

a．诊断为什么？

b．该妊娠期对胎儿的危险是什么？

c．对母亲的主要危险是什么？

This woman presents at 14 weeks' gestation with a widespread vesicular rash.

a．What is the diagnosis?

b．What is the risk to the fetus at this stage of pregnancy?

c．What is the main maternal risk?

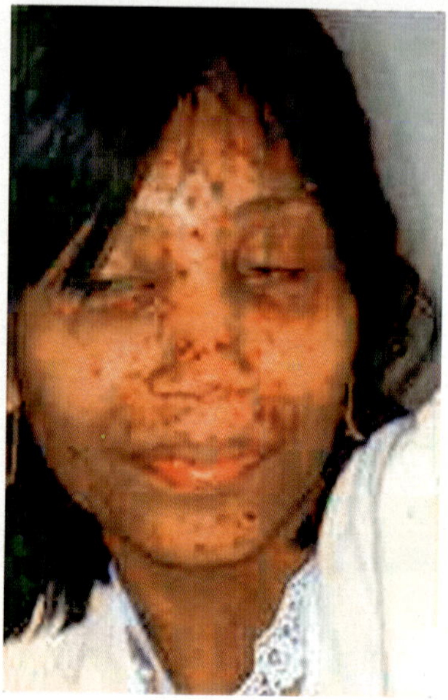

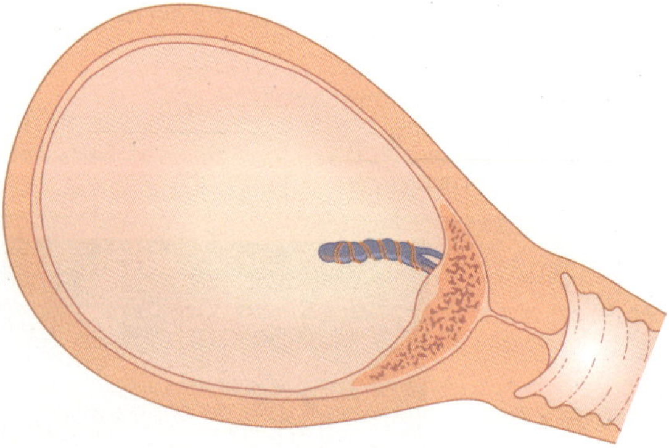

25．该图显示的是异常的胎盘植入。

a．诊断为什么？分级为什么？

b．列出该病的两种临床表现。

c．列出该病的三种高危因素。

This line drawing shows an abnormal placental implantation.

a．What is the diagnosis and grade?

b．Name two ways in which this can present.

c．Name three risk factors for this problem.

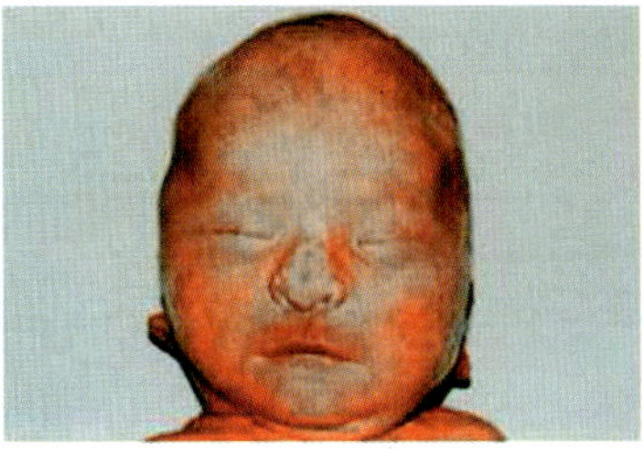

26．该死产儿有鼻和耳畸形。
a．此种面部异常称为什么？
b．引起此外貌的原因是什么？
c．尸检时肺部检查可发现什么？

This stillborn infant was found to have a malformed nose and abnormal ears.
a．What name is given to this pattern of facial dysmorphism?
b．What causes this appearance?
c．What was found on examination of the lungs at postmortem?

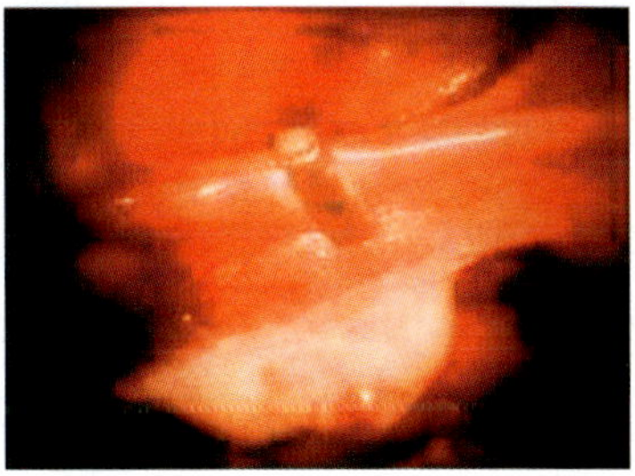

27．该图摄于腹腔镜检查时。
a．现已实施的是哪一步骤？
b．列出该步骤的两个并发症。
c．如在剖宫产手术过程中实施该步骤，其失败率是多少？

This image was taken at the time of laparoscopy.
a．What procedure has been performed?
b．Name two complications of this procedure.
c．What is the failure rate of this procedure if it is performed at caesarean section?

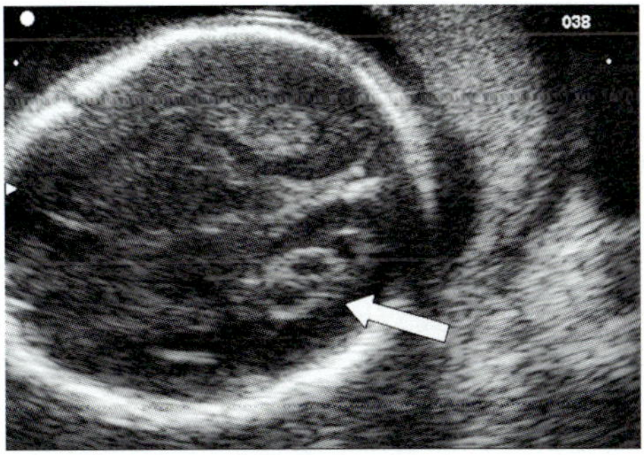

28．该超声图显示的是妊娠 20 周时通过胎儿头部的横断面。
a．箭头所示的是何种异常？
b．与此相关的最常见的染色体畸形是什么？
c．该病在正常妊娠中的发生率是多少？

This ultrasound scan shows a cross-section through the fetal head at 20 weeks' gestation.
a．What abnormalities are shown by the arrow?
b．Which chromosomal abnormalities are most commonly found in association with these?
c．How common are they in normal pregnancies?

29. 该新生儿有明显的产伤。

a. 该婴儿是如何分娩的?

b. 第二产程中该患儿的胎方位是什么?

c. 列出能发生在此分娩方式中的其他三种产伤。

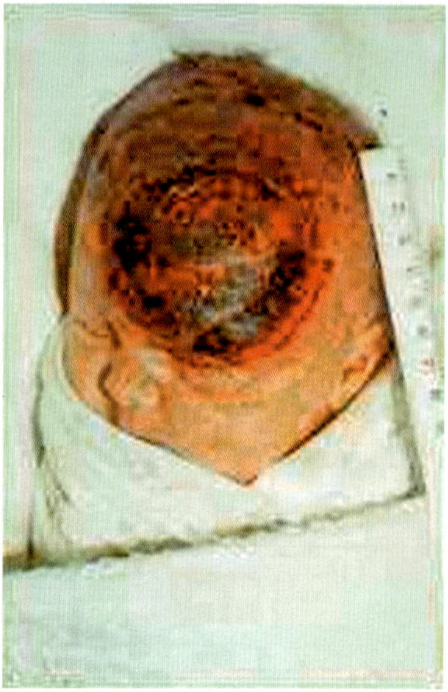

This newborn baby has suffered a significant birth injury.

a. How was this baby delivered?

b. What was the position of the fetal head during second stage?

c. Name three other injuries that can occur with this mode of delivery.

30. 该新生儿于妊娠 39 周出生，体重 4.6kg。

a. 用何术语描述该新生儿的外观?

b. 造成此现象发生的潜在母体因素是什么?

c. 列出三个很可能发生的新生儿并发症。

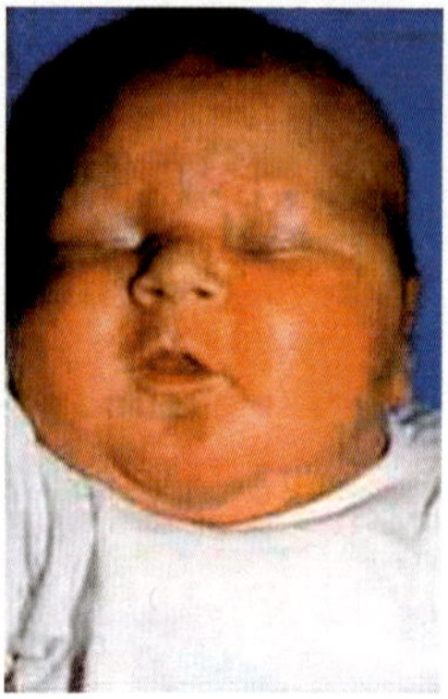

This newborn baby weighed 4.6 kg at 39 weeks' gestation.

a. What term is used to describe this appearance?

b. What underlying maternal condition has caused this to occur?

c. Name three neonatal complications that are more likely.

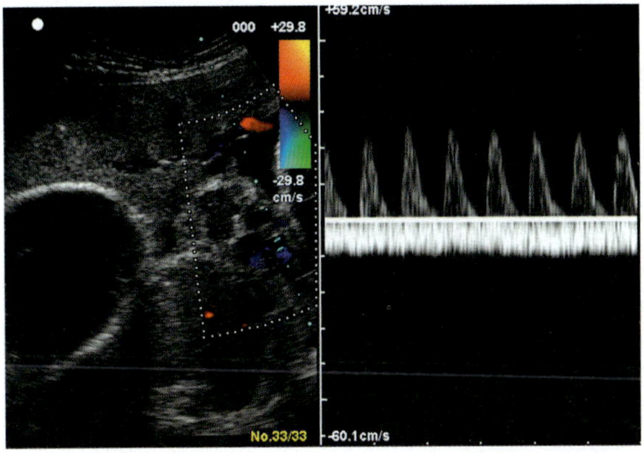

31．该图为妊娠 35 周生长受限胎儿的脐动脉多普勒记录图像。
a．该图说明了什么问题？
b．产生该现象最可能的原因是什么？
c．你如何处置该病例？

This umbilical artery Doppler recording was performed on a growth-restricted fetus at 35 weeks' gestation.
a．What does it show?
b．What is the likely cause of this?
c．How would you manage this case?

32．此新生儿为 4 天龄。
a．用何术语描述该新生儿的外观？
b．列出两种能导致该症状的性传播疾病。
c．分别列出对婴儿和对产妇的两种治疗方案。

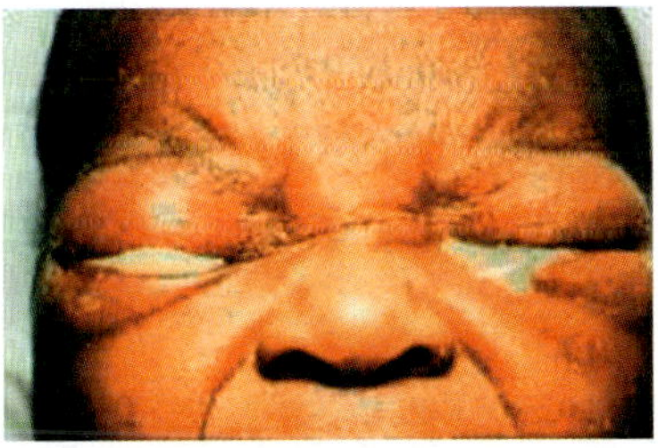

This newborn infant is 4 days old.
a．What is the term given to this appearance?
b．Name two sexually transmitted diseases that can cause it.
c．Name two management strategies for the baby and two for the mother.

33．此先天畸形在分娩后即出现。
a．这称为什么？
b．列出两种可以在该婴儿身上发现的两种情况。
c．最初的治疗是什么？

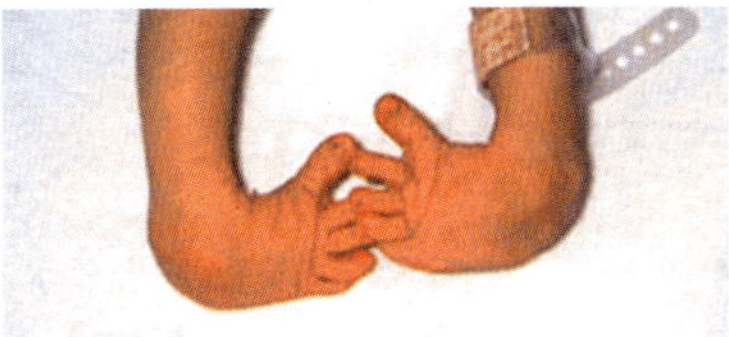

This congenital abnormality was noted immediately after delivery.
a．What is it called?
b．Name two conditions that might also be found in the baby.
c．What is the initial management?

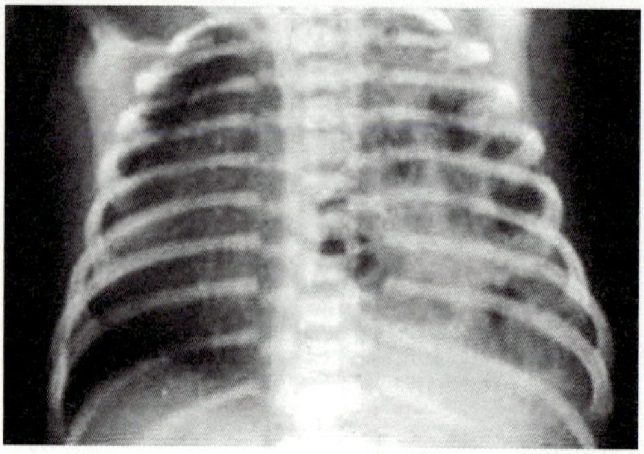

34．该片为出现呼吸窘迫的足月儿分娩后立即拍摄的 X 线胸片，图中显示心脏右移，通气很困难。

a．诊断为什么？

b．妊娠过程中行超声检查可发现哪些特征性表现？

c．如果是一个独立的疾病，患儿的存活率是多少？

This neonatal chest X-ray was performed on a term baby with respiratory distress immediately after delivery. The heart was found to be shifted to the right and ventilation proved to be very difficult.

a．What is the diagnosis?

b．What are the characteristic ultrasound findings during pregnancy?

c．If this is an isolated lesion, what proportion of these babies will survive?

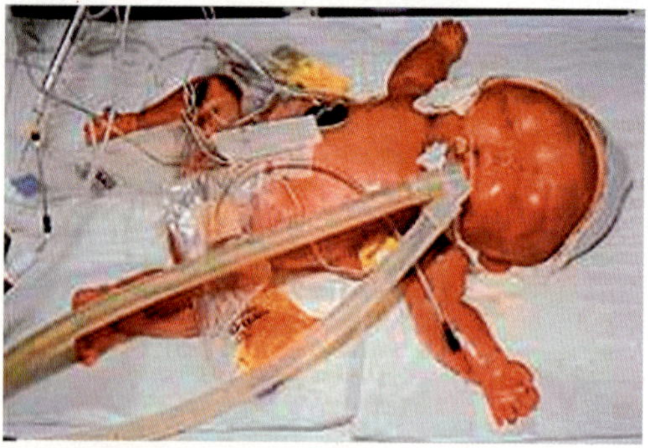

35．该新生儿表现为浮肿、心衰、腹水和肺水肿。

a．该表现称为什么？

b．50 年前该表现最常见的原因是什么？

c．列出另外四种病因。

This newborn infant is oedematous and has cardiac failure, ascites and pulmonary oedema.

a．What is this appearance called?

b．What was the most common cause 50 years ago?

c．Name four other causes.

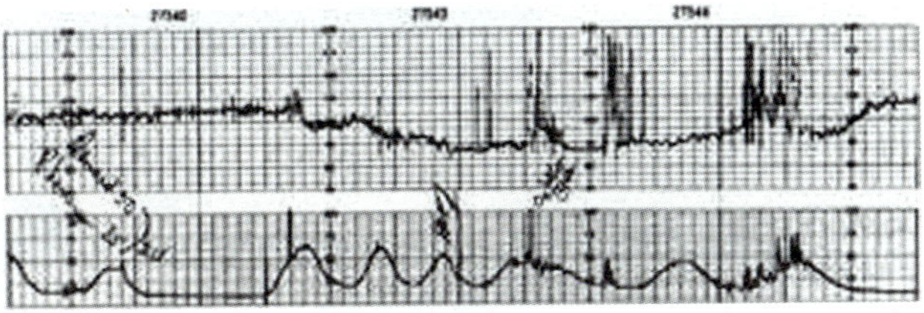

36．图为给予催产素的产程中产妇的胎心产力图，胎心基线为140次/分。

a．通过此图你能发现何种异常?

b．最可能的原因是什么?

c．你应采取哪三种急救措施?

This cardiotocogram (CTG) is taken from a woman in labour receiving oxytocin. The baseline heart rate has been 140 beats/min during the day.

a．What abnormality is seen on this CTG?

b．What is the most likely cause?

c．What three first-aid measures would you perform?

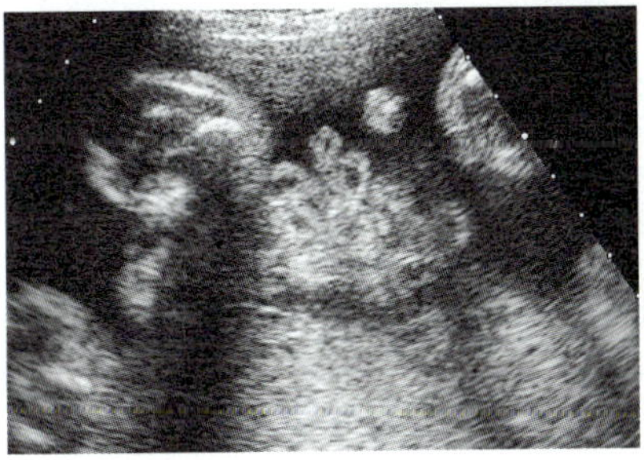

37．此图显示的是妊娠20周时常规产前超声检查，图示的是肠管自由漂浮于羊膜腔中。

a．诊断为什么?

b．最主要的鉴别诊断为什么?

c．列出这两种情况的两条鉴别要点。

This image was taken at the time of a 20-week routine detailed ultrasound scan. It shows loops of bowel floating free in the amniotic cavity.

a．What is the diagnosis?

b．What is the main differential diagnosis?

c．Name the two features that distinguish these two conditions.

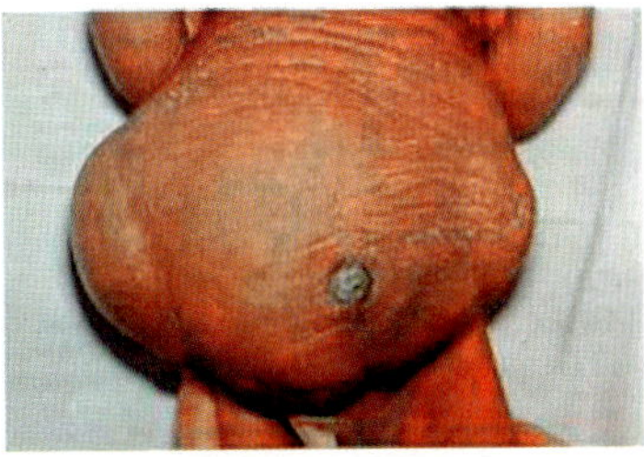

38．图为新生儿的腹部图片。

a．该表现称为什么?

b．引起该现象最常见的病因是什么?

c．最重要的后果是什么?

This is an image of a newborn abdomen.

a．What is this appearance called?

b．What condition most commonly gives rise to this appearance?

c．What is the most important consequence?

39．此新生儿出生即有脚趾部分截断。

a．引起此种畸形最可能的原因是什么？

b．列出该致畸因素可能引起的另外三种先天缺陷。

c．再次妊娠发生该畸形的风险是多少？

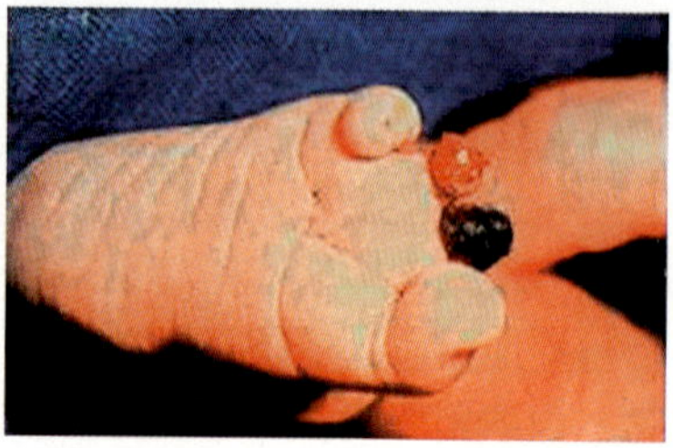

This newborn infant was born with partially amputated toes.

a．What is the most likely cause for this abnormality?

b．Name three other congenital defects that can be caused by the same process.

c．What is the recurrence risk for a future pregnancy?

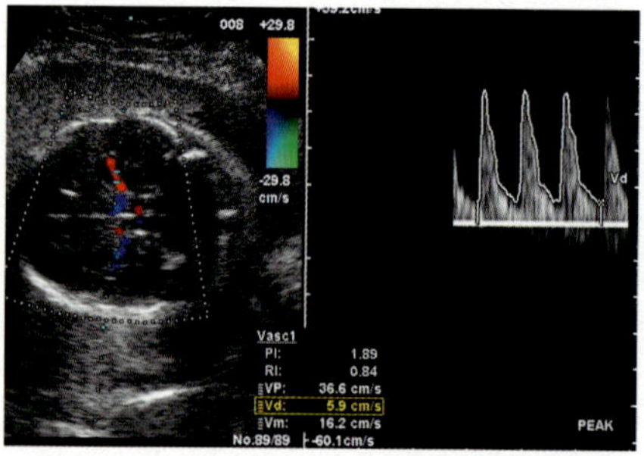

40．该图显示的是产前多普勒检查。

a．研究的是哪个胎儿血管？

b．在严重生长受限胎儿血流阻力发生什么情况？

c．在贫血胎儿该血管的血流如何？

This image shows an antenatal Doppler waveform study.

a．Which fetal blood vessel is being studied?

b．What happens to the resistance to blood flow in a severely growth-restricted fetus?

c．What happens to the blood flow in this vessel in anaemic fetuses?

41．此对双胞胎于妊娠 36 周出生。

a．如何描述他们的生长情况？

b．列出两种可以导致该现象的情况。

c．列出小胎儿出生后可能发生的四种并发症。

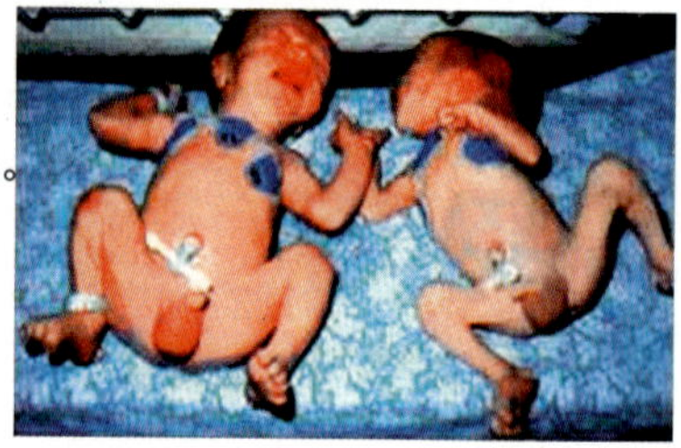

This pair of twins was born at 36 weeks' gestation.

a．How would you describe their growth?

b．Name two conditions that could lead to this appearance.

c．Name four complications the smaller twin might experience after birth.

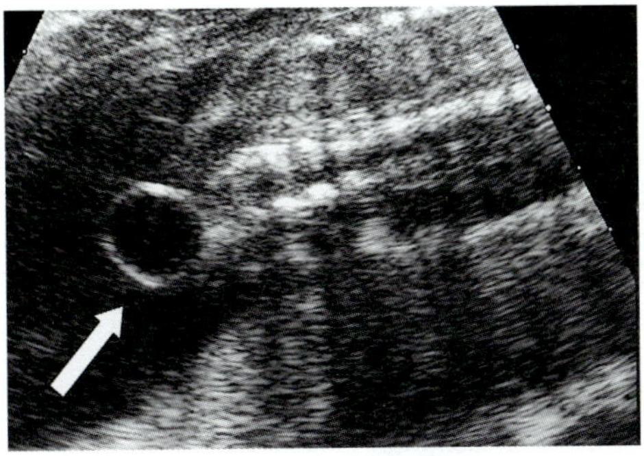

42．该超声图摄于妊娠 20 周。
a．白色箭头所示的是何种畸形？
b．另外列出两个与该畸形相关的特征。
c．若不经过预防性治疗，再次妊娠发生该畸形的危险有多大？

This ultrasound image was taken at 20 weeks' gestation.
a．What abnormality is the white arrow pointing to?
b．Name two other features that can be found in association with this defect.
c．What is the recurrence risk in a future pregnancy without any preventative treatment?

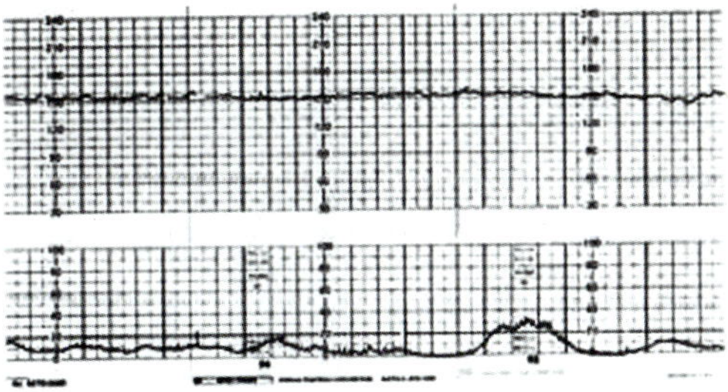

43．该图为妊娠 39 周孕妇的胎心图。该孕妇主诉胎动减少 3 天，轻度腹部紧缩感，胎心基线为 140 次 / 分，临床给予处置前胎心图如此又持续一个小时。
a．如何描述该胎心图？
b．如何处置该患者？
c．如行脐动静脉血气分析，你认为会发现什么？

This cardiotocogram (CTG) is taken from a woman at 39 weeks' gestation who complained of reduced fetal movements for 3 days prior to admission and mild tightenings. The baseline is 140 beats/min and the CTG continued like this for another hour before action was taken.
a．How would you describe this CTG?
b．How would you manage the case?
c．What would you expect to find on blood gas evaluation of the umbilical artery and vein?

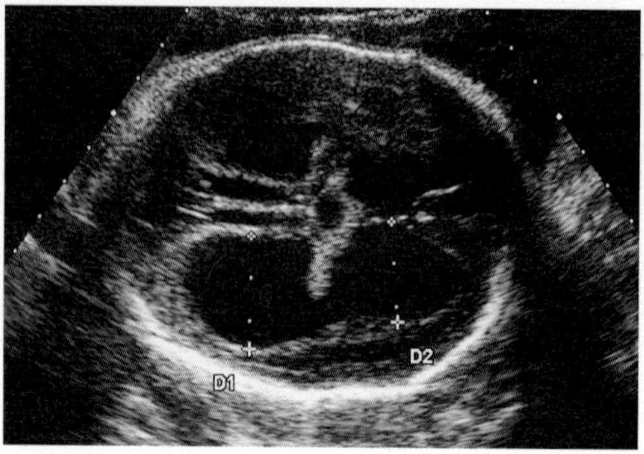

44．图为妊娠 21 周常规超声检查。

a．测径器测量的是何结构？

b．该表现称为什么？

c．列出三种原因。

This scan was performed routinely at 21 weeks' gestation.

a．What structures are the calipers measuring?

b．What is this appearance called?

c．Name three causes.

45．该图为新生儿前脑冠状面超声图像。

a．从该扫描中可发现何异常？

b．写出两个可导致该情况的妊娠并发症。

c．写出该患儿的两种结局。

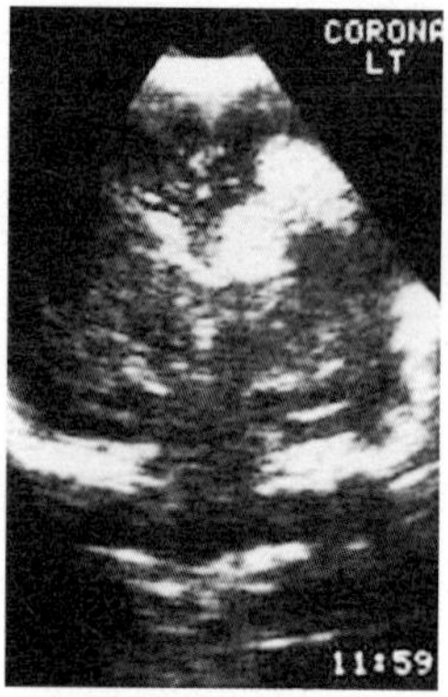

This ultrasound picture shows a coronal section through a newborn forebrain.

a．What abnormality is visible on this scan?

b．Name two pregnancy complications that can lead to this.

c．Name two consequences for the baby.

46．该新生儿经阴道分娩，因其母亲筋疲力尽导致第二产程延长。

a．该婴儿是如何经阴道分娩出的?

b．写出采用该分娩方式的另外两个指征。

c．采用该分娩方式可引起哪三种并发症?

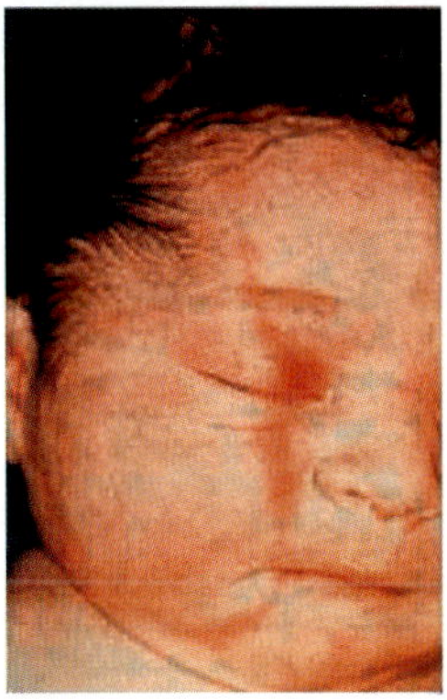

This baby was born vaginally following a prolonged second stage of labour due to maternal exhaustion.

a．How was this baby delivered?

b．Name two other indications for this procedure.

c．What three complications can result from this mode of delivery?

47．这些染色体处于细胞分裂中期，取材自绒毛活检样本的单细胞。

a．你如何报告该胎儿的染色体核型?

b．此种染色体异常称为什么?

c．写出该病的五个特征。

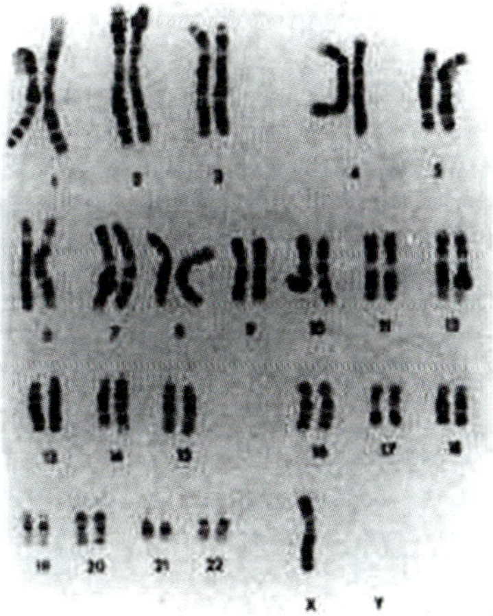

This spread of chromosomes in metaphase was taken from a single cell at chorionic villus sampling.

a．How would you report the fetal karyotype?

b．What name is given to this chromosomal abnormality?

c．Name five features of this condition.

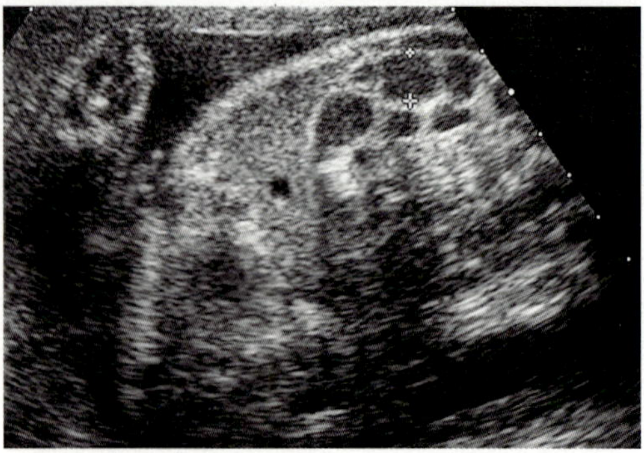

48．该超声图显示的是胎儿肾的纵切面。

a．如何描述此肾？

b．哪两个征象可以确认胎儿生成胎尿？

c．如对侧肾正常，最可能的诊断为什么？

This ultrasound image shows a fetal kidney in longitudinal view.

a．How would you describe this kidney?

b．What two features on scan would reassure you that the fetus is producing urine?

c．What would be the most likely diagnosis if the contralateral kidney appears normal?

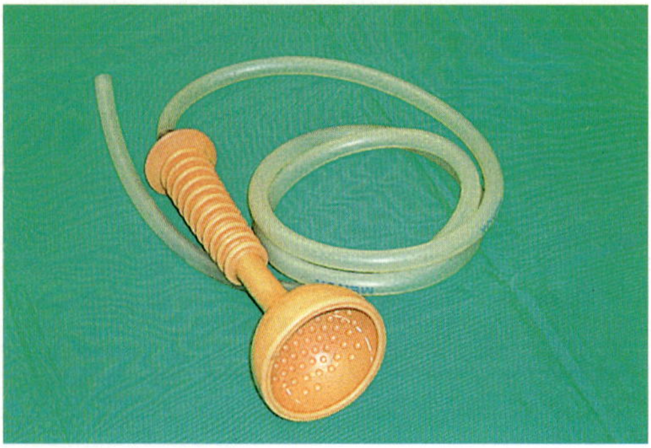

49．此器具通常在产房可见。

a．此器具称为什么？

b．此器具可否用于持续性枕后位导致的第二产程延长？证明你的回答。

c．在胎儿的何种医学情况是此器具使用的禁忌证？

This instrument is commonly found on the labour ward.

a．What is this instrument?

b．Can it be used for failure to progress in second stage due to a persistent occipitoposterior position? Justify your answer.

c．Which medical conditions in the fetus contraindicate its use?

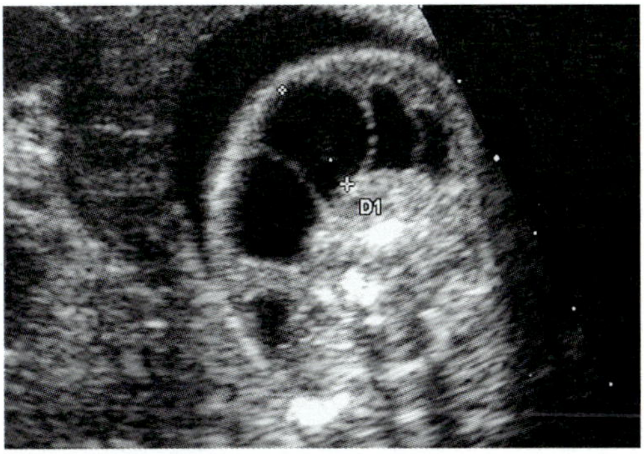

50．该超声图显示的是通过妊娠 16 周胎儿颈部的横切面。

a．图中显示的是何种异常？

b．列举一个可导致该表现的疾病。

c．你将提供进行什么附加的检查？

This ultrasound image shows a cross-section through the fetal neck at 16 weeks' gestation.

a．What abnormality is shown here?

b．Name one condition that can give rise to this appearance.

c．Which additional investigation would you offer?

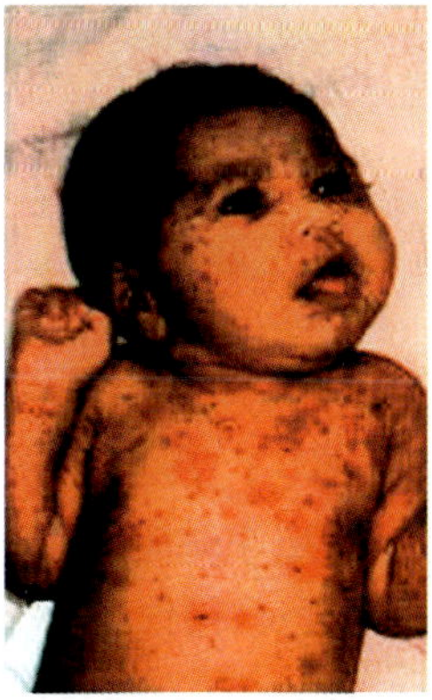

51．此新生儿表现为广泛分布的疱疹。

a．哪两种由母体传播的常见病毒能引起此症状？

b．写出感染这些病毒的新生儿的四种后果。

c．哪类药物用于治疗被感染的新生儿？

This newborn baby has a widespread vesicular rash.

a．Which two common viral infections transmitted from the mother may be responsible?

b．Name four consequences to the newborn of infection with these viruses.

c．Which drug is used to treat neonates with these infections?

52．图为 4 天龄婴儿的腹部 X 线平片，该婴儿于妊娠 28 周出生。

a．最可能的诊断为何？

b．列出早产的其他三个并发症。

c．如何降低这些并发症的发生率？

This abdominal X-ray was taken from a 4-day-old baby born at 28 weeks' gestation.

a．What is the likely diagnosis?

b．Name three other complications of prematurity.

c．How can the incidence of these complications be reduced?

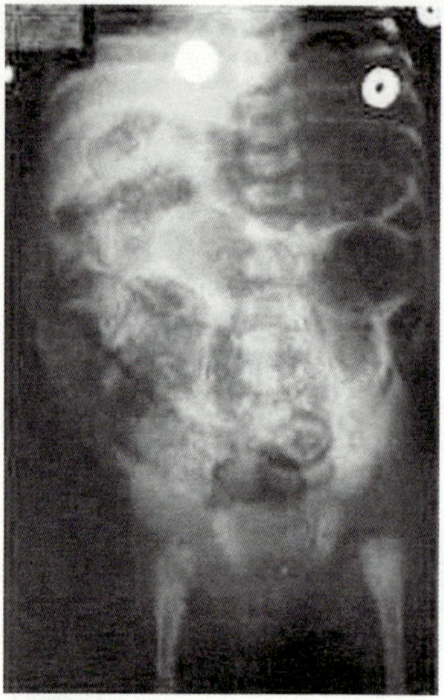

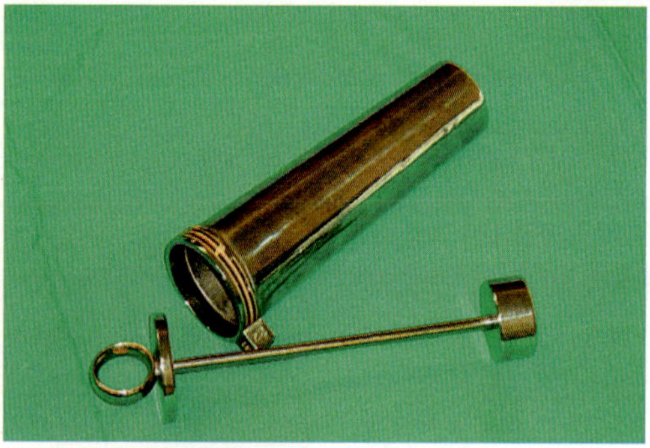

53．这是分娩室内常见的工具。

a．这个工具叫做什么？

b．它用于何种操作？

c．进行该操作的适应证是什么？

This instrument is commonly found in the labour suite.

a．What is this instrument?

b．For which procedure is it used?

c．What is the indication for this procedure?

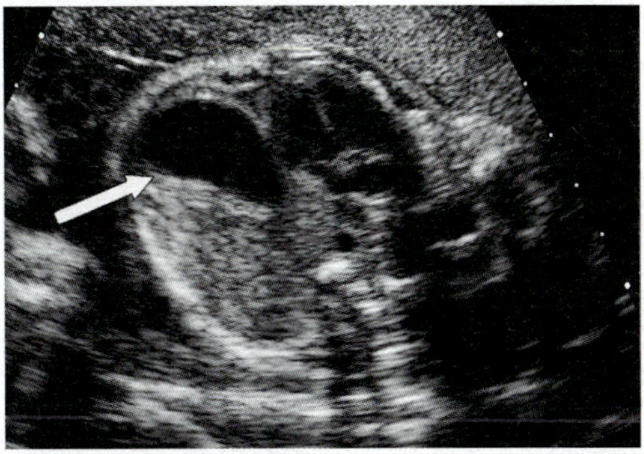

54. 此超声图显示的是通过胎儿胸部的横切面。

a. 箭头所指的是何结构?

b. 诊断为什么?

c. 如无其他畸形，该病的总体存活率是多少?

This ultrasound image shows a transverse section through a fetal chest.

a. Which structure is indicated by the arrow?

b. What is the diagnosis?

c. What is the overall survival rate for this condition if there are no other abnormalities in the baby?

55. 此新生儿出生时发现有严重的皮肤瘢痕化。

a. 何种母婴间感染可引起该现象?

b. 何种产前治疗可以降低胎儿损害的发生率?

c. 列出两种此种感染可能引起的其余先天畸形。

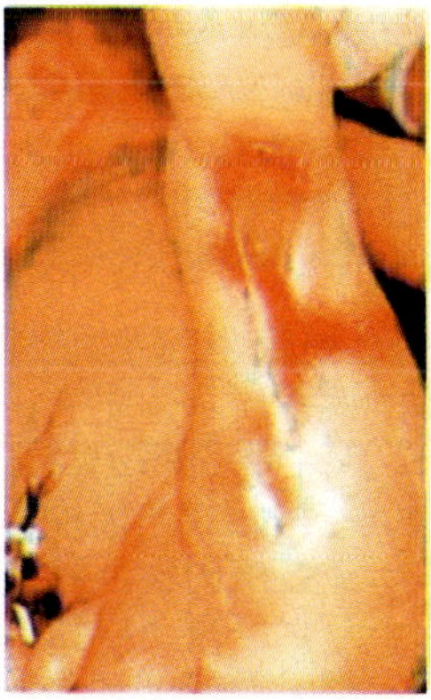

This baby was found to have severe skin scarring at delivery.

a. Which fetomaternal infection may cause this appearance?

b. Which antenatal intervention may reduce the incidence of fetal damage?

c. Name two other congenital abnormalities that may result from this fetal infection.

56. 这个肾及输尿管取于 23 周终止妊娠的胎儿，对侧肾有同样外观。

a. 如何描述此肾？

b. B 超检查时可能发现羊水量有何异常？

c. 尸检报告中可能会提及胎肺有什么改变？

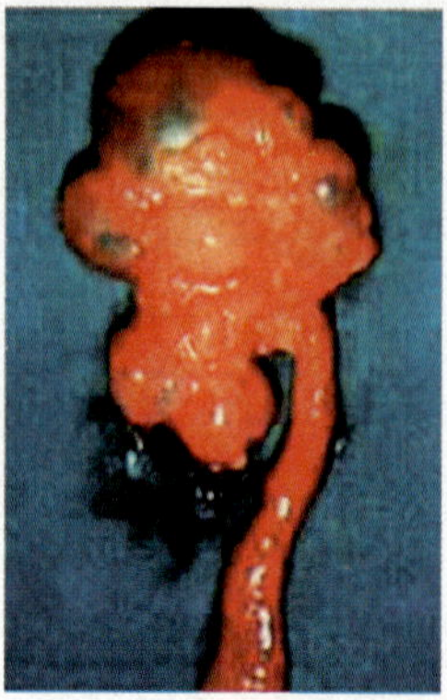

This kidney and ureter were dissected from a fetus after the pregnancy was terminated at 23 weeks' gestation. The other kidney had the same appearance.

a. How would you describe this kidney?

b. What abnormality of liquor volume might have been found on ultrasound scan?

c. What might the postmortem report have said about the fetal lungs?

57. 这是一个 15 周胎儿腹部的超声图像。

a. 通过胎儿腹壁疝出的结构是什么？

b. 诊断为什么？

c. 何种染色体异常最可能与此发现有关？

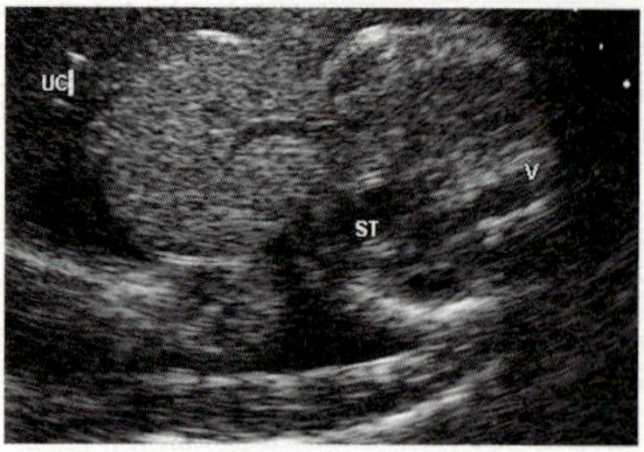

This is an ultrasound scan of a fetal abdomen at 15 weeks' gestation.

a. What structure is herniating through the fetal abdominal wall?

b. What is the diagnosis?

c. Which chromosomal abnormality is most commonly associated with this finding?

58. 该新生儿是唐氏综合征患儿。

a. 此图所示的是唐氏综合征的哪一种细微的特征？

b. 何种常规产前检查可用于筛查妊娠时的此种情况？

c. 写出妊娠 20 周时超声检查有助于诊断的 6 个征象。

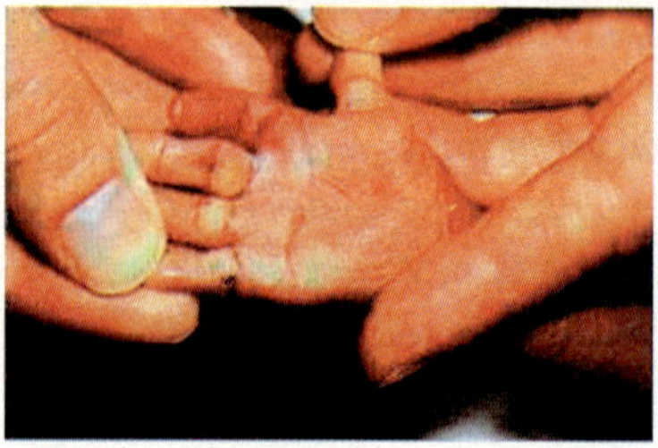

This newborn infant has Down syndrome.

a. Which subtle feature of Down syndrome is shown here?

b. What routine screening tests are available for this condition in pregnancy?

c. Name six features on a 20-week scan that point to the diagnosis.

59．该新生儿于妊娠39周出生，体重2.3kg，其母亲由于有高血压及蛋白尿而引产。

a．如何描述该婴儿？

b．其潜在的病理改变如何？

c．写出你有可能发现的与诊断有关的三个超声征象。

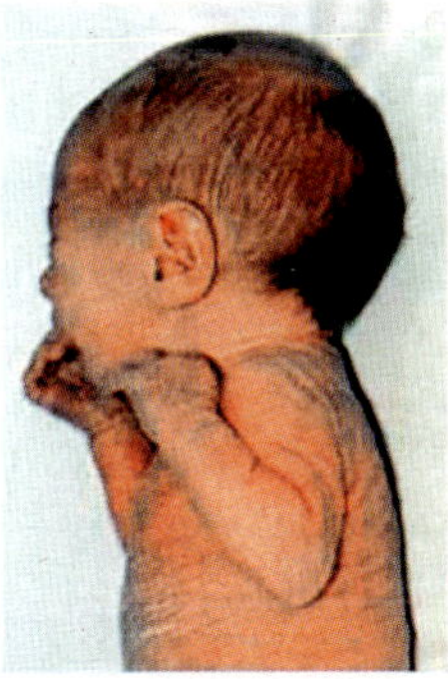

This baby was born weighing 2.3 kg at 39 weeks' gestation. His mother was induced for hypertension and proteinuria.

a．How would you describe this baby?

b．What is the underlying pathology?

c．Name three ultrasound features you might expect to find with this diagnosis.

60．该婴儿有非常短以及变形的长骨。

a．描述此类先天畸形的术语是什么？

b．写出妊娠期间有助于诊断的两种检查方法。

c．此类患儿的主要死因是什么？

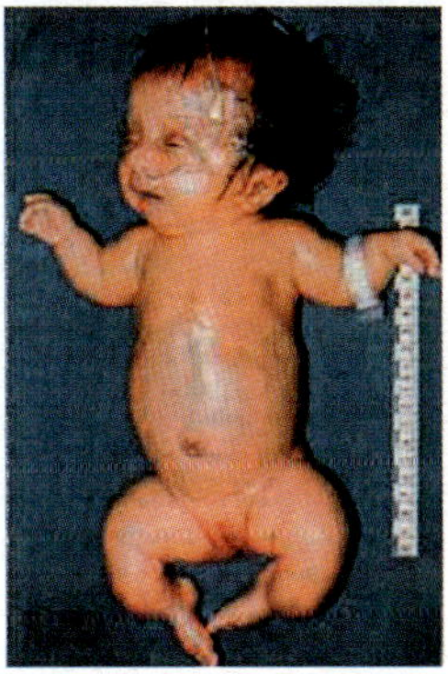

This baby has very short and deformed long bones.

a．What is the term given to this group of congenital abnormalities?

b．Name two investigations that help make the diagnosis during pregnancy.

c．What is the main reason these babies die?

61．该患儿母亲拒绝做任何产前检查。

a．此图所示的是何种畸形？

b．写出该患儿将来可能面对的四种问题。

c．写出该病现出生时发病率下降的两个原因。

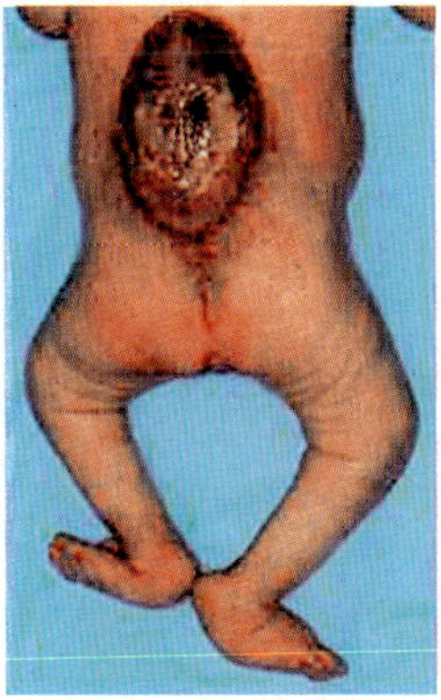

This baby was born to a woman who declined antenatal screening.

a．What abnormality is shown here?

b．Name four problems that this child might face in later life.

c．What are the two reasons for the falling incidence of this condition at birth?

62．该患儿有产伤。
a．这一发现称为什么？
b．最可能的分娩方式是什么？
c．该患儿最可能出现什么后果？

This baby has suffered birth trauma.

a．What is this finding called?
b．What was the most likely mode of delivery?
c．What condition is the neonate more likely to develop as a consequence of this?

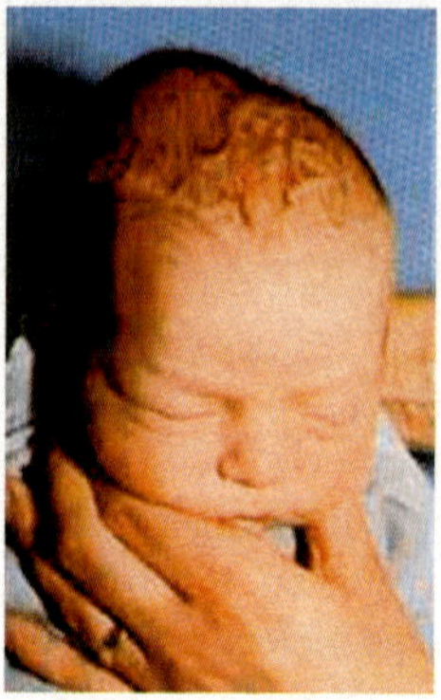

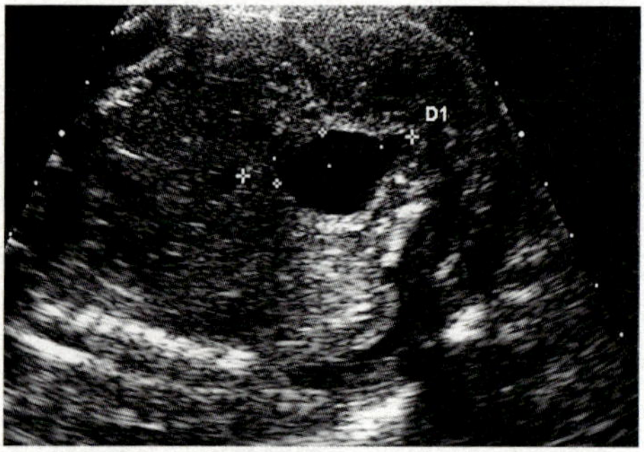

63．该超声图示的是胎儿增大的膀胱纵切面，胎儿为男性。
a．诊断为什么？
b．该情况的主要后果是什么？
c．可考虑行何种产前治疗？

This ultrasound scan shows an enlarged bladder in longitudinal view. The fetus is male.

a．What is the diagnosis?
b．What are the main consequences of this condition?
c．What antenatal therapeutic intervention might be considered?

64．图为婴儿刚出生时所拍。
a．图中所示的是何体征？
b．该体征提示什么？
c．写出导致该现象的四种可能原因。

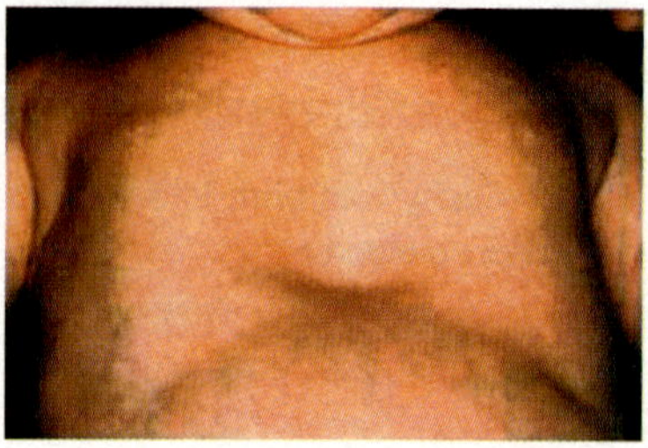

This is an image of a baby taken soon after delivery.

a．What physical signs are demonstrated here?
b．What do they indicate?
c．Name four possible causes for this appearance.

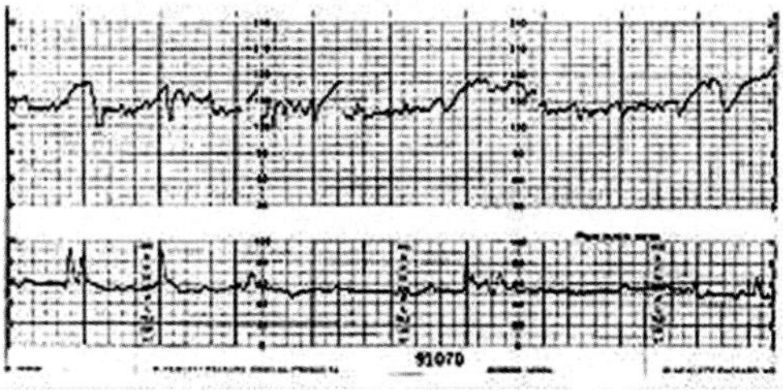

65．图为妊娠 40 周低危妇女产程早期的胎心产力图。胎心基线为 140 次 / 分。

a．如何描述此图？

b．该产妇需要继续监护吗？

c．临产时还可以用什么可替代的方法监护胎儿？

This cardiotocogram (CTG) is taken from a low-risk woman at 40 weeks' gestation in early labour. The baseline rate was 140 beats/min.

a．How would you describe it?

b．Should monitoring be continued?

c．What alternative method of fetal monitoring can be used to monitor the fetus in labour?

66．图为一经产妇自发临产时的产程图。

a．图中所示的是何种产程异常？

b．写出该情况的三个原因。

c．如继续分娩该主要的风险是什么？

This is a partogram taken from a multiparous woman in spontaneous labour.

a．What abnormal pattern of labour is illustrated here?

b．Name three causes for this.

c．What is the main risk if labour is allowed to continue?

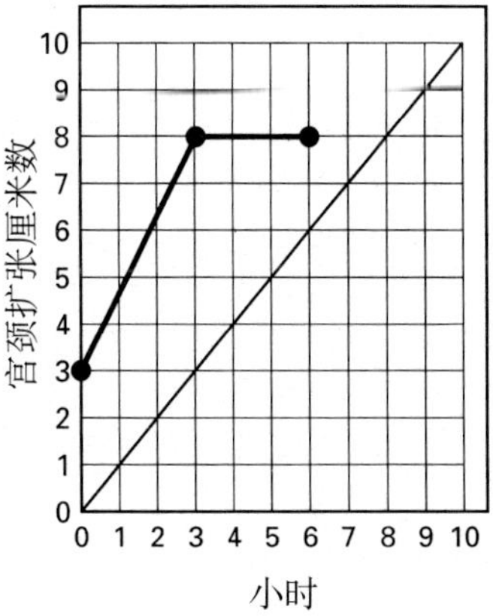

67．该孕妇主诉图中所示区域感觉异常、麻木。

a．诊断为什么？

b．累及了哪个神经？

c．你将提供哪两种治疗？

This pregnant woman complains of paraesthesia and numbness in the distribution shown in the picture.

a．What is the diagnosis?

b．Which nerve is involved?

c．What two treatments would you offer?

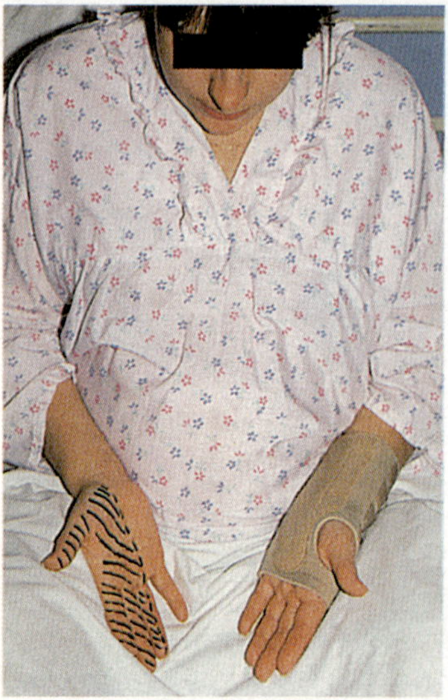

68．该妇女就诊于医疗 / 产科联合诊所。

a．她患的是何病？

b．为确诊应做何血液检查？

c．写出与此病相关的四种妊娠期并发症。

This woman attends a joint medical/obstetric clinic.

a．What condition does she suffer from?

b．What blood tests might you perform to confirm the diagnosis?

c．Name four complications associated with this condition in pregnancy.

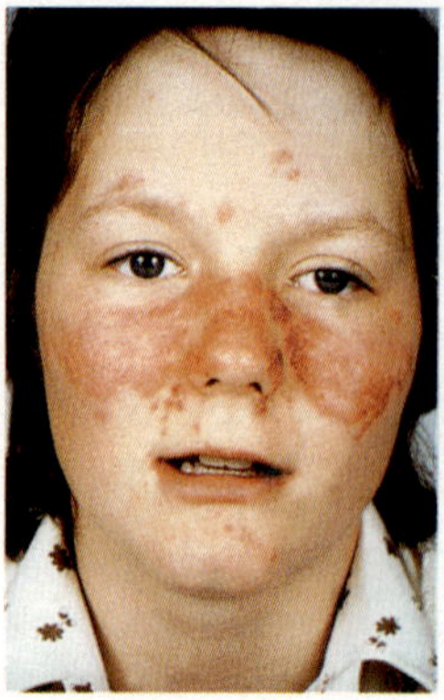

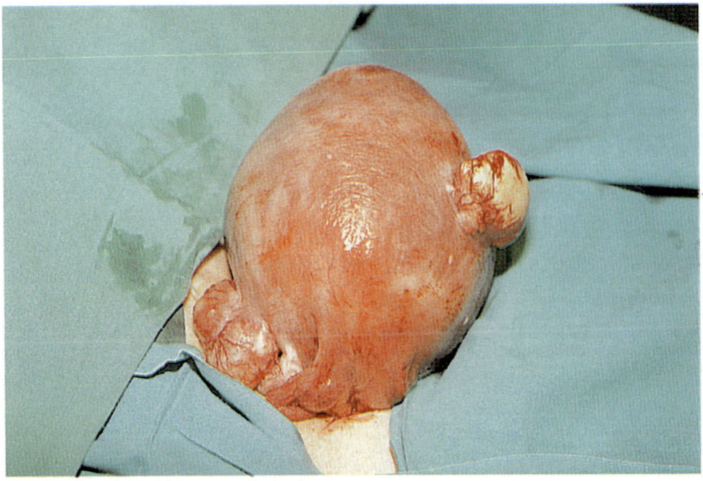

69．图为剖宫时的子宫表现。

a．附着于子宫上的结构为什么？

b．写出该疾病妊娠期间的三种并发症。

c．可否在剖宫产术中将其切除？

This was the appearance of a term uterus at caesarean section.

a．What are the structures attached to the uterus?

b．Name three complications of these in pregnancy.

c．Would you remove them at the time of the caesarean delivery?

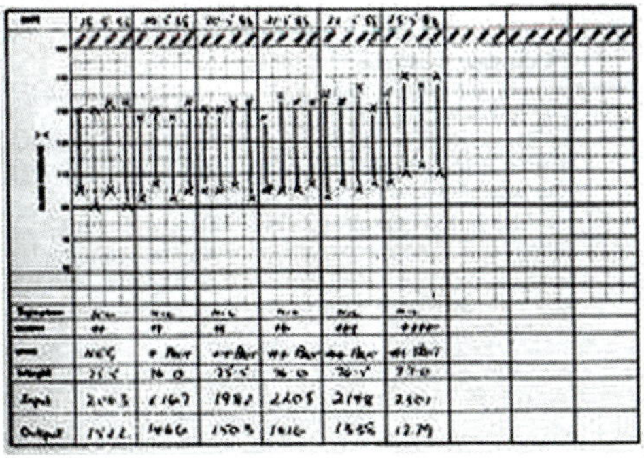

70．图为一妊娠足月初产妇的监测图。

a．最可能的诊断为什么？

b．写出应行的 5 种检查。

c．确定的治疗是什么？

This is the maternal observations chart from a primiparous woman admitted at term.

a．What is the likely diagnosis?

b．Name five investigations that should be carried out.

c．What is the definitive treatment?

InFocus

问题

71．图为剖宫产术后 6 周产妇的 CT 图像。

a．图中所示的是何结构？

b．图中连线所示的是何产科测量？

c．该检查对评估再次妊娠的分娩方式有价值吗？

This CT scan was performed 6 weeks after delivery by caesarean section.

a．What structure has been imaged, and which view are we seeing?

b．Which obstetric measurements are shown by the dotted lines?

c．Is this test of any value in managing future pregnancies?

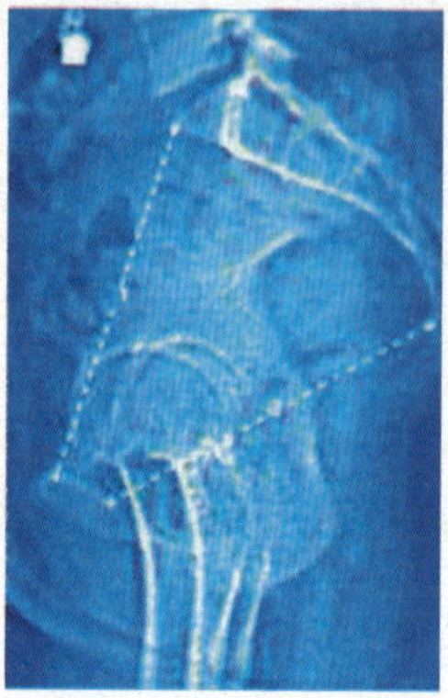

72．该临产足月孕妇有外阴疼痛和挛缩。

a．诊断为什么？

b．决定该患分娩方式的重要因素是什么？

c．经阴道分娩对胎儿有何危险？

This woman presented at term with vulval soreness and contractions.

a．What is the diagnosis?

b．What information is critical in deciding mode of delivery?

c．What risks does a vaginal delivery pose to the baby?

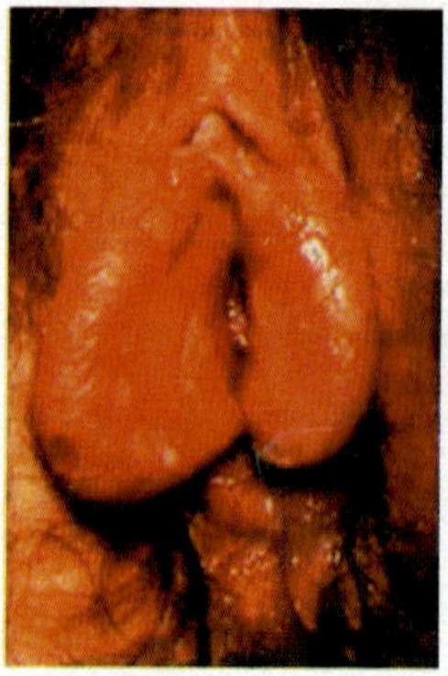

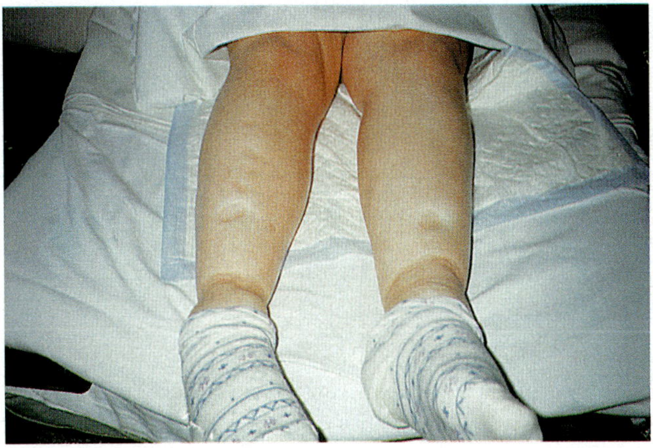

73．该孕妇现为妊娠 36 周。
a．图示的是何体征?
b．写出该患在检查时 4 种其他的重要特征。
c．写出你将做的五个检查。

This woman is at 36 weeks' gestation.
a．What physical sign is evident from this image?
b．Name four other important features on examination of this patient.
c．Name five investigations that you would organize.

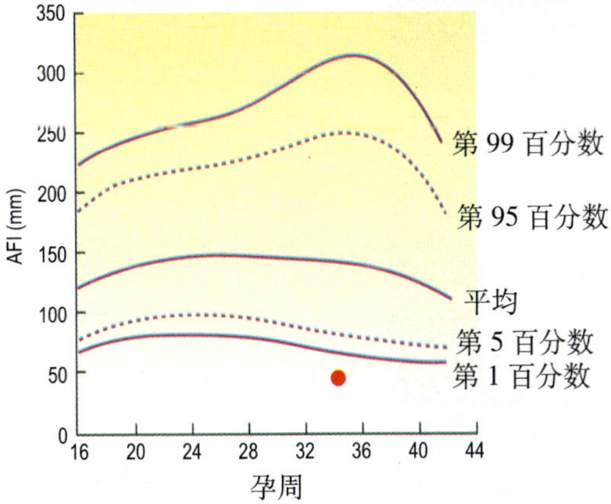

74．仔细观察此羊水指数图。
a．它表现为何种异常?
b．写出此种情况的三个原因。
c．写出扫描可发现的三个特征。

Study this amniotic fluid index (AFI) chart.
a．What abnormality is represented here?
b．Name three causes for this.
c．What three other features would you examine on scan?

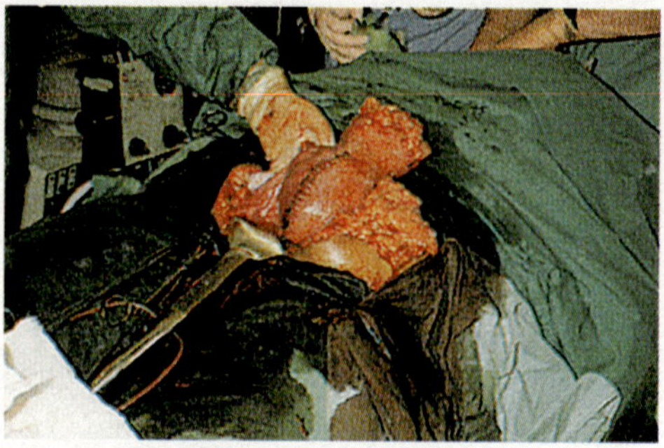

75．图示的是剖宫产术结束时的子宫。

a．进行的是何种剖宫产术？

b．写出比常规剖宫产术后更易出现的一个即时并发症和一个远期并发症。

c．写出这个手术的两个有效指征。

This image shows a uterus at the end of a caesarean section.

a．What type of caesarean section has been performed?

b．Name one immediate and one long-term complication that are more likely than after a normal caesarean section?

c．Name two valid indications for this operation.

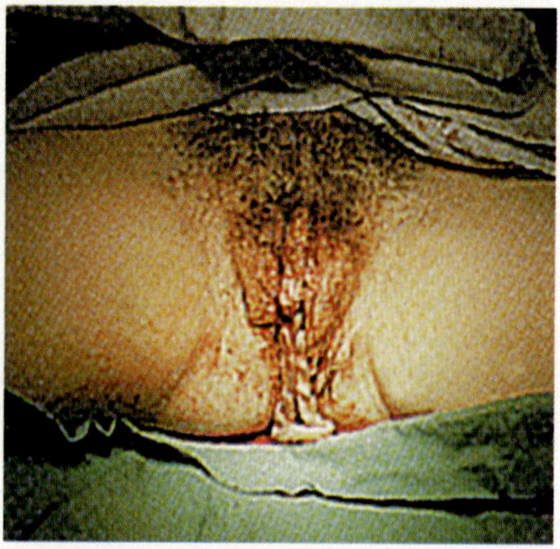

76．该产妇由接生婆陪同急入院，该产妇自然破膜后由其陪同。

a．图示的是什么问题？

b．写出四个易发因素。

c．一旦患者入院而宫口尚未开全，胎儿仍存活，应采取哪两种措施？

This woman has been rushed in from home by her midwife who attended her following spontaneous membrane rupture.

a．What problem is shown here?

b．Name four predisposing factors.

c．What are the two measures that should be taken once the patient is in hospital if the cervix is not fully dilated and the fetus is alive?

77. 该小男孩与其怀孕的母亲就诊于产前诊所，小男孩有咳嗽，面色潮红。

a. 他患有哪种感染疾病？

b. 你如何确诊是否其母亲也感染同一病毒？

c. 这对她的妊娠有何危险？

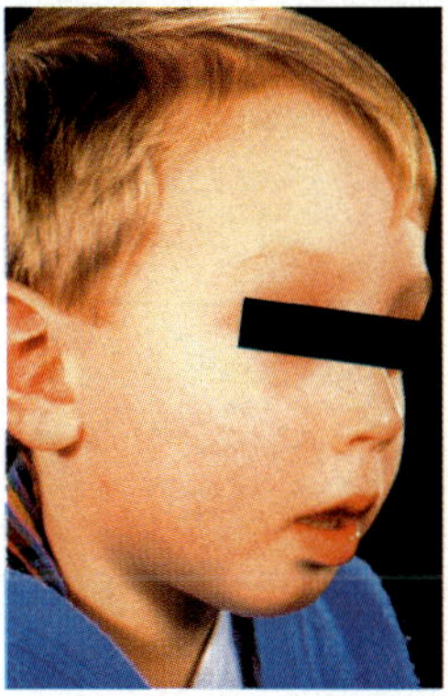

This young boy attended an antenatal clinic with his pregnant mother. He has a cough and very red cheeks.

a. What is the diagnosis for his infectious illness?

b. How would you ascertain if his mother is at risk of contracting the same viral illness?

c. What risks does this pose to her pregnancy?

78. 图示的是胎头横切面。

a. 此为何种检查？

b. 该检查对胎儿有危害吗？

c. CT 检查可作为替代检查吗？

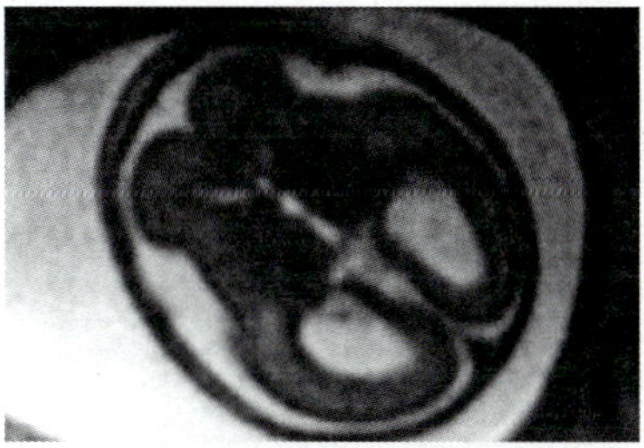

This image shows a transverse section through a fetal head.

a. What type of investigation has been performed?

b. Does it involve any risk to the fetus?

c. Is a CT scan a viable alternative?

79. 这些细胞取自羊水。

a. 此为何种分子学检查？

b. 此检查可以发现何种异常？

c. 这些细胞是正常的吗？论证你的观点。

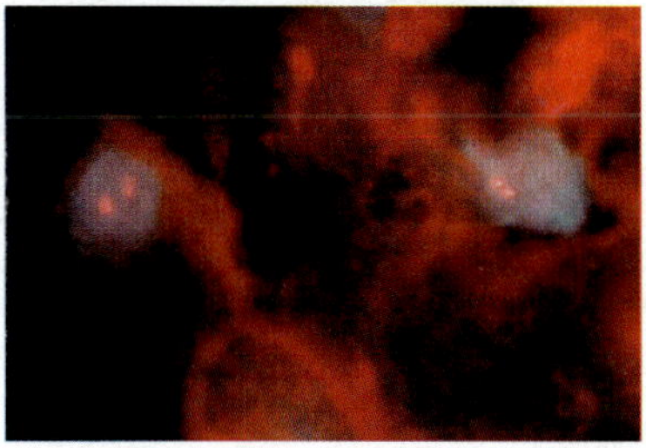

These cells are derived from amniotic fluid.

a. What molecular test has been performed?

b. What kind of abnormalities is it able to detect?

c. Are these cells normal? Justify your answer.

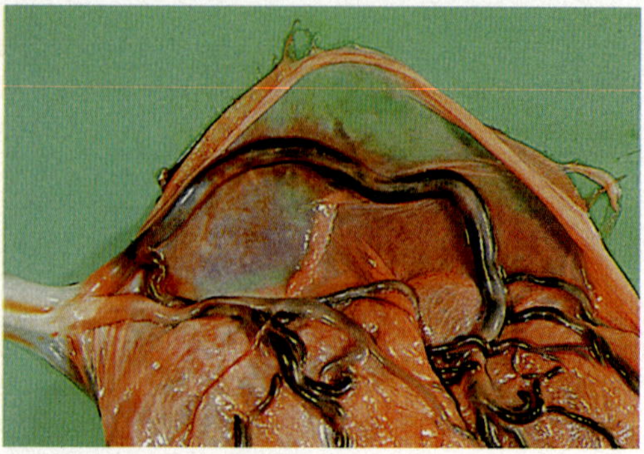

80. 图为助产士仔细检查刚娩出的胎盘。

a. 此现象称为什么？

b. 它有什么意义？

c. 分娩过程中可能出现什么问题？

Following delivery this placenta was examined closely by the midwife.

a. What is this appearance called?

b. What significance may it have?

c. How might this problem present in labour?

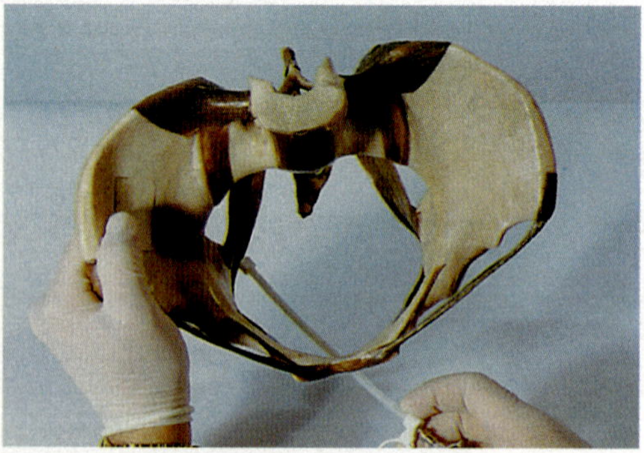

81. 图示的是骨盆。

a. 图中所指的是什么结构？

b. 哪个神经临近此结构？

c. 为什么此神经在产科比较重要？

This image shows the bony pelvis.

a. Which structure is being pointed to?

b. Which nerve passes close to this point?

c. Why is this of importance in obstetrics?

时间	进餐与胰岛素量	毛细血管血糖值
0800 h		9.3 mmol/L (167.4 mg/dL)
0905 h	早餐和18U短效胰岛素	
1000 h		3.0 mmol/L (54.0 mg/dL)
1230 h	午餐和24U短效胰岛素	5.6 mmol/L (100.8 mg/dL)
1235 h		
1530 h		7.2 mmol/L (129.6 mg/dL)
1800 h		4.8 mmol/L (86.4 mg/dL)
1805 h	晚餐和26U短效胰岛素	
2000 h		6.9 mmol/L (124.2 mg/dL)
2200 h		5.6 mmol/L (91.8 mg/dL)
2230 h	宵夜和16U中效胰岛素	

孕32周的糖尿病患者的血糖和胰岛素概况

82．图示的是妊娠 32 周合并糖尿病患者的血糖值，此图概括了该患者上周的病情。

a．如何调整睡前长效胰岛素的用量?

b．如何调整早晨胰岛素的用量?

c．测量何指标以反应长期血糖控制情况?

Study this blood glucose profile of a diabetic patient at 32 weeks' gestation. It is representative of her profiles for the preceding week.

a．What would you do with the evening dose of long acting insulin?

b．How would you alter her morning insulin dose?

c．How would you measure her longer-term control?

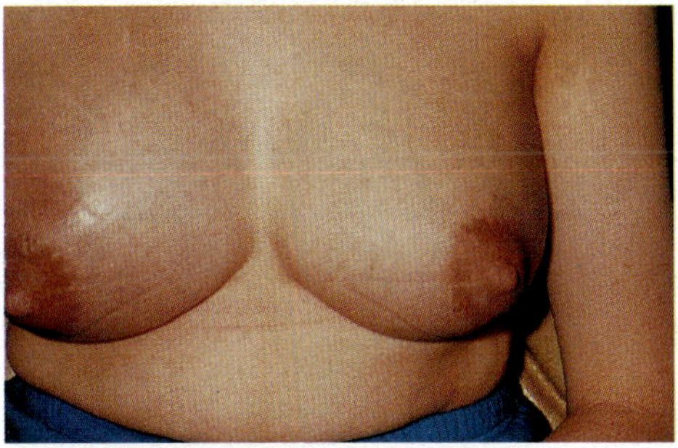

83．该产妇产后 8 天出现哺乳痛。

a．诊断为什么?

b．常见的病原菌有哪两种?

c．写出三条处理措施。

This woman presents with painful breastfeeding 8 days after delivery.

a．What is the diagnosis?

b．Which two species of microorganism are commonly responsible?

c．Name three components of the management.

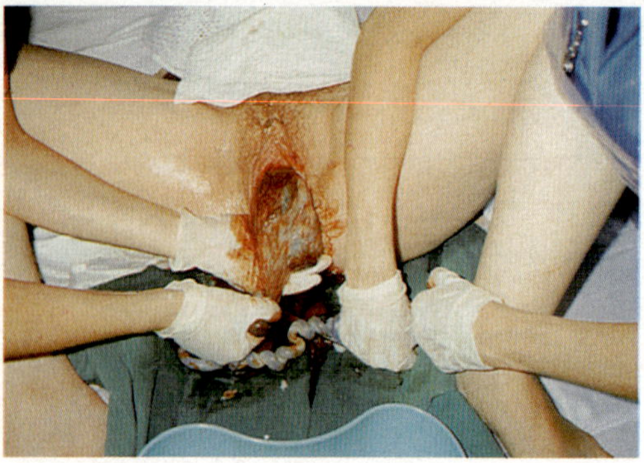

84．此图表示的是第三产程。

a．图中所使用的是何方法？

b．如操作不当，可能出现哪两种并发症？

c．写出此方法无效的可能原因。

This image was taken during the third stage of labour.

a．What is the name of the technique which has just been used?

b．Name two complications that can occur if it is done incorrectly.

c．What is the reason this may be unsuccessful?

85．图示的是临产时因产科并发症而切除的子宫。

a．该子宫有何异常？

b．写出两个易患因素。

c．写出临产时该情况可能出现的四种原因。

This hysterectomy was performed following a complication in labour.

a．What uterine problem is shown here?

b．Name two predisposing factors.

c．Name four ways in which it may present in labour.

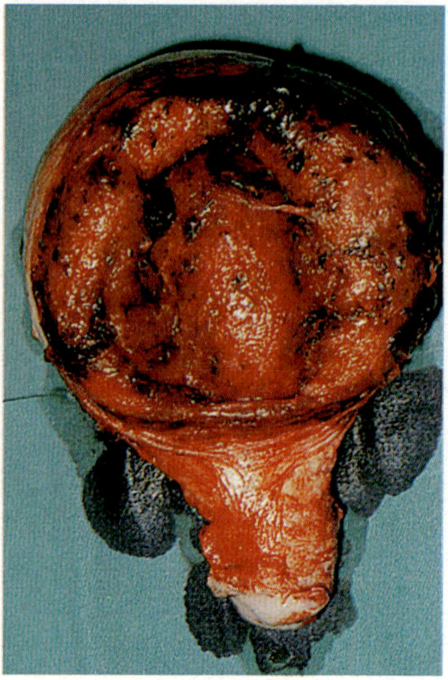

1．a．羊水过多。
b．妊娠期糖尿病、胎儿畸形（例如小肠闭锁、先天膈疝）、双胎输血综合征、病毒感染、同种免疫。
c．腹部不适、子宫收缩感。触诊子宫大于相应妊娠周数、胎儿扪及不清。

a．Polyhydramnios.
b．Diabetes in pregnancy, structural abnormalities (e.g. bowel atresias, congenital diaphragmatic hernia), twin-twin transfusion syndrome, viral infections, isoimmunization.
c．Abdominal discomfort and preterm uterine tightenings. On palpation the uterus would be large-for-dates and the fetal parts difficult to feel.

2．a．异位妊娠。尽管血 hCG > 1500IU/L 界限（宫腔内应该可见妊娠囊），但宫腔内空虚。此外， 附件区可见一包块。
b．前次宫外孕、输卵管手术史、既往盆腔感染史、助孕技术、宫内节避孕器。
c．外科手术可以是开腹手术，最好是腹腔镜手术。输卵管可保留（输卵管切开术），也可全部切除（输卵管切除术）。较小的异位妊娠病灶有时也可用甲氨蝶呤治疗。

a．Ectopic pregnancy. The uterus is empty despite an hCG value well above the 1500 IU/L threshold at which an intrauterine gestation sac should be seen. Furthermore, there is a mass in the adnexal region.
b．Previous ectopic pregnancy, tubal surgery, previous pelvic infection, assisted conception, intrauterine contraceptive devices.
c．Surgical management can be open, but preferably laparoscopic. The tube can be conserved (salpingotomy) or removed entirely (salpingectomy). Small ectopics can sometimes be treated medically with methotrexate.

3．a．妊娠滋养细胞疾病（葡萄胎）。
b．胎盘有多囊或落雪状图像。
c．该患者应就诊于最近的滋养细胞疾病专科中心，连续监测血清或尿 hCG 是必要的，如其水平未降至零，则需进一步的刮宫或化疗。

a．Gestational trophoblastic disease (molar pregnancy).

b．A multicystic or 'snowstorm' appearance in the placenta.

c．The patient would need to be registered with the nearest specialist trophoblast centre. Serial monitoring of serum/urine hCG measure-ments would be necessary. If levels failed to fall to zero, then further curettage or chemotherapy would be indicated.

4．a．顶臀径（crown-rump length,CLR）。

b．采用 CLR 估算妊娠周数的误差为± 5 天。

c．双顶径及股骨长。

a．Crown-rump length (CRL).

b．The error is ± 5 days using the CRL to date a pregnancy.

c．The biparietal diameter and femur length.

5．a．卵黄囊。

b．阴道超声下，卵黄囊最早可在妊娠 5 周时见到，通常于妊娠 12 周消失。

c．它对胚胎的营养、生物合成及造血起重要作用。

a．The yolk sac.

b．It is first visible at 5 weeks' gestation with a transvaginal scan and has usually gone by 12 weeks.

c．It plays a major role in embryonic nutrition, biosynthesis and haemopoiesis.

6．a．双顶径。

b．脉络丛。

c．产生脑脊液。

a．The biparietal diameter.

b．The choroid plexus.

c．It produces cerebrospinal fluid.

7．a．小脑。

b．A 图中所示的是正常小脑（两个小脑半球、小脑蚓部）。

c．B 图中所示的是神经管缺陷时的“香蕉”形小脑，其他与脊柱裂相关的颅部超声图像包括柠檬形头及小脑延髓池消失。

a．The cerebellum.

b．Image A shows a normal cerebellum (two hemispheres and a midline vermis).

c．Image B shows a 'banana'-shaped cerebellum associated with neural tube defects. Other cranial ultrasound features associated with spina bifida include a 'lemon'-shaped head and an effaced cisterna magna.

8．a．该超声图中可见四个羊膜囊，提示四胎妊娠。其中两个羊膜比较厚，有 λ 征。另有一个羊膜非常薄，且没有 λ 征。这说明四胎中有一对是单羊膜囊双胎，还有一对是“独生子”。
b．辅助生育（试管婴儿）。
c．流产、早产、胎儿生长受限、先兆子痫、胎儿畸形、双胎输血综合征、先露异常，需行剖宫产。

a．This scan shows four amniotic sacs, suggesting a quadruplet pregnancy. Two of the membranes are thick and have lambda signs. One of the membranes is much thinner and there is no lambda sign. This suggests that there is a pair of monochorionic twins and two 'singletons'.
b Assisted conception (in vitro fertilization).
c．Miscarriage, preterm labour, fetal growth restriction, pre-eclampsia, fetal anomalies, twin-twin transfusion syndrome, malpresentation and need for caesarean delivery.

9．a．颈部半透明度（nuchal translucency，NT）。
b．检查 NT 的最常见原因为筛查唐氏综合征。
c．NT 筛查在大约妊娠 13 周之后就不能使用了，该法至今未广泛使用。二倍体或三倍体血清学筛查应在所有妊娠妇女的妊娠 15 ~ 19 周时进行，尽管该法作为唐氏综合征的筛查方法不如 NT 筛查敏感。

a．The nuchal translucency (NT).
b．The most common reason for NT scanning is to screen for Down syndrome.
c．NT scanning cannot be performed after approximately 13 weeks' gestation and is still not widely available. Double or triple serum screening should be offered to all pregnant women at 15-19 weeks' gestation, although it is less sensitive as a screening test for Down syndrome than NT scanning.

10．a．无脑儿（神经管缺陷的一种形式）。
b．妊娠 15 ~ 19 周行血清学筛查对开放性神经管缺陷敏感性超过 90%。在妊娠 20 周行常规超声检查可检查出 98% 以上的该畸形。
c．无脑儿常表现为羊水过多，很可能因为神经功能异常导致胎儿吞咽羊水减少。

a. Anencephaly (a form of neural tube defect).

b. Serum screening at 15-19 weeks has a greater than 90% sensitivity for detection of open neural tube defects, and routine detailed scanning at 20 weeks' gestation detects more than 98% of these abnormalities.

c. Anencephalic pregnancies are often complicated by polyhydramnios, possibly due to a failure of fetal drinking secondary to disturbed neurological function.

11. a. Edward 综合征。

b. 18 三体。

c. 与 18 三体综合征相关的其他畸形包括先天性心脏病（特别是室间隔缺损）、脐疝（见于 25% 的患者）、神经管缺陷、膈疝、船形足。

a. Edward syndrome.

b. Trisomy 18.

c. Other abnormalities commonly associated with trisomy 18 include congenital heart disease (in particular ventricular septal defect), omphalocele (found in 25%), neural tube defects, diaphragmatic hernia and rocker-bottom feet.

12. a. 脐疝。

b. 羊水检查或绒毛活检分析染色体核型。大约 25% 与染色体异常相关。

c. 18 三体或 13 三体是最常见的脐疝非整倍体。

a. Exomphalos (omphalocele).

b. Fetal karyotyping by either amniocentesis or chorionic villus sampling. Approximately 25% are associated with chromosomal abnormalities.

c. Trisomies 18 and 13 are the most common aneuploidies found with exomphalos.

13. a. 双泡征。

b. 十二指肠闭锁导致增大的充满液体的胃和近端十二指肠由幽门处分隔开。

c. 该情况 30% 见于唐氏综合征（21 三体综合征）。

a. The 'double-bubble' sign.

b. Duodenal atresia results in an enlarged fluid-filled stomach and proximal duodenum, separated by the pylorus.

c. Down syndrome (trisomy 21) is found in 30% of cases.

14．a．基线变异减少（消失）、晚期减速，无加速。

b．为病理性的（比如超过一处异常）。

c．新鲜的胎粪。此胎心产力图高度提示胎儿缺氧和酸中毒。极有可能胎儿已经反应性排出新鲜胎粪。

a．Reduced (absent) baseline variability, late decelerations and absence of accelerations.

b．Pathological (i.e. more than one abnormal feature).

c．Fresh meconium. This CTG is highly suggestive of fetal hypoxia and acidosis. It is very possible that this fetus has passed fresh meconium in response.

15．a．Turner 综合征（45，XO）。

b．身材矮小、颈蹼、心脏畸形（双瓣的主动脉瓣、主动脉缩窄）、肾畸形（如马蹄肾）、条状卵巢（导致第二性征发育不良）。

c．水囊瘤（颈部后外侧淋巴聚集）。

a．Turner syndrome (45, XO).

b．Short stature, neck webbing, cardiac abnormalities (bicuspid aortic valve, coarctation of the aorta), renal anomalies (e.g. horseshoe kidney) and streak ovaries (causing failure of secondary sexual development).

c．A cystic hygroma (collections of lymph in the posterolateral aspect of the neck).

16．a．左侧面神经麻痹。

b．很可能是产钳助产，正常新生儿偶可见特发性面神经麻痹。

c．不是。预后良好，大多数患儿数天内症状自然消失。

a．Left facial nerve palsy.

b．Forceps delivery is most likely, although unexplained facial nerve palsies are occasionally seen after normal births.

c．No. The prognosis is very good, with the vast majority settling spontaneously within a few days.

17．a．缺氧 - 缺血性脑病（hypoxic ischaemic encephalopathy，HIE）。

b．脑电图。

c．中至重度（HIE Ⅱ级、Ⅲ级）患儿有 50% ~ 90% 的风险发生神经损害。

a. Hypoxic ischaemic encephalopathy (HIE).
b. Electroencephalogram.
c. Babies at the moderate to severe end of the spectrum of HIE (grades II and III) have a 50-90% risk of neurodevelopmental damage.

18. a. 坏死性肠炎。
b. 至少分娩前 48 小时给予产妇糖皮质激素（地塞米松或倍他米松）。
c. 静脉应用抗生素和补液，禁食、水。

a. Necrotizing enterocolitis.
b. Administration of steroids (dexamethasone or betamethasone) to the mother at least 48 h before delivery.
c. Intravenous antibiotics and fluids. Nil intake by mouth.

19. a. 枕部脑膨出。
b. 神经管缺陷。
c. 超声和 MRI。

a. Occipital encephalocele.
b. Neural tube defects.
c. Ultrasound and MRI.

20. a. 胎儿水肿。
b. A：腹壁水肿；B：腹水。
c. 同种免疫、染色体异常、病毒感染、血液从胎儿流向母体、心脏畸形（如心律失常）、骨骼发育异常、双胎输血综合征、先天性代谢缺陷病、血红蛋白变异。

a. Fetal hydrops.
b. A, abdominal wall oedema; B, ascites.
c. Isoimmunization, chromosomal abnormalities, viral infections, fetomaternal haemorrhage, cardiac abnormalities (e.g. arrhythmias), skeletal dysplasias, twin-twin transfusion, inborn errors of metabolism, haemoglobinopathies.

21. a. 内眦赘皮、虹膜 Brushfield 斑、眼裂外侧上斜。
b. 唐氏综合征（21 三体综合征）。
c. 大多数唐氏综合征是特发性的，再发危险为百分之一，除非该妇女的年龄（与再发危险有关）高于此。罕见的易位型唐氏综合征可能由于亲代染色体平衡易位所致，再发的风险显著升高。

a. Epicanthic folds, Brushfield's spots (on the iris) and upward-slanting palpebral fissures.

b. Down syndrome (trisomy 21).

c. Most cases of Down syndrome are spontaneous. The recurrence risk is quoted as 1 in 100, unless the woman's age-related risk is higher than this, in which case it is used instead. Rare forms of translocation Down syndrome may result from a parental balanced translocation. The recurrence risk is then significantly higher.

22. a. 脐动脉多普勒波形记录与测量。

b. 此波形与通过胎盘胎儿面的血流阻力相关。舒张末期出现前向血流意味着胎盘抵抗没有严重地增加。

c. 先兆子痫的发生是由于胎盘欠佳引起的。子宫床母体螺旋动脉的不充分再造使其成为高阻血管。这将进而影响到胎盘胎儿面的发展，也引起更大的血流抵抗。

a. Umbilical artery Doppler waveform recording and measurement.

b. This waveform correlates with resistance to blood flow through the fetal side of the placenta. The presence of end-diastolic forward flow means that placental resistance is not severely elevated.

c. Pre-eclampsia occurs because of suboptimal placentation. Inadequate remodelling of maternal spiral arteries in the uterine bedleaves them as high-resistance vessels. This in turn impacts on the development of the fetal side of the placenta, also causing greater resistance to blood flow.

23. a. Erb 麻痹。

b. 胎肩娩出时外牵引过度导致 C5、C6 及 C7 臂丛神经根拉伸或撕脱伤。

c. 孕妇患糖尿病（妊娠期糖尿病或妊娠前即发生糖尿病）是肩难产的危险因素（导致 Erb 麻痹），不依赖于胎儿大小。

a. Erb's palsy.

b. Stretching or avulsion of the C5, C6 and C7 nerve roots of the brachial plexus due to excessive lateral traction at the time of delivery of the fetal shoulders.

c. Maternal diabetes mellitus (pre-existing or gestational) is a risk factor for shoulder dystocia (and therefore Erb's palsy), independent of fetal size.

24. a. 水痘（水痘 - 带状疱疹）。
b. 在妊娠 20 周前感染的孕妇所生婴儿患先天水痘综合征的风险是 1% ~ 2%（表现为小头畸形、癫痫发作、神经发育迟缓、四肢发育不全及瘢痕）。近分娩期的感染有潜在的导致神经严重损害的新生儿水痘的危险。
c. 可能发生水痘性肺炎，被认为导致妊娠期死亡率危险增加。

a. Chickenpox (varicella zoster).
b. Maternal infection before 20 weeks' gestation carries a 1-2% risk of congenital varicella syndrome (microcephaly, seizures, neurode velopment delay, limb hypoplasia and scarring). Infections close to delivery carry a risk of potentially very damaging neonatal chickenpox.
c. Chickenpox pneumonitis may occur with adult infections and is thought to carry a greater mortality risk in pregnancy.

25. a. Ⅳ级（重度）前置胎盘（即胎盘完全覆盖胎盘内口）。
b. 产前或产时出血、胎位异常、胎先露不能衔接。
c. 既往前置胎盘史、前次剖宫产、子宫畸形、多胎妊娠、多产。

a. Grade Ⅳ (major) placenta praevia (i.e. covering the internal cervical os).
b. Antepartum or intrapartum haemorrhage, abnormal lie, failure of engagement of the presenting part.
c. Previous placenta praevia, previous caesarean section, uterine anomalies, multiple gestations, high parity.

26. a. Potter 面容。
b. 胎儿较长时间地暴露于自妊娠早期开始的羊水量过少，羊水量过少是由于胎儿肾发育不全、多囊肾或胎膜早破时间过长导致。
c. 肺发育不全。严重的羊水减少阻碍宫腔内肺扩张和生长，导致肺发育不全。

a. Potter's facies.
b. Prolonged fetal exposure to very low liquor volumes from an early gestation as a result of renal agenesis, polycystic or dysplastic kidneys or prolonged preterm ruptured membranes.
c. Pulmonary hypoplasia. Severely reduced levels of amniotic fluid prevent lung expansion and growth in utero, leading to inadequate pulmonary development.

27. a. Filshie 夹绝育术。
    b. 并发症包括绝育失败（1/300）和后悔。如用腹腔镜实施该手术仍有脏器损伤的可能性。
    c. 绝育术可在剖宫产时一并实施，通常是切除双侧部分输卵管，结扎末端，绝育失败率较高（1/200）。

    a. Filshie clip sterilization.
    b. Complications include failure (1 in 300) and regret. If it is done laparoscopically there is also a risk of visceral injury during the procedure.
    c. Sterilization can be performed at the time of caesarean section and is usually carried out by removing segments of each tube and ligating the ends. The failure rate is higher (1 in 200).

28. a. 脉络丛囊肿。
    b. 主要与 18 三体综合征（Edward 综合征）有关，然而也可能与 21 三体综合征（唐氏综合征）有微小的联系。
    c. 可见于 1% 的正常胎儿。

    a. Choroid plexus cysts.
    b. It is most closely associated with trisomy 18 (Edward syndrome). However, it also probably has a weak association with trisomy 21 (Down syndrome).
    c. 1% of normal fetuses.

29. a. 胎头吸引。
    b. 杯罩的位置在胎头前方说明胎儿是枕后位。可能是施行分娩的操作者将胎儿体位变成枕后位。
    c. 其他产伤包括胎头血肿、帽状腱膜下出血、小脑幕与静脉窦撕裂、结膜下及视网膜出血。黄疸也很常见。

    a. Ventouse delivery.
    b. The site of the cup placement over the anterior aspect of the head indicates that the fetus must have been in an occipitoposterior position. It is likely that the individual performing the delivery incorrectly took the position to be occipitoanterior.
    c. Other injuries include cephalohaematomas, subgaleal haemorrhage, tentorial and venous sinus tears and subconjunctival and retinal haemorrhages. Jaundice is also more common.

30. a. 巨大儿。
b. 孕妇糖耐量受损或糖尿病。
c. 新生儿低血糖、呼吸窘迫、低血钙、红细胞增多症、黄疸。

a. Macrosomic.
b. Maternal impaired glucose tolerance or diabetes mellitus.
c. Neonatal hypoglycaemia, respiratory distress, hypocalcaemia, polycythaemia and jaundice.

31. a. 缺乏舒张末期血流（absent end-diastolic flow，AEDF）。
b. 由于胎盘疾病导致的胎盘血流阻抗增加。
c. AEDF 的出现是围生期发病率和死亡率升高的标志。如出现在妊娠末期则通常提示需终止妊娠，择期剖宫产比引产更安全。

a. Absent end-diastolic flow (AEDF).
b. Increased resistance to blood flow through the placental bed secondary to placental disease.
c. AEDF is a marker of increased perinatal morbidity and mortality. At this relatively advanced gestation it would usually indicate the need for delivery. In a compromised fetus, planned caesarean birth may be safer than an induced vaginal delivery.

32. a. 新生儿眼炎。
b. 衣原体和淋球菌均可引起此种表现。
c. 行眼部微生物拭子检查，然后使用含抗生素的眼药水。产妇及其丈夫应在泌尿生殖诊所行三次微生物拭子检查，且密切随访。

a. Ophthalmia neonatorum.
b. Chlamydia and gonorrhoea can both cause this appearance.
c. Microbiological swabs from the eyes followed by antibiotic eye drops. Triple swabs should be taken from the woman and her partner at a genitourinary clinic and contact tracing should be carried out.

33. a. 两侧畸形马蹄内翻足（“畸形足”）。
b. 足畸形可单独发生，也可与染色体或单基因疾病以及不明原因的多发畸形综合征相关。其中以 18 三体综合征、神经肌肉失调最引人注意。
c. 轻度病例只用物理疗法即可。在这种重度病例首先应术前做系列的固定，以助挛缩组织伸展。将韧带变松和肌腱拉长以允许骨骼复位。

a．Bilateral talipes equinovarus ('club foot').

b．Talipes can occur in isolation but is also associated with many chromosomal and single gene disorders, as well as multiple malformation syndromes of uncertain cause. Trisomy 18 and neuromuscular disorders are of particular note.

c．Mild cases can be treated by physiotherapy alone. In a case of this severity, serial casting is first performed to help stretch contracted tissues prior to surgery. Ligaments are released and tendons lengthened to allow bony repositioning.

34．a．先天性膈疝。

b．大多数病例中，妊娠 20 周行超声检查可发现心脏右偏，左胸腔内可见肠管。如胸腔内肠梗阻，可导致羊水过多。这有可能出现相应临床症状。

c．大约 70%。即使没有其他先天畸形或非整倍体综合征，一部分患儿可因继发肺发育不全而不能实施手术。那些做手术的患者结局好得多，大多数患儿存活。

a．Congenital diaphragmatic hernia.

b．Cardiac deviation to the right and visualization of bowel contents in the chest on the left can be seen at a 20-week routine scan in most cases. Polyhydramnios can result if the bowel in the chest becomes obstructed. This may have presented clinically.

c．Approximately 70%. Even in the absence of other congenital abnormalities or aneuploidy, a proportion of infants will not make it to surgery due to secondary pulmonary hypoplasia. Of those that do, the outlook is much more favourable, with the majority surviving.

35．a．胎儿水肿。

b．Rh D 同种免疫。

c．心脏结构异常、心律失常、染色体异常、由其他原因导致的胎儿贫血（比如血红蛋白病、慢性胎儿向母体出血）、单基因病、病毒感染、代谢紊乱。

a．Hydrops fetalis.

b．Rhesus D isoimmunization.

c．Cardiac structural abnormalities and arrhythmias, chromosomal abnormalities, fetal anaemia from other causes (e.g.haemoglobinopathies, chronic fetomaternal haemorrhage), single gene disorders, viral infections and metabolic disorders.

36. a．持续性心动过缓。
 b．催产素使用过量导致的子宫过度刺激。
 c．嘱产妇左侧卧位，撤掉催产素，给予宫缩抑制剂（如静点利托君或特布林皮下给药），如心动过缓仍持续存在，胎儿则应立即娩出。

 a．Prolonged bradycardia.
 b．Uterine hyperstimulation secondary to excessive oxytocin.
 c．Turn the woman into left lateral, turn off the oxytocin and administer a tocolytic (e.g. ritodrine intravenously or terbutaline subcutaneously). The baby will need to be delivered urgently if the bradycardia persists.

37. a．腹裂。
 b．脐疝（脐膨出）。
 c．大多数脐疝外包绕包膜（而腹裂没有），且肠内容突向脐带底部。腹裂时脐带通常插入腹裂左侧腹壁。

 a．Gastroschisis.
 b Exomphalos (omphalocele).
 c．A membrane surrounds most omphaloceles (unlike gastroschisis) and the bowel contents herniate into the base of the umbilical cord. The cord usually inserts into the abdominal wall to the left side of a gastroschisis.

38. a．杏梅腹综合征。
 b．男婴尿道的后尿道瓣膜可能阻断尿流，导致巨大的膀胱扩张，这使宫内胎儿腹壁显著扩张。如膀胱破裂或尿道梗阻解除，胎儿腹壁又缩小，遂出现这种特征性表现。
 c．由于逆行性阻力过大导致发育不良的改变，不可逆的肾损害很可能已经发生。

 a．Prune belly syndrome.
 b．Posterior urethral valves within the urethra of a male fetus may obstruct flow of urine, causing massive bladder dilatation. This grossly distends the abdominal wall in utero. If the bladder ruptures, or if the outflow obstruction is overcome, the abdominal wall deflates, leaving this characteristic appearance.
 c．Irreversible renal damage is likely to have occurred because of excessive retrograde pressure causing dysplastic changes.

39. a．羊膜索综合征。

b．无脑畸形、脑膨出、面裂、断肢、指融合、前腹壁缺陷。

c．很低，尽管有病例报道称此与某些遗传性结缔组织病有关。

a．Amniotic band syndrome.

b．Anencephaly, encephalocele, facial clefts, limb amputations, fusion of digits and anterior abdominal wall defects.

c．Very low, although cases have been reported in association with certain inherited connective tissue disorders.

40. a．大脑中动脉（middle cerebral artery,MCA）。

b．生长受限胎儿代偿机制引起脑血流阻抗降低。大脑中动脉的多普勒波形可表现为低阻形，直至接近胎儿死亡点时该处波形反转。

c．在贫血胎儿中，大脑中动脉内最大血流速度增加超过正常范围。

a．The middle cerebral artery (MCA).

b．Compensatory mechanisms in a growth-restricted infant cause a reduction in resistance to blood flow through the brain. The waveform in the MCA takes on a low-resistance profile until a point close to fetal death, at which point this pattern reverses.

c．In anaemic fetuses, the maximum velocity of blood flow within the MCA increases outside of the normal range.

41. a．不协调。

b．子宫胎盘功能不足在多胎妊娠中很常见，可能引起双胎生长不均衡。此外，在单绒毛膜双胎妊娠中，双胎输血综合征可导致受血胎儿过大而供血胎儿过小。

c．生长受限的新生儿发生围生期窒息、胎粪吸入综合征、坏死性小肠结肠炎、低体温、低血糖、黄疸的危险更高。

a．Discordant.

b．Uteroplacental insufficiency is more common in multiple gestations and may result in unequal growth patterns between the two fetuses. Alternatively, in monochorionic twin pregnancies, twin-twin transfusion syndrome may produce a larger 'recipient' twin and smaller 'donor' twin.

c．A growth-restricted newborn is at greater risk of perinatal asphyxia, meconium aspiration syndrome, necrotizing enterocolitis, hypothermia, hypoglycaemia and jaundice.

42. a. 腰骶部脊膜膨出（脊柱裂）。
 b. 超声检查还可发现柠檬形头、阿 - 希畸形（香蕉形小脑、小脑延髓池消失）、畸形足。
 c. 神经管缺陷是多基因遗传。再发危险为 2% ~ 3%。如服用大剂量叶酸片（每日 5mg）可使危险率下降到 1%。
 a. Lumbosacral meningocele (spina bifida).
 b. Other common ultrasound features include 'lemon'-shaped skull, Arnold-Chiari malformation ('banana' cerebellum and effacement of cisterna magna) and talipes.
 c. Neural tube defects demonstrate polygenic inheritance. The recurrence risk after one affected pregnancy is 2-3%. This can be reduced to less than 1% by taking periconceptual high-dose folic acid (5 mg daily).

43. a. 病理性的。基线变异幅度小于 5 次 / 分，没有加速（即无反应型）。但胎心基线值正常，且未出现减速。
 b. 急诊剖宫产。
 c. 根据病史及该胎心产力图，很有可能在脐动、静脉中发现严重的酸中毒。
 a. Pathological. The baseline variability is <5 beats/min, and there are no accelerations (unreactive). There are no decelerations and the baseline rate is normal.
 b. Emergency caesarean section.
 c. It would be very likely with this history and this CTG to find a severe metabolic acidosis in both the umbilical artery and vein.

44. a. 侧脑室角部。
 b. 脑室扩张。与头围增加相关的这种发现的术语为脑积水。
 c. 染色体异常、神经管缺陷、先天感染（巨细胞病毒、弓形虫）、先天性水管狭窄以及一些不太常见的畸形综合征。有可能发生正常的预后，特别是那些非常临界的病例。
 a. The horns of the lateral ventricles.
 b. Ventriculomegaly. Hydrocephalus is a term reserved for this finding in association with increased head circumference.
 c. Chromosomal abnormalities, neural tube defects, congenital infections (cytomegalovirus and toxoplasmosis), congenital stenosis of the aqueduct and a host of less common malformation syndromes. A normal outcome is possible, especially with very borderline cases.

45. a. 脑室内出血（侧脑室内的白色区域即为出血）。

b. 早产，生长受限胎儿是发生此并发症的高危情况，特别伴有围生期缺氧和酸中毒发生时。

c. 取决于脑室内出血的严重程度，结局可以无影响，也可以是脑积水，甚至是永久性的神经发育受损。

a. Intraventricular haemorrhage (blood is seen as the white areas in the lateral ventricles).

b. The preterm and growth-restricted infant is at greater risk of this complication, in particular if superadded perinatal hypoxia or acidosis occurs.

c. Depending on the severity of the intraventricular haemorrhage, the consequences range from none to hydrocephalus and permanent neurodevelopmental damage.

46. a. 产钳助产。

b. 可疑或证实了的胎儿窘迫（如胎心产力图异常／出现新鲜胎粪／胎儿头皮血 pH 低）或因母体医学原因禁用 Valsalva 手法（顶推）（如浆液动脉瘤、近期有颅内出血、心脏畸形、视网膜剥离）。

c. 面部擦伤、面神经麻痹、颅骨骨折、母体软组织损伤。

a. Forceps delivery.

b. Suspected or confirmed fetal compromise (CTG abnormalities/fresh meconium/low scalp pH value) or maternal medical reasons contraindicating the Valsalva manoeuvre (pushing) (e.g. berry aneurysms, recent intracranial bleeds, cardiac abnormalities, retinal detachments).

c. Facial bruising, facial nerve palsy, skull fracture, maternal soft tissue damage.

47. a. 45，XO

b. Turner 综合征。

c. 身材矮小、大动脉挛缩、条状卵巢、不育、肾畸形。

a. 45, XO.

b. Turner syndrome.

c. Short stature, coarctation of the aorta, streak ovaries, infertility, renal anomalies.

48. a. 多囊。
   b. 可见膀胱，且羊水量正常水平。
   c. 多囊发育不良肾（multicystic dysplastic kidney, MCDK）。大多数遗传性囊性肾累及双侧肾（如婴儿和成人多囊肾疾病）。早期梗阻是引起 MCDK 的可能原因之一。双侧 MCDK 预后不良。

   a. Multicystic.
   b. The visualization of the bladder and normal levels of amniotic fluid.
   c. Multicystic dysplastic kidney (MCDK). Most inherited cystic renal conditions involve both kidneys (e.g. infantile and adult polycystic kidney disease). Early obstruction is one possible cause for MCDK. Bilateral MCDK carries a poor prognosis.

49. a. 硅胶胎头吸引器。
   b. 不能。当胎儿是枕后位时，胎头吸引器的设计不容许其置于弯曲点。需要特殊制造的枕后吸引器来进行旋转的胎头吸引术助娩。
   c. 易于发生胎儿出血的医学情况是绝对禁忌证。如血友病或胎儿血小板减少（如继发于同种免疫性血小板减少或母体先天性血小板减少）就是例子。

   a. Silastic ventouse cup.
   b. No. The design of this ventouse cup does not allow for its placement over the flexion point when the fetus is in an occipitoposterior position. Specially constructed 'OP' cups are required for a rotational ventouse delivery.
   c. Medical conditions that predispose to fetal bleeding problems are strict contraindications. Haemophilia or fetal thrombocytopenia (e. g. secondary to alloimmue thrombocytopenia or maternal idiopathic thrombocytopenia) are examples.

50. a. 水囊瘤。
   b. Turner 综合征（45，XO）是最常见原因。Noonan 综合征、Robert 综合征、多翼状胬肉综合征是其他更少见的原因。
   c. 染色体组型分析（羊膜腔穿刺术或绒毛活检）。

   a. Cystic hygroma.
   b. Turner syndrome (45, XO) is the most common cause. Noonan, Robert's and multiple pterygium syndromes are other much less common causes.
   c. Karyotyping (amniocentesis or chorionic villus sampling).

51．a．单纯疱疹及水痘 - 带状疱疹。
   b．肝脾大、血小板减少、脑膜脑炎、肺炎及 DIC。在存活者中长期神经发育受损常见。
   c．阿昔洛韦。

   a．Herpes simplex and varicella zoster.
   b．Hepatosplenomegaly, thrombocytopenia, meningoencephalitis, pneumonitis and disseminated intravascular coagulation. Long-term neurodevelopmental damage is common amongst survivors.
   c．Aciclovir.

52．a．坏死性小肠结肠炎。
   b．早产后呼吸窘迫综合征、脑室内出血、脑室周围白质软化、慢性肺疾病、早产视网膜病。
   c．至少产前 48 小时给予糖皮质激素（倍他米松或地塞米松）。

   a．Necrotizing enterocolitis.
   b．Respiratory distress syndrome, intraventricular haemorrhage, periventricular leukomalacia, chronic lung disease, retinopathy of prematurity.
   c．Administration of antenatal steroids (betamethasone or dexamethasone) at least 48 h before delivery.

53．a．羊膜镜。
   b．用于分娩过程中的胎儿血样采集。
   c．指征为当产程时胎心产力图为病理性的（即有 2 处或 2 处以上的异常特征）。胎心产力图提示胎儿酸中毒和缺氧的假阳性率很高。分娩过程中单纯依靠胎心产力图作为判定胎儿状态好坏与否的指征，会由于假想的胎儿窘迫导致过多不必要的剖宫产。

   a．Amnioscope.
   b．Fetal blood sampling during labour.
   c．This procedure is indicated when a CTG becomes pathological in labour (i.e. it has two or more abnormal features). The CTG carries a high false-positive rate for fetal acidosis and hypoxia. Relying solely on the CTG during labour as an indicator of fetal well-being would result in excessive numbers of unnecessary caesarean sections for presumed fetal compromise.

54. a. 胎儿胃。
 b. 先天性膈疝。
 c. 如无其他畸形，肺发育不全是此情况中最主要的存活限制因素。如果新生儿能够有满意的氧和，则结局会很好，大约有70% 的存活率。不能够获得足够的通气与非常差的预后相关。

 a. Fetal stomach.
 b. Congenital diaphragmatic hernia.
 c. Pulmonary hypoplasia is the main limiting factor for survival in this condition if there are no other anomalies. If the neonate can be oxygenated satisfactorily then the outlook is quite good, with approximately 70% survival rates. Failure to achieve adequate ventilation is associated with an extremely poor prognosis.

55. a. 水痘。
 b. 对于暴露的无免疫的孕妇免疫球蛋白静脉给药以降低母儿感染率。
 c. 先天水痘综合征中还可表现的畸形有：小头畸形、肢体发育不全、眼部缺陷。

 a. Varicella zoster (chickenpox).
 b. Giving intravenous immunoglobulin to exposed non-immune pregnant women reduces maternal and fetal infection rates.
 c. Other anomalies found with the congenital varicella syndrome include microcephaly, limb hypoplasia and eye defects.

56. a. 多囊。
 b. 羊水过少。
 c. 如果肾功能明显降低导致严重减少或消失的羊水量，宫内胎儿肺不张则很可能引起肺发育不全。

 a. Multicystic.
 b. Oligo- or anhydramnios.
 c. If renal function was reduced enough to result in very low or absent liquor volumes, then the inability of the fetal lungs to expand in utero is likely to have caused pulmonary hypoplasia.

57. a. 肝。
 b. 脐疝。
 c. 最通常见于 18 三体，也可见于 13 三体。

a. Liver.

b. Exomphalos (omphalocele).

c. Trisomy 18 most commonly, but also trisomy 13.

58. a. 通贯手。

b. 妊娠 11 ~ 13 周行颈半透明度筛查。妊娠早期联合检查包括颈半透明度检查和生化检查。妊娠 15 ~ 19 周根据要测量的标志物的多少行二倍体、三倍体或四倍体血清学生化检查。检查所有这些变量被称为“整体”检验。

c. 心脏畸形（特别是房室间隔缺损）、十二指肠闭锁、小肠发生回波、颈褶厚于 6mm、指／趾弯曲、股骨短、肾性骨盆扩张、脉络丛囊肿。

a. Single palmar crease.

b. Nuchal translucency scanning at 11-13 weeks. The addition of first trimester biochemistry to the nuchal scan results in the 'combined' test. Serum biochemistry at 15-19 weeks is known as the 'double', 'triplc' or 'quadruple' test, depending on how many markers are measured. Measuring all these variables is called the 'integrated' test.

c. Cardiac defects (especially atrioventricular septal defect), duodenal atresia, echogenic bowel, ≥ 6 mm nuchal fold, clinodactyly, short femur, sandal gap and possibly renal pelvic dilatation and choroid plexus cysts.

59. a. 生长受限。

b. 继发于先兆子痫的子宫胎盘功能不足。

c. 腹围、头围比例不称。连续检查发现腹围增长缓慢。羊水过少，脐动脉多普勒波形中出现阻抗增加波形。

a. Growth-restricted.

b. Uteroplacental insufficiency secondary to pre-eclampsia.

c. Asymmetry between abdominal circumference (AC) and head circumference measurements. Slowing of the progression of AC values over serial scans. Oligohydramnios and raised resistance patterns in the umbilical artery Doppler waveforms.

60. a. 骨骼发育不良。

b. 超声检查、分子遗传学检查。

c. 由于胸腔狭小，出现肺发育不全、呼吸窘迫。

a. Skeletal dysplasias.

b. Ultrasound and molecular genetics.

c. Pulmonary hypoplasia and respiratory distress due to a small chest.

61. a. 腰骶段脊髓脊膜膨出（脊柱裂）。

b. 运动神经受损（可能是轮椅束缚），膀胱、肠管失禁，脑积水（可能需要外科手术分流，并导致神经发育迟缓）。

c. 围受孕期叶酸应用的增加可减少该病的实际发生率。几乎全球性地筛查母体血清中甲胎蛋白及妊娠 20 周时常规做超声检查，这意味着绝大多数的妊娠受影响的夫妻可以有终止妊娠的选择。

a. Lumbosacral myelomeningocele (spina bifida).

b. Motor problems (may be wheelchair-bound), bladder and bowel incontinence and hydrocephalus (which may need to be surgically shunted and may result in neurodevelopmental delay).

c. The increased use of folic acid around the time of conception has reduced the actual incidence of these conditions. Almost universal detection through maternal serum α-fetoprotein testing and routine detailed scanning at 20 weeks means that most couples with an affected pregnancy have a choice regarding termination.

62. a. 胎头血肿。

b. 很可能是胎头吸引助娩。

c. 最可能是黄疸，因为血肿中的红细胞分解生成过多的胆红素。

a. Cephalohaematoma.

b. This is more likely with a ventouse delivery.

c. Jaundice is more likely because of the increased bilirubin resulting from haemolysis of the red cells within the haematoma.

63. a. 后尿道瓣膜（膀胱壁肥厚而扩张，伴有“锁孔样”后尿道扩张）。

b. 肾管压力增加通常会引起某种程度肾盂肾盏扩张，通常会导致肾实质发育异常及功能降低。羊水量可显著减少，继发肺发育不全。

c. 如羊水量在妊娠 32 周前减少，而胎儿肾功保存，应对宫内胎儿通过膀胱留置猪尾形导管以缓解梗阻。

a. Posterior urethral valves (dilated thick walled bladder with 'keyhole' posterior urethral expansion).

b. Increased pressure in the renal tract usually causes some degree of pelvicalyceal dilatation and commonly results in dysplastic changes in the renal parenchyma and reduced function. A marked reduction in amniotic fluid is probable, followed by secondary pulmonary hypoplasia.

c. If liquor volumes decline before 32 weeks' gestation and fetal renal function is preserved, then pigtail catheters may be sited through the bladder in utero to bypass the obstruction.

64. a. 肋下及胸骨回缩。

b. 呼吸窘迫。

c. 肺透明膜病（与早产有关）、新生儿暂时呼吸急促、先天肺炎、气胸、肺发育不全。

a. Subcostal and sternal recession.

b. Respiratory distress/compromise.

c. Hyaline membrane disease (associated with prematurity), transient tachypnoea of the newborn, congenital pneumonia, pneumothorax, pulmonary hypoplasia.

65. a. 有反应型（正常的）。正常的基线上有加速，变异良好。无减速。

b. 不需要。低危产妇分娩时不需要持续监护胎心。

c. 胎儿监护应在分娩时继续采用，即每隔 15 分钟使用 Pinard 听诊器或手提式多普勒听一次胎心。第二产程中应在每次宫缩后听胎心。羊水引流的颜色也是分娩期监护胎儿的方法，但不敏感。

a. Reactive (normal). There are accelerations on a normal baseline with good variability. There are no decelerations.

b. No. Low-risk women do not need to be continuously monitored by CTG in labour.

c. Fetal monitoring should be continued in all labours, namely by intermittent auscultation every 15 min with a Pinard stethoscope or hand-held Doppler. In second stage, the fetal heart should be auscultated after every contraction. The colour of the liquor draining is another (insensitive) method of intrapartum fetal surveillance.

66. a. 继发停滞。
    b. 宫缩乏力、真性头盆不称、胎位异常（如枕后位）、先露异常（如面先露、肩先露、额先露）。
    c. 如梗阻不能克服，继发停滞可能最终导致经产孕妇子宫破裂。在这种情况下应用催产素时必须严密监护。

    a. Secondary arrest.
    b. Dysfunctional uterine activity, true cephalopelvic disproportion, malposition (e.g. occipitoposterior) or malpresentation (e.g. face, shoulder or brow).
    c. If an obstruction is not overcome, then secondary arrest may finally result in uterine rupture in a multiparous patient. Great care must therefore be taken in using oxytocin in this situation.

67. a. 腕管综合征。
    b. 正中神经。
    c. 如有疼痛，应予夹板固定，给予一般的止痛剂。妊娠期间给利尿剂无作用，需要手术治疗的很少见。

    a. Carpal tunnel syndrome.
    b. Median nerve.
    c. Splinting and simple analgesics if there is pain. There is no role for diuretics in pregnancy, and the need for surgery is very rare.

68. a. 系统性全身性红斑狼疮。
    b. 基线全血计数，肾生化检查。自身抗体也需要检查。
    c. 妊娠期狼疮的后果取决于脏器受累的程度、疾病活动水平、哪种自身抗体存在。如发现抗 Ro 和抗 La 抗体，可引起胎儿心脏传导阻滞。抗磷脂抗体和狼疮抗凝物与下列风险增加有关：流产、破膜、胎儿生长受限、先兆子痫、母体血栓、肾受损及高血压。

    a. Systemic lupus erythematosus.
    b. Baseline full blood count and renal biochemistry should be performed. An autoantibody profile should also be requested.
    c. The effect of lupus on pregnancy depends on the extent of visceral organ involvement, levels of disease activity and which autoantibodies are present. Anti-Ro and anti-La antibodies, if found, may cause fetal heart block. Anticardioplin antibodies and lupus anticoagulant are associated with an increased risk of miscarriage, abruption, fetal growth restriction, pre-eclampsia and maternal thrombosis, as are renal involvement and hypertension.

69. a. 浆膜下肌瘤。

b. 肌瘤在妊娠期通常增大。如瘤体增长快于其血供，则可能发生一种称为红色变性的过程。这引起剧烈腹痛，如带蒂肌瘤扭转能引起的疼痛。粘膜下肌瘤阻塞子宫下段，引起先露异常。肌瘤还可导致原发产后出血。

c. 不能。剖宫产时行肌瘤外科切除术有危险，最好避免，因其出血汹涌，难以控制。

a. Serosal fibroids.

b. Fibroids often enlarge in pregnancy. If they outgrow their blood supply, then a process called red degeneration may occur. This can cause significant pain, as can torsion of a pedunculated fibroid. Submucous fibroids may obstruct the lower part of the uterus and cause malpresentation. Fibroids predispose to primary postpartum haemorrhage.

c. No. Myomectomy at the time of caesarean section is hazardous and best avoided. Bleeding can be torrential and difficult to control.

70. a. 先兆子痫（妊娠期蛋白尿高血压疾病）。

b. 肾功检查、24 小时尿蛋白定量、肝功检查、超声检查胎儿及血小板计数。

c. 胎儿胎盘娩出。

a. Pre-eclampsia (proteinuric hypertension of pregnancy).

b. Renal function tests, 24 h urine collection for total protein estimation, liver function tests, fetal ultrasound and platelet count.

c. Delivery of the fetus and placenta.

71. a. 女性骨盆侧位片（骨盆测量）。

b. 上面那条线称为“真结合径”，测量的是骨盆入口前后径。下面那条线测量的是骨盆出口同样径线。

c. 没有。骨盆测量过去曾用于妊娠期进行以预测成功的臀位经阴道分娩可能性。急诊剖宫产的产妇通常行骨盆测量以提示再次的分娩方式。高质量的证据表明在这两种分娩中骨盆测量并非有用的检查。

a. A lateral view of the female pelvis (pelvimetry).

b. The upper dotted line is called the 'true conjugate' and measures the anteroposterior diameter at the inlet. The lower dotted line measures the same, at the outlet.

c. No. Pelvimetry was previously performed during pregnancy to help predict the chances of successful breech vaginal delivery. Women having an emergency caesarean section often underwent pelvimetry to help advise about future deliveries. Good-quality evidence shows that pelvimetry is not a helpful investigation in either of these scenarios.

72. a. 外阴疱疹。

b. 是首次发病（原发疱疹）还是再发？

c. 如为再发病例，经阴道分娩新生儿的新生儿疱疹发病率很低，因已从母体获得抗体从而获得被动免疫。原发疱疹发生于妊娠 30 周后的任何时间即为剖宫产手术指征，因经阴道分娩感染胎儿的几率很高。

a. Vulval herpes.

b. Is this the first ever attack (primary herpes) or a recurrence?

c. If this represents a recurrence, then the risk of neonatal herpes following a vaginal delivery is very low because of passive immunity from maternal antibodies. Primary herpes occurring any time after 30 weeks is an indication for caesarean section because transmission rates to the fetus born vaginally are much higher.

73. a. 凹陷性外周水肿。

b. 血压、反射、是否存在阵发性抽搐、上腹部压痛以及子宫大小。

c. 如要考虑到先兆子痫发生的可能性，母体检查应包括 24 小时尿蛋白定量、中段尿培养、肝肾生化检查（包括尿酸盐）、全血细胞计数、出凝血时间。胎儿检查应包括 CTG、生长参数、羊水量、脐动脉多普勒波形测定。

a. Pitting peripheral oedema.

b. Blood pressure, reflexes, presence of clonus, upper abdominal tenderness and uterine size.

c. If there is concern regarding the possibility of pre-eclampsia, maternal investigations should include 24-h urine collection for protein, midstream urine culture, liver and renal biochemistry (including urate), full blood count and occasionally clotting profile. Fetal investigations include CTG, growth parameters, liquor volume and umbilical artery Doppler waveform measurements.

74．a．羊水过少。
b．子宫胎盘功能不足（如先兆子痫）、破水、严重的胎儿双肾畸形。
c．胎儿生长参数及脐动脉多普勒对确定胎盘病理有帮助。异常肾扩张或多囊肾提示是肾原因导致。但破膜的诊断必须根据临床做出。

a．Oligohydramnios.

b．Uteroplacental insufficiency (e.g. pre-eclampsia), rupture of membranes and severe bilateral fetal renal abnormalities.

c．Fetal growth parameters and umbilical artery Doppler should help to identify a placental pathology. Abnormally dilated or multicystic kidneys will point to a renal cause. The diagnosis of ruptured membranes must be made clinically.

75．a．古典式剖宫产（纵向切口）。
b．古典式剖宫产术中出血较多，再次妊娠时子宫破裂危险增加。
c．不能充分通过子宫下段（如子宫肌瘤、严重粘连、胎盘低置）。妊娠足月前伴羊水过少的胎位异常。

a．Classical caesarean section (vertical incision).

b．Blood loss is greater with classical caesarean section and the risk of uterine rupture is higher in a subsequent pregnancy.

c．Inadequate access to the lower segment (e.g. fibroids, severe adhesions and placenta percreta) and malpresentations with reduced liquor at preterm gestations.

76．a．脐带脱垂。
b．早产、胎位异常、羊水过多、多胎妊娠、头高位人工破膜。
c．术者手入阴道内，手握成杯状轻持脐带，手指压先露部使其不下降，以减轻脐带受压。产妇膝胸卧位直至可实施急诊剖宫产术为止。

a．Cord prolapse.

b．Prematurity, malpresentations, polyhydramnios, multiple gestations and artificial rupture of membranes with a 'high head'.

c．The cord should be gently held in a cupped hand in the vagina with the fingers pressing on the presenting part to relieve any pressure on it. The woman should adopt the 'knees-to-chest' position until emergency caesarean section can be performed.

77. a. 拍打面颊综合征（传染性红斑），由细小病毒 B12 引起。
b. 大多数成人细小病毒 B12 感染无症状。血清学 IgM 抗体升高提示近期母体感染。IgG 抗体通常提示既往感染。
c. 细小病毒 B12 感染胎儿可引起再障危象，导致胎儿贫血、水肿、胎死宫内。

a. Slapped cheek syndrome (erythema infectiosum). Caused by parvovirus B12.
b. Many adult parvovirus B12 infections are asymptomatic. Serological testing for IgM antibodies raised against parvovirus would recognize a recent maternal infection. IgG antibodies usually indicate past maternal infection.
c. Fetal infection with parvovirus B12 can cause an aplastic crisis, resulting in fetal anaemia, hydrops and intrauterine fetal death.

78. a. 胎儿核磁共振。
b. 目前未有证据表明 MRI 对妊娠有危害。
c. 不能。CT 使胎儿高度暴露于电离辐射中，妊娠早期可使发生先天畸形的危险增加，在后期则影响胎儿生长、神经发育及日后患恶性肿瘤危险。

a. Fetal MRI.
b. There is no evidence that MRI harms pregnancies.
c. No. CT scanning involves very high fetal exposures to ionizing radiation which early on in pregnancy may increase the risk of congenital abnormalities and later may have an impact on growth, neurological development and future risk of malignancy.

79. a. 羊膜穿刺术后的荧光原位杂交。
b. 染色体数目异常（如三倍体）。
c. 该细胞是正常细胞，因为每个细胞有 2 个标记。只有当这是 Y 染色体探针时它才是一个正常细胞。

a. Fluorescent in situ hybridization (FISH) following amniocentesis.
b. Abnormalities of chromosome number (e.g. trisomies).
c. This cell is normal because there are two signals per cell. Only if this were a Y chromosome probe would it be an abnormal cell.

80. a. 前置血管。
b. 走行于羊膜内的血管参与部分胎儿循环。如这些血管破裂，胎儿将失血过多。
c. 自然破膜或人工破膜后是由前置血管引起胎儿出血的最危险的时机。出现阴道流血、胎心异常，但母体未出现休克。

a. Vasa praevia.

b. The vessels running through the membranes form part of the fetal circulation. If they tear, fetal exsanguination can occur very quickly.

c. The time of highest risk for fetal bleeding due to vasa praevia occurs when the membranes rupture spontaneously or if artificial rupture is performed. Vaginal bleeding occurs and the fetal heart tracing becomes abnormal in the absence of maternal shock.

81. a. 坐骨棘。

b. 阴部神经。

c. 第二产程时由产科医生行阴部神经阻滞，该麻醉方法操作简单、起效快、安全，有助于产钳助产或修补扩张的阴道及会阴裂伤。

a. The ischial spine.

b.. The pudendal nerve.

c. A pudendal nerve block can be easily carried out by an obstetrician in second stage to provide fast-acting and safe analgesia sufficient for a forceps delivery or repair of an extensive vaginal and perineal tear.

82. a. 增加其剂量。早餐前血糖水平过高，通常反映夜间胰岛素不足。

b. 减量。早餐后血糖水平稍低。但低血糖症的预兆在妊娠期很少发生，甚至长期患有糖尿病的患者可能仍然不会发生预兆。

c. 查糖化血红蛋白（HbA_{1c}），其值小于 7% 意味近期血糖控制合理。

a. Increase it. The fasting glucose level in the morning is too high and usually reflects inadequate insulin overnight.

b. Decrease it. The post breakfast blood glucose is a little low. Warnings of hypoglycaemia are less pronounced in pregnancy and even a long-standing experienced diabetic may nevertheless be caught out by this.

c. By measuring glycosylated haemoglobin (HbA_{1c}). A value less than 7% suggests reasonable recent sugar control.

83. a. 乳腺炎。
b. 葡萄球菌、链球菌。
c. 应鼓励产妇吸空一侧乳房内乳汁后再用另侧乳房哺乳。氟氯西林为经验的治疗选择。乳头拭子或挤出的乳汁能够做微生物培养及药敏试验。非甾体抗炎药可用于止痛。专家指导产妇正确的哺乳技巧能够减少乳头疼痛的机会及同样问题的复发。

a. Mastitis.
b. *Staphylococcus* and *Streptococcus species.*
c. The woman should be encouraged to express milk from that side and to continue breastfeeding with the other. Flucloxacillin is the empiric treatment of choice. Nipple swabs or expressed milk can be sent for microbiological culture and sensitivity testing. Non-steroidal anti-inflammatory drugs can be used for analgesia. Expert help with breastfeeding technique should reduce the chances of sore nipples and recurrences of the same problem.

84. a. 控制性脐带牵引。
b. 如脐带牵引过度可导致子宫外翻，特别是宫缩不良时。此产科并发症引起重度心动过缓性休克，尽快纠正宫底位置可以纠正。如该技术实施不当，可导致胎盘母体面绒毛小叶残留。
c. 尽管实施控制性脐带牵引术，胎盘粘连发生率是 1% ～ 2%。手术室内徒手操作应在全麻或局麻下进行。极少出现胎盘病态粘连而不能剥离，甚至于徒手。子宫切除术经常是必要的。

a. Controlled cord traction.
b. Uterine inversion can occur if excessive cord traction is used, particularly if the uterus is somewhat atonic. This obstetric complication causes profound bradycardic shock, which is corrected by replacing the uterine fundus as soon as possible. Placental cotyledons may be retained if this technique is poorly performed.
c. 1-2% of placentas remain adherent to the uterine wall despite controlled cord traction. They are removed manually in theatre under regional or general anaesthesia. Much less commonly the placenta is morbidly adherent and cannot be removed, even manually. A hysterectomy is usually necessary.

85．a．子宫破裂。

b．前次剖宫产（特别是古典式剖宫产）或其他全层子宫损伤史（如肌瘤核除术或刮宫时穿孔）。经产妇梗阻性分娩、不当的催产素使用是其他的原因。

c．表现为持续剧烈的耻骨上疼痛、产妇虚脱、分娩时阴道流血、血尿、严重的或突然的 CTG 异常。

a．Uterine rupture.

b．Previous caesarean section (especially classical) and any other full-thickness uterine damage (e.g. myomectomy or perforation at the time of curettage). Obstructed labour in multiparous women and the injudicious use of oxytocin are other causes.

c．It may present as severe continuous suprapubic pain, maternal collapse, intrapartum vaginal bleeding, haematuria or profound and sudden CTG abnormalities.

专业词汇英中对照

A

abdominal circumference(AC)	腹围
abdominal pain,ectopic pregnancy	腹痛，异位妊娠
abdominal repair,caesarean section	腹部缝合，剖宫产
abdominal wall defects	腹壁缺陷
abscess,breast,	脓肿，乳房
absent end diastolic flow(AEDF)	舒张末期血流缺如
acceleration,in cardiotocography	加速，在胎心图上
achondroplasia	软骨发育不全
aciclovir	阿昔洛韦
alcohol	酒精
α -fetoprotein screening(AFP)	甲胎蛋白
amnihook	羊膜钩
amniocentesis	羊膜穿刺术
amnioscope	羊膜镜
amniotic bands	羊膜索
amniotic fluid index(AFI)	羊水指数
amniotic fluid volume(AFV)	羊水量
ampicillin	氨比西林
anaemia	贫血
fetal	胎儿
folic acid deficiency	叶酸缺乏
iron deficiency	缺铁
pregnancy	妊娠
puerperium	产褥
analgesia	镇痛
caesarean section	剖宫产
episiotomy	会阴切开术
labour	分娩
epidural see epidural anaesthesia	硬膜外麻醉
non-pharmacological	非药物性的
pharmacological	药物性的
twin birth	双胎分娩
anal sphincter tears	肛门括约肌撕裂

anencephaly	无脑儿
answers	答案
antenatal care	产前检查
aims of care	检查目的
booking (first visit)	预约(初次检查)
diabetes mellitus	糖尿病
examinations	检查
history taking,maternal	病史采集，产妇
twin pregnancy	双胎妊娠
visit numbers and timing	检查次数及周期
antenatal screening	产前筛查
antepartum fetal assessment	产前胎儿评估
blood tests	血液化验
chromosomal analysis	染色体核型分析
diabetes mellitus	糖尿病
Down syndrome	唐氏综合征
fetal imaging	胎儿成像
antepartum haemorrhage	产前出血
venous thromoembolic disease	静脉血栓栓塞性疾病
anticonvulsants	抗惊厥药
anti-D immunoglobin	抗 D 免疫球蛋白
antihiatamines	抗组胺药
antihypertensives	抗高血压药
antiretrovirals	抗逆转录病毒约
aorta,coarctation	主动脉，缩窄
Apgar score	阿普加评分
Arnold-Chiari malformation	Arnold-Chiari 畸形
Aromatherapy	芳香疗法

B

barrier contraception	屏障避孕法
baseline rate,cardiotocography	胎心率基线，胎心图
variability	胎心变异
biochemical screening tests, fetal health assessment	生化筛查试验，胎儿健康评估
biophysical profile scoring(BPS)	胎儿生物物理评分
biophysical testing, fetal health assessment	生物物理试验，胎儿健康评估

biparietal diameter	双顶径
birthing ball	分娩球
birthing partner	陪伴分娩
birthing pool	分娩池
bladder	膀胱
distension	扩张
herniation	疝
blastocyst	胚泡
blighted ovum（anembryonic pregnancy）	枯萎孕卵（无胚胎妊娠）
blood pressure	血压
antenatal examination	产前检查
hypertension	高血压
measurement	测量
see also hypertension	*参见*高血压
blood sampling,fetal *see* fetal blood sampling(FBS)	采血，胎儿*见*胎儿血样
bone deformities	骨畸形
booking,first visit	预约，初次检查
brachial nerve injuries	臂丛神经损伤
bradycardia,fetal	心动过缓，胎儿
brain defects	脑缺陷
breast,antenatal changes	乳房，产前改变
breast abscess	乳房脓肿
breast feeding	母乳喂养
complications	并发症
contraception	避孕
drug excretion	药物代谢
HIV	人类免疫缺陷病毒
ovulation	排卵
breech presentation	臀先露
birth injury	产伤
Brushfield's spots	布鲁什菲尔德斑
Bupivacaine	布比卡因

C

caesarean section（CS）	剖宫产术
birth injuries	产伤

breech presentation	臀先露
classical(vertical incision)	古典剖宫产(纵切口)
complications	并发症
indications	适应证
procedure	步骤
sterilization	绝育
technique	方法
twins	双胎
campomelic dysplasia	躯干发育异常
cardiac arrhythmias,fetal	心律失常，胎儿
cardiotocography	胎心图
classification	分类
contractions	子宫收缩
fetal asphyxia	胎儿窘迫
pathological	病理的
reactive	反应型
carpal tunnel syndrome	腕管综合征
cephalohaematoma	头部血肿
cervical funneling	宫颈漏斗状
cervica length scanning,preterm labour	宫颈长度扫描，早产
cervica lesions	宫颈损伤
cervica suture	宫颈缝合
chickenpox *see* varicella zoster	水痘*见*水痘 / 带状疱疹
chignon	毛孢子菌病 / 拜格耳病
Chlamydia	衣原体
Chlamydia trachomatis	沙眼衣原体
chloasma,during pregnancy	妊娠期，黄褐斑
choriocarcinoma	绒癌
chorionic villi	绒毛
chorionic villus sampling	绒毛活检
choroid plexus	脉络丛
cysts	囊肿
chromosomal abnormalities	染色体异常
chromosomal analysis	染色体核型分析
exomphalos	脐疝
hydatidiform mole	葡萄胎
intrauterine growth restriction	宫内生长受限
Turner syndrome	Turner 综合征

club foot(bilateral talipes equinovarus)	畸形足(双侧马蹄内翻足)
coarctation of aorta	主动脉缩窄
combined oral contraceptive pill(COCP)	复方口服避孕药
‘complete’mole	“完全性”葡萄胎
conception	受孕
conceptus，four-cell stage	孕体，四细胞期胚胎
condoms	避孕套
congenital abnormalities	先天畸形
diabetes mellitus	糖尿病
twin pregnancy	双胎妊娠
congenital infections	先天感染
congenital varicella syndrome	先天水痘综合征
conjoined twins	联体双胎
contraception,post-pregnancy	避孕，妊娠后
barrier methods	屏障避孕法
hormonal methods	激素避孕法
intrauterine contraceptive devices	宫内节育器
sterilization	绝育
crowing	胎头着冠
crown-rump length(CRL)	顶臀长
CT scanning,fetal	胎儿 CT 扫描
Cyst（s),choroid plexus	脉络丛囊肿
cystic hygroma	水囊状淋巴管瘤
cytomegalovirus（cmv)	巨细胞病毒

D

decelerations,cardiotocography	减速，胎心图
early	早期
late	晚期
variable	变异
deep vein thrombosis	深静脉血栓形成
delivery	分娩
anterior shoulder	前肩
forceps	产钳
intrauterine growth restriction	宫内生长受限
placenta	胎盘
preterm rupture of membranes	胎膜早破

delivery *(cont'd)*	分娩（续）
twins	双胎
vacuum/ventouse	胎头吸引
vaginal breech	臀位阴道分娩
dermatomyositis	皮肌炎
diabetes mellitus（DM)	糖尿病
Erb's palsy	Erb 麻痹
fetal risks	对胎儿的危害
gestational	妊娠期的
pre-existing	预先存在的
diaphragmatic hernia	膈疝
ultrasound findings	超声检查发现
diaphragms	膈
diastrophic dysplasia	骨畸形发育不良
digoxin	地高辛
direct endoscopy(fetoscopy)	直接内镜检查(胎儿镜检查)
disseminated intravascular coagulation	弥漫性血管内凝血
Doppler ultrasound	多普勒超声
antepartum fetal health assessment	产前胎儿健康评估
continuous FHR monitoring	持续胎心监护
ductus venosus blood flow	静脉导管血流
middle cerebral artery blood flow	大脑中动脉血流
umbilical artery blood flow	脐动脉血流
'double' bubble sign	双泡征
'double' test	双检测
Down syndrome（trisomy 21）	唐氏综合征（21 三体综合征）
α -fetoprotein （AFP） screening	甲胎蛋白筛查
choroid plexus cysts	脉络丛囊肿
facial features	面部特征
karyotype	核型
nuchal translucency screening	颈半透明度筛查
palmar creases	掌褶
recurrence risk	复发危险
drug abuse	药物滥用
Duffy antibodies	Duffy 抗体
duodenal atresia	十二指肠闭锁
dysmenorrhoea	痛经

E

ectopic pregnancy	异位妊娠
ectopic vesicae	异位膀胱
eczema	湿疹
Edward syndrome（trisomy 18）	Edward 综合征（18 三体综合征）
associated anomalies	联合畸形
choroid plexus cysts	脉络丛囊肿
karyotype	核型分析
emboli，pulmonary	栓子，肺
encephalocele，occipital	脑膨出，枕骨的
endometritis	子宫内膜炎
endoscopy,direct(fetoscopy)	内镜检查，直接（胎儿镜检查）
entonox	一氧化二氮—氧混合气
epidural anaesthesia	硬膜外麻醉
complications	并发症
contraindication	禁忌证
technique	方法
episiotomy	会阴切开术
repair	缝合
Erb's palsy	Erb 麻痹
diabetes mellitus	糖尿病
ergometrine	麦角新碱
erythema infectiosum	传染性红斑
erythromycin	红霉素
examinations	检查
antenatal	产前
hypertensive mother	高血压孕妇
postnatal	产后
exomphalos	脐疝
diferential diagnosis	鉴别诊断
screening	筛查
expected date of delivery(EDD)	预产期
external cephalic version	外转胎位术

F

facial nerve palsy	面神经麻痹

facial pigmentation	面部色素沉着
fallopian tube	输卵管
ectopic pregnancy	异位妊娠
fertilization	受精
removal	切除
sterilization	绝育
fertilization	受精
fetal alcohol syndrome	胎儿酒精综合征
fetal biopsy	胎儿活检
fetal blood sampling(FBS)	胎儿血样采集
equipment	仪器
during labour	分娩过程中
rhesus disease	Rh 病
fetal goiter	胎儿甲状腺肿
fetal heart rate（FHR） monitoring	胎心监护
continuous	持续的
intrapartum	产时
see also cardiotocography	见胎心图
fetal skin electrodes	胎儿经皮电极
injury	损伤
α -fetoprotein screening（AFP）	甲胎蛋白筛查
fetoscopy(direct endoscopy)	胎儿镜检查(直接内镜检查)
fetus	胎儿
anaemia	贫血
ascites	腹水
birth trauma	产伤
cardiac arrhythmias	心律失常
congenital abnormalities	先天畸形
congenital infections	先天感染
growth restricted *see* intrauterine growth restriction	生长受限*见*宫内生长受限
head rotation	胎头旋转
hypoxia	缺氧
monitoring	监护
antepartum health assessment	产前健康评估
intrapartum	产时
oedema	水肿
pleural effusion	胸腔积液

screening *see* antenatal screening	筛查*见*产前筛查
triploid	三倍体
flecainide	氟卡尼
flucloxacillin	氟氯西林
fluorescence in situ hybridization(FISH)	荧光免疫杂交
folic acid deficiency anaemia	叶酸缺乏性贫血
folic acid supplements	补充叶酸
neural tube defects	神经管缺陷
forceps delivery	产钳助娩
complications	并发症
of head ,caesarean section	头，剖宫产术
indications	适应证
procedure	步骤
vaginal breech delivery	臀位经阴道分娩
forceps mark	产钳标记

G

gastrointestinal system	胃肠系统
anomalies	畸形
obstruction	梗阻
pregnancy changes	妊娠改变
gastroschisis	腹裂
Gaucher disease	戈谢病
genital herpes	生殖器疱疹
German measles(rubella)	风疹
gestational age estimation	孕龄估算
gestational diabetes	妊娠期糖尿病
gestational trophoblastic disease (molar pregnancy)	妊娠滋养细胞疾病（葡萄胎妊娠）
gestation sac	妊娠囊
goiter,fetal	胎儿甲状腺肿
gonorrhoeae	淋病
griseofulvin	灰黄霉素
group B streptococcus	B 族链球菌
growth restriction *see* intrauterine growth restriction(IUGR)	宫内生长受限*见* IUGR
gum hypertrophy	齿龈增生

H

Haematoma	血肿
– vaginal	阴道的
– wound	损伤
haemorrhage	出血
– antepartum	产前
– hepatic	肝的
– intraventricular	心室的
– postpartum *see*	产后
postpartum haemorrhage	见产后出血
– subconjunctival	结膜下的
haemorrhoids	痔
head circumference	头围
heart rate monitoring,fetal *see* fetal heart rate（FHR） monitoring	胎心监护
heparin	肝素
hernia,diaphragmatic *see* diaphragmatic hernia	疝，膈的，见膈疝
herpes simplex infection	单纯疱疹病毒感染
herpes zoster	带状疱疹
history taking,maternal	病史采集，孕妇的
holoprosencephaly	前脑无裂畸形
human chorionic gonadotrophin(HCG)	人绒毛膜促性腺激素
– Down syndrome	唐氏综合征
– ectopic pregnancy	异位妊娠
human immunodeficiency virus（HIV）	人类免疫缺陷病毒
hydatidiform mole	葡萄胎
hydrocephalus	脑积水
hydrocortisone	氢化可的松
hydronephrosis	肾积水
hydrops fetalis	胎儿水肿
– non-immune	非免疫性的
– parvovirus	细小病毒
– rhesus disease	Rh 病
– Turner syndrome	Turner 综合征
hypertension	高血压
– management	治疗

pre-existing	预先存在的
pregnancy induced	妊娠期高血压疾病
see also pre-eclampsia	*见*子痫前期
hypochromia	血红蛋白过少
hypoglycaemia	低血糖
hypoproteinaemia	低蛋白血症
hypoxic ischaemic encephalopathy（HIE）	缺血缺氧性脑病

I

Implantation	植入
inefficient uterine activity	无效的子宫活动
infections	感染
congenital	先天的
sexually transmitted	性传播的
uterine	子宫
wound	损伤
see also individual diseases	*见*个体疾病
inferior vena cava filter	下腔静脉过滤器
insulin	胰岛素
intrauterine contraceptive devices	宫内节育器
intrauterine growth restriction（IUGR）	宫内生长受限
diagnosis	诊断
fetal measurement	胎儿测量
management	处理
neonatal complications	新生儿并发症
smoking	吸烟
intrauterine pressure catheter	宫内压力导管
iron deficiency anaemia	缺铁性贫血
iron supplementation	补充铁剂
ischial spine	坐骨棘

J

jaundice	黄疸
jejunal atresia	空肠闭锁

K

karyotyping *see* chromosomal analysis	染色体核型分析

Kell antibodies	Kell 抗体
kick chart	胎动图
Kleihauer test	Kleihauer 试验
Klumpke's palsy	克隆普克麻痹

L

labetalol	拉贝洛尔
labour	分娩
active management	积极治疗
analgesia	镇痛
first stage	第一产程
induction	引产
monitoring	监护
onset	开始
preterm	早产
primary dysfunctional	原发宫缩乏力
progress of	进展
secondary arrest	继发停滞
second stage	第二产程
third stage	第三产程
twin pregnancy	双胎妊娠
lacerations,facial	裂伤，面部
lambda sign	λ 征
last menstrual period（LMP）	末次月经
limb reduction deformities	短肢缺陷畸形
limbs,hypoplasia	肢体，发育不全
linea nigra	妊娠时色素沉着的腹白线
liquor	羊水
assessment	估定
preterm rupture of membranes	胎膜早破
Listeria monocytogenes	单核细胞增多性利斯特杆菌
listeriosis	利斯特杆菌
liver biopsy,fetal	肝活检，胎儿
lower motor neuron injury	下运动神经损伤

M

macrocytosis	巨细胞病毒

macrosomia,diabetes mellitus	巨大儿，糖尿病
malpresentation	先露异常
mastitis	乳腺炎
maternity records	产妇记录
Mauriceau-smellie-veit manoeuvre	莫 - 斯 - 韦三氏手法
mean pool diameter（MPD）	平均羊水池径线
meconium	胎粪
meconium aspiration	胎粪吸入
median nerve compression(carpal tunnel syndrome)	正中神经受压(腕管综合征)
membrane rupture,artificial	人工破膜
meningocele *see* spina bifida	脑膜膨出*见*脊柱裂
meningomyelocele *see* spina bifida	脊膜脊髓膨出*见*脊柱裂
menorrhagia	月经过多
methotrexate	甲氨蝶呤
methyldopa	甲基多巴
microcephaly	小头畸形
microcytosis	小红细胞症
microphthalmia,rubella-induced	小眼畸形，风疹病毒引起
midstream urine sample	中段尿培养
Mirena	曼月乐
miscarriage	流产
complete	完全
incomplete	不全
inevitable	难免
listeriosis	利斯特杆菌
missed	稽留
threatened	先兆
molar pregnancy(gestational trophoblastic disease)	葡萄胎妊娠 (妊娠滋养细胞疾病)
monoamniotic twins	单羊膜囊双胎
monoclonal antibody assay	单克隆抗体
monozygotic twins	单卵双胎
Montgomery's tubercles	蒙氏结节
MRI scans,fetal	胎儿核磁扫描
multicystic dysplastic kidney（MCDK）	多囊发育不良肾
multiple pterygium syndrome	多发翼状胬肉综合征
myelomeningocele *see* spina bifida	脊膜脊髓膨出*见*脊柱裂

myomectomy	子宫肌瘤切除术

N

Naegele's rule	内格利规律
naloxone	纳洛酮
National Institute of Clinical Excellence(NICE)guidelines, antenatal appointments	NICE 指导方针，产前预约
necrotizing enterocolitis	坏死性小肠结肠炎
Neisseria gonorrhoeae	淋球菌
neonatal depression	新生儿窘迫
neonatal herpes	新生儿疱疹
neonatal respiratory depression	新生儿呼吸窘迫
nerve injuries	神经损伤
brachial	臂丛神经
median nerve	正中神经
neural tube defects(NTD)	神经管缺陷
diabetes mellitus	糖尿病
MRI scans	核磁扫描
screening	筛查
nifedipine	硝苯地平
non-rotational forceps	非旋转产钳
Noonan syndrome	努南综合征
nuchal translucency measurement	颈部半透明度检查

O

obstetric cholestasis	妊娠胆汁淤积症
oedema	水肿
fetal	胎儿
perineal	会阴的
pitting peripheral	外周凹陷性
pulmonary	肺的
oligohydramnios	羊水过少
omphalocele *see* exomphalos	脐疝
ophthalmia neonatorum	新生儿眼炎
opiates	阿片制剂
oral glucose tolerance test（OGTT）	口服葡萄糖耐量试验
osteogenesis imperfecta	成骨不全

ovulation,post pregnancy	排卵，妊娠后
ovum	卵子
blighted (anembryonic pregnancy)	枯萎孕卵（无胚胎妊娠）
oxytocin	催产素
side effects	副作用

P

pain	疼痛
ectopic pregnancy	异位妊娠
perineal	会阴的
relief *see* analgesia	缓解疼痛 / 镇痛
palmar creases	掌褶
palsy	麻痹
Erb's *see* Erb's palsy	Erb 麻痹
facial nerve	面神经
Klumpke's	克隆普克
phrenic nerve	膈神经
partial mole	部分性葡萄胎
partogram	产程图
parvovirus infection	细小病毒感染
Patau syndrome(trisomy 13)	帕塔综合征(13 三体综合征)
pelvimetry	骨盆测量
pelvis	骨盆
pemphigoid gestationins	妊娠性类天疱疮
penicillin	青霉素
perineal bruising	会阴裂伤
perineal pain	会阴疼痛
perineal tears	会阴撕裂
Placenta	胎盘
biopsy,chorionic villus sampling	活检，绒毛活检
bleeding from	自……出血
delivery	娩出
insufficiency	机能不足
neoplasia	肿瘤形成
separation	剥离
trophoblastic diseas	滋养细胞疾病
placental abruption	胎盘早剥
placental cotyledons	胎盘母体面绒毛小叶

placental praevia	前置胎盘
podophyllin	鬼臼树脂
polyhydramnios	羊水过多
polymorphic eruptions	多形态疹
porencephaly	脑穿通畸形
posterior urethral valves	后尿道瓣膜
postnatal examination	出生后检查
posypartum haemorrhage	产后出血
deep vein thrombosis	深静脉血栓形成
primary	原发的
Potter's facies	Potter 面容
pre-eclampsia	子痫前期
complications	并发症
see also hypertension	*见*高血压
pregnancy	妊娠
anembryonic(blighted ovum)	无胚胎妊娠(枯萎孕卵)
bleeding in	出血
care in	检查
see also antenatal care	*见*产前检查
cholestasis of	胆汁淤积
dermatoses	皮肤病
diagnosis	诊断
early	早期
see also antenatal screening	*见*产前筛查
diseases in	疾病
see also individual diseases	*见*个体疾病
early	早期
ectopic	异位的
‘high-risk’	“高危”
molar	葡萄胎
multiple	多胎
normal	正常
physiological changes	生理改变
signs of	体征
prematurity	早产
prenatal diagnosis *see* amtenatal screening	产前诊断*见*产前筛查
preterm birth	早产
consequences	结局

preterm rupture of membranes	胎膜早破
progestogen-based intrauterine system (Mirena)	宫内孕激素控释系统(曼月乐)
progestogenic implants	孕激素埋植
progestogen-only pill	单纯孕激素避孕药
prostaglandin E_2	前列腺素 E_2
prune belly syndrome	梨状腹综合征
prurigo	痒疹
pruritic folliculitis	瘙痒性毛囊炎
psoriasis	银屑病
pudendal nerve block	阴部神经阻滞
puerperal sepsis	产后败血症
puerperuim	产褥期
complications	并发症
pulmonary emboli	肺栓子
pulmonary hypoplasia	肺发育不全
purpura,thrombocytopenic	血小板减少性紫癜

Q

'quadruple' test	四倍体检测
questions	问题

R

rectal examination,episiotomy repair	直肠指检，会阴切开缝合术
rectal tears	直肠撕裂
renal dysplasia	肾发育不全
renal tract anomalies	泌尿道畸形
respiratory distress syndrome	呼吸窘迫综合征
retinoid	类维生素 A
retroplacental clots	胎盘后凝血块
rhesus (Rh) disease	Rh 病
rhesus sensitization	Rh 致敏
amniocentesis	羊膜穿刺术
Robert's syndrome	罗伯特综合征
rotational forceps	旋转产钳
rubella (German measles)	风疹
rubella vaccination	风疹疫苗接种

S

salpingectomy	输卵管切除术
salpingotomy	输卵管切开术
scalp abrasions	头皮擦伤
screening *see* antenatal screening	筛查*见*产前筛查
serosal fibroids	浆膜纤维瘤
sexually transmitted infection	性传播感染
‘shared’ care	“共享”检查
shingles	带状疱疹
short-limbed dwarfism	短肢性侏儒
shoulder tip pain,ectopic pregnancy	肩痛，异位妊娠
‘show’	见红
skeletal abnormalities	骨骼畸形
skin	皮肤
antenatal changes	产前改变
episiotomy repair	会阴切开缝合术
pregnancy	妊娠
skull defects	颅骨缺陷
‘banana’ shaped	“香蕉”形
lemon-shape	柠檬形
slapped cheek stndrome	传染性红斑综合征
smoking	吸烟
sphygmomanometer	血压计
spina bifida	脊柱裂
folic acid supplements	补充叶酸
'lemon-shaped' head	“柠檬形”头
motor problems	运动障碍
ultrasound features	超声特征
sterilization	绝育
complications	并发症
female	女性
male	男性
sternal recession	胸骨凹陷
steroids	皮质类固醇
preterm rupture of membranes	胎膜早破
striae gravidarum	妊娠纹
subcostal recession	肋骨下凹陷
submucous fibroids	粘膜下纤维瘤

substance abuse	精神性药物滥用
suction and curettage,trophoblastic disease	吸刮术，滋养细胞疾病
suction machine	吸引器
surgery	手术
abdominal wall defects	腹壁缺陷
ectopic pregnancy	异位妊娠
miscarriage	流产
see also caesarean section	*见*剖宫产
swab tests	拭子试验
preterm rupture of mambranes	胎膜早破
sexually transmitted diseases	性传播疾病
symphysiofundal height	耻上宫底高度
syphilis	梅毒
systemic lupus erythematosus	系统性红斑狼疮
systemic sclerosis	系统性硬化病

T

tachycardia,fetal	心动过速，胎儿
talipes equinovarus,bilateral(club foot)	马蹄内翻足，双侧(畸形足)
tentorial tear	小脑幕撕裂
testes,undescended	睾丸未降至阴囊
tetracycline,fetal teeth staining	四环素，四环素牙
thalidomide	沙利度胺
thanatophoric dwarfism	致死性侏儒症
thrombocytopenia purpura	血小板减少性紫癜
tocolysis	宫缩抑制 / 保胎
toxoplasmosis	弓形虫病
tracheo-oesophageal atresia	气管—食管闭锁
tracheo-oesophageal fistula	气管—食管瘘
traction	牵引
ventouse cups	胎头吸引器
transcutaneous nerve stimulation	经皮神经刺激
Treponema pallidum	梅毒螺旋体
‘triple’ bubble	三泡
‘triple’ test	三倍体检测
Trisomy 13(Patau syndrome)	13 三体综合征(帕塔综合征)
Trisomy 18 *see* Edward syndrome	18 三体综合征（*见*爱德华综合征)

Trisomy21 *see* Down syndrome	21 三体综合征(见唐氏综合征)
trophoblastic disease	滋养细胞疾病
'true conjugate'	“真结合径”
Turner syndrome	Turner 综合征
in female	女性
twins	双胎
complications	并发症
conjoined	联体
discordant growth	生长不协调
dizygotic	双卵双胎
monoamniotic	单羊膜囊
monozygotic	单卵双胎
twin-twin transfusion syndrom	双胎输血综合征

U

ultrasound	超声
antenatal	产前
diaphragmatic hernia	膈疝
Doppler *see* Doppler ultrasound	多普勒*见*多普勒超声
duodenal atresia	十二指肠闭锁
EDD determination	预产期
intrauterine growth restriction	宫内生长受限
‘late dating’	晚于预期的
miscarriage	流产
neural tube defects	神经管缺陷
placental snowstorm	胎盘“落雪征”
twins	双胎
umbilical cord	脐带
clamping/cutting	钳夹，切断
entanglement	缠绕
fetal blood sampling	胎儿血样
position during labour	分娩时方位
prolapse	脱垂
traction	牵引
caesarean section	剖宫产
umbilical pigmentation	脐带色素沉着
umbilical vein,fetal blood sampling	脐静脉，胎儿血样
umbilicus defects	脐带缺陷

undescended testes	隐睾
urinalysis	尿液分析
urinary obstruction	尿路梗阻
ursodeoxycholic acid	熊去氧胆酸
uterine atony	子宫弛缓
uterine hyperstimulation	子宫过刺激
uterine inversion	子宫内翻
uterine repair,caesarean section	子宫缝合，剖宫产术
uterine rupture	子宫破裂
uterine size,antenatal examination	子宫大小，产前检查
uteroplacental insufficiency	子宫胎盘功能不足
uterus,hypotonic	低张子宫

V

vacuum delivery	吸引助娩
vaginal examination	阴道检查
episiotomy repair	会阴切开缝合术
preterm rupture of membranes	胎膜早破
vaginal haematoma	阴道血肿
Valsalva manoeuvre	咽鼓管捏鼻鼓气法
varicella immnunoglobulin（VZIG）	水痘免疫球蛋白
varicella zoster(chickenpox)	带状疱疹(水痘)
fetal infection	胎儿感染
maternal infection	母体感染
varicose veins	静脉曲张
vasa praevia	前置血管
venous thromboembolic disease	静脉血栓栓塞性疾病
ventouse cups	胎头吸引
injure	产伤
ventriculomegaly	脑室扩张

Y

yolk sac	卵黄囊